I've Told Someone

A Transgendered Tale

Tricia Dale

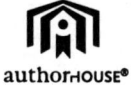

authorHOUSE®

AuthorHouse™ UK Ltd.
1663 Liberty Drive
Bloomington, IN 47403 USA
www.authorhouse.co.uk
Phone: 0800.197.4150

Published by AuthorHouse   09/27/2013

ISBN: 978-1-4567-8597-0 (sc)
ISBN: 978-1-4567-8598-7 (e)

Preface

We Are what We Are

> We face life though it's sometimes
> sweet and sometimes bitter,
> Face life, with a little guts and lots of glitter.
> Look under our frocks: Girdles and jocks,
> Proving we are what we are!

Chesterfield, Thursday 26th December 2007

Iain Writes:

The one thing that's constantly been with me all my life is that I love, no adore, dressing as a member of the opposite sex. It was clearly there before I was born since my earliest recollection of childhood is being told off by my Father for putting on my Mother's stage dress (she was a singer, her stage name was Margaret Dale, which is why I am called Tricia Dale). I wonder now how I managed to get it on! I also remember as a boy playing silly dress up games. I was desperate to play the part of a girl. My friends would say I couldn't as I was a boy and I would accept it. If only I knew then....

As I got older and reached puberty, I realised that the little thing between my legs was not just for what I thought and wasn't always so little. For some reason, most likely because of the person I am, I become sexually aroused by imagining my feminine self rather than girls (or boys). I only looked at girls in magazines because I wanted to be the girl in the magazine. I daren't let anybody know but I secretly wanted them to. I think that is the way society worked on me up until puberty and during it. If I had been allowed and allowed myself to grow up as a girl I'm pretty certain I would have the normal sexual appetite of a girl. However, as I have since learnt; what is normal?

The trouble is that I wasn't (and am still not) ever worried about being a man. I could do it, I could hack it; I was popular, I was good at sports especially football and cricket. Inside however my dreams started to become more erotic as I progressed through puberty. I should have been dating girls. That was a real problem though because I'd look at a girl and think how much I wanted to be her, to wear what she wore, to smell how she smelt, just to have the opportunity to be feminine. I did go on some dates but I just wasn't committed enough. Although the girls were lovely I had no real desire to be with them, I just wanted to be one of them. At this stage of my life I didn't think about whether I fancied boys at all. Had I allowed myself to dress as I would like though that may have been different. If I saw a very pretty girl with a guy I'd just think how wonderful it would be if I could be her; not lucky him.

So I went to University having been successful at school and still playing sport to a very good level. Inside me this desire to be feminine, to look and feel like a woman; but externally I would do everything not to show my true feelings. I was seen through at University and had options to develop my feminine side which I refused point blank. I did have girlfriends but I couldn't make love to them as a man would. Underneath I suppose I wanted to be underneath. I fought and fought for the one thing I shouldn't have fought for. So I left University with a degree but no acceptance of who I really was; so I carried on fighting.

I started a job in computing and threw myself into sport, particularly cricket, and beer. I was still trying to cover up what was inside, trying to be macho and to some extent it succeeded. Men would treat me as one of them but as soon as I met a woman, she would read that there was something different about me. I didn't think, kiss or act as any other man she had met before. I was in no way the predator she was used to and was desperate for her to take control. It was extremely difficult for me to get past a first date - and as for sex? Well you now know the problems I had with that.

I did get one or two chances to dress up, at themed parties - but the ache I felt when I took off my clothes and make-up hardly made it worthwhile, added to which I looked awful. So in my mind at the time I was succeeding as a man but as a girl? I had no clothes of my own and wasn't particularly happy. I moved into a flat with a mate, a wonderful guy who knew nothing then but does now and is so scared, so the opportunities became less and less. Under cover, under the covers, things were becoming more and more compelling. I couldn't resist the transgender phone lines which were available at the time and loved to read about t-girls in newspapers but couldn't bring myself to buy a transgender magazine. I might out myself. I was also starting to learn about my submissive side.

Then I met the girl of my dreams, trying desperately to forget the fact that I was the girl of my dreams. We knew each other as friends earlier so the transition wasn't too hard. I was very much in love and did think that I had got rid of the biggest burden of my life. Inside me I was determined to make it work. Sex was so difficult though, as soon as I got on top there was nothing there. We managed, thanks to her determination, and eventually produced twin girls to go with her other daughter. So I had a ready made family and I was WAS going to be a Father to them. I still love them to bits. Sexually things went further downhill after the twins were born, though I wouldn't describe it as a particularly steep decline. I did play the dutiful Father and feel my femininity helped in bringing them up. I was and still am much closer to them than most men manage. So I was stuck in a rut. No dressing, no clothes, much love for my children; but still many thoughts deep down which were becoming even deeper. But then ......

The Internet reached me and I realised I wasn't alone. I couldn't believe it. Thousands and thousands of people who were similar to me, desperate to be what they were but equally desperate to hide it. So I started to talk to them, and I started to learn, and I couldn't resist any longer. Later that year, it was 1995, my Father died. This totally destabilised me and I was at a loss at what to do. I haven't yet mentioned my parents, but they were so lovely, they brought me up perfectly, and my feelings were nothing to do with them. I still love them both dearly. My Mother knows what I am but never wants to see me as Tricia; after all I am her only son. But...... she is old and I don't, seriously don't, want to scare or hurt her.

I told my partner, there was no other way, I had to - it was really getting to me. I always thought it would get easier to live with my secret, but it got harder and harder. She was at first supportive and we went to get a wig fitting and went to Manchester; with me dressed on a couple of occasions. Ultimately though neither of us could cope. My transgender ways were coming home, and would roost, and she simply could not accept me as the person I was when we initially met. We have, and are still, together for the children but ultimately we lead separate lives. We both wanted our freedom but still love the children and would hate any harm to come to them. I think we are working well together to ensure they are happy.

Manchester, Friday 27th December 2007

Tricia Writes

I have played around with being me for about six months on and off and have noticed changes happening. Now both Iain and I have decided that Tricia is going to come out of her shell for real.

This is it!

But if I am going to become my true self I have to be fair to my old self. I'll try my best.

I am very proud of my other person. He is caring, kind, honest, trustworthy, open, considerate and principled. I suspect he is a somewhat nicer person than myself. He works hard with little reward and adores his family. I suppose I would say that as he let me into the world, but I do believe it. In some respects we are as different as chalk and cheese. He is a deep thinker who worries and churns things over in his mind for days, whereas I act on the spur of the moment. He is very quite and shy whereas I am much more open and up front. I am struggling to properly express this at the moment having been locked in Iain's psyche for so long but I know that over time this will change. He couldn't care a jot about what he looks like (hardly surprising as he wants to look like me) whereas I am obsessed with it. I love reading the fashion magazines and websites, he prefers serious newspapers and novels. I suppose he is complex and I am flippant. He cares too much about the world; I know I care too much about my appearance.

We do get on very well but I have noticed that the more Iain allows me into his life, the more our qualities merge, it seems to work. It seems to make us both more flexible. Most of the time it is correct to ponder before making decisions but sometimes you have to just do it, you have to immediately choose which way to go; I come into my own then. I also notice that sometimes at work Iain will send cheeky emails (actually it's me!) that are a bit risky or I will come out and make a cheeky or camp comment in the most surprising circumstances. I need to be careful though, I don't want to harm him. We do have our little battles, and for the time being Iain is winning most of the important ones, at least from a moral perspective. For example, I would like Iain's picture in this book, because I want to be open and honest. Iain has thus far forbidden me however because he wishes to protect his children and his job. I guess that makes him a bit more of a realist. I am well aware that my head is sometimes in the clouds. I think this all may change over time and it will be interesting to see if it does.

I suppose you are wondering why Iain has let me into his life, especially since I am so proud of him. Well I'm afraid he had no choice. For years and years he thought he did but ultimately he could not resist me. I have been constantly with him, gnawing away, every day getting stronger and stronger. I was the forbidden fruit, I was Pandora's box but was I? Could I really come out as become my true self; everywhere and to everybody? That is my aim.

So there you have it, my other side, my better side? Iain. I do love him and don't want to harm him or his close circle of family, colleagues and friends. But do I regret anything? My life could have been so different if had I accepted who I was initially. Actually though I don't. I have a lovely family, now grown up who know nothing about the real me.

But it is now my time and I'm not going to let the grass lie. Tricia will come out and will become who she wishes to be. But how to tell people? So awkward.

What follows is how it happened.....

Introduction

Wilkommen

Leave your troubles outside.
So life is disappointing? Forget it!
We have no troubles here! Life is beautiful ....
The girls are beautiful ....

The story itself is part fact, part fiction (I'll leave you to decide) and happened over the last few years. I've changed the ages of the main characters to reflect where I feel they fit in at the moment, more about that later, and have slightly twisted what actually happened to fit in with the story line.

Initially (the first few chapters) I was very poor at dressing so the gay village in Manchester where I was practicing became a school. My hotel room became my dormitory.

Other things in the early chapters:

School uniform = dressed
Fizzy pop = beer
Cream cakes = use your imagination
Tuck shop = our local pub
Big girls club = Gay nightclub often frequented by girls like me.
The sweets which make you giggle are merely poppers, not drugs

All character names in the story are correct (obviously femme names for us girls) unless Tina and I have nicknames for people – when I use the nickname. Tina is my best friend and we are at about the same stage in our development. Tina lives in Manchester (at T-Girl Towers) which is about two miles from the gay village. I have since moved in to live with her at weekend but initially used hotels. We learn different things from each other which fast-tracks our development. The sub-text of the story is about two of us getting stronger and more confident as girls, growing up in fact.

The third main character is George/Georgina a 6 foot 2 inch schoolgirl with a passion for pink socks. The three of us are pretty much inseparable and do many things together, often with hilarious consequences.

There are plenty of other varied and different characters to meet: Sonia, my favourite hooker Antonia, Megan and Becky (aka wife and wife) who are partners, Paula with the ample charms, Mark/Morticia who is lapsed and Glenda, and Monica who is an American to name but a few. Many men also pop up from time to time, often repeatedly. Whenever I go to Manchester, and that is pretty much every weekend, I meet someone new.

I must also mention the guys working behind the bar at the pub. Steve, Lee, Paul and Marie are tremendous fun (yes, even Paul, even though he never smiles), always make us welcome and look after us – which is very important. It can be dangerous out there! Also many thanks to Jay who looks after me in the nightclub when I'm quite often the worse for ware; although I'm always the best for what I'm wearing.

The chapters themselves for the main are in three parts. There is the bit written by me at the start. I tend to write this while I am in Manchester so it's fresh in my mind. This is why it is not very long. I just want to get on with living my new life not writing about it. Then there is a song, which will always have some relevance to the story (however tenuous) then there is the main part, written by Iain when he is back home in Chesterfield and has some time. It's therapeutic for him to do this and keeps me in him during the week.

So don't take everything at face value but it all happened. Iain has great fun writing it and we both want you to enjoy reading it hence the explanation.

Have you noticed that every song is a transgendered song?

Hugs,
Trish xx

Oh, and by the way, I beg you, open your eyes!

Chapter 1

Somewhere Over the Rainbow

So this is it. After fifty years I am determined to come out everywhere as Tricia. That means family knowing, work knowing, dressing in public, going on buses and trains, shopping as a girl, everything. Am I stupid or what? The trouble is its within me, its always been within me but I've suppressed it. I had been up to Manchester a few times so before so know the lay of the land and indeed the lays of the land. This is for real and its dead scary.

I hadn't been to Manchester for a while as I was trying to make this ridiculous decision. Could I take my male side through all this? He would find it very hard. My time was running out however and I decided it was now or never. It is wonderful to be back though, and to meet up with old friends and make some new. By the way, I'm sure its possible to get there.

> Somewhere over the rainbow
> Way up high
> There's a land that I heard of
> Once in a lullaby

In which our heroine returns to school, buys some summer clothes, meets up with her pals, and becomes aware of some mistakes she has made.

After two weeks at home feeling very unwell, Tricia was jolly glad to be going back to school. She was going to meet her best chum Tina again and Tina's chum Georgina. There would be so much to talk about, so many yummy goodies to eat and so much fizzy pop to drink. She was therefore in a very happy mood when Matron showed her to her room. It was brill, plenty of room for two girls and a double bed so scrummy that she had to dive into it. She wondered who she was going to share it with this time.

But no time for play girl, she thought to herself. Time to get up and get out into the big City before meeting her pals. It was now summer, the sun was shining and Tricia needed a new satchel and summer blazer. She was pleased to go shopping in the big City, but sad that she didn't have enough time to put on her school uniform. She was very proud of her school.

Shopping done, Tricia met up with her chums at the tuck shop. It served delicious ginger pop which all the girls loved. What was more, nice boys were allowed to buy pop as well. (Tricia thought about how much she had changed since last year when boys didn't matter at all) .Oh how the girls chatted, so glad to be back together again and how the ginger pop went down. It was so lovely to be back with Tina and Georgina, and Tricia was so happy.

Then one of the teachers, Josh, came in. Tricia had heard about him but had never been in his class. Georgina and Tina had however, and told Tricia about the yummy cream cakes and sweets which made you giggle he gave you if you went for extra tuition. Tricia was thirsting for knowledge and thought she would like some private lessons. By now though it was getting late and the youngest girl Georgina, who was twelve, but a very old twelve, had to leave before lights out.

Tricia and Tina were very excited however because they were old enough to go to the big girls club. Josh wanted to come too but by then he had drunk so much ginger pop he was nearly bursting and the girls were frightened he wouldn't be allowed in. They were all very pleased when they managed to smuggle him past the senior prefects.

Tina and Tricia loved the big girls club. Boys were allowed in if they behaved (though not many seemed to) and lots of old schoolgirls came back to visit. Everybody listens to music, talks, dances and has lots of fizzy pop. The girls stuck with Josh because he told them he had enough cream cakes for them both and plenty of the sweets which made you giggle. At the end of the evening they decided to go back to Tricia's dorm for some extra tuition - but then disaster struck. Tricia had not specified to Matron that she was well enough to have visitors so Josh and Tina couldn't come in. Instead they went back to T-Girl Towers where Tina stayed and, so Tina said, had a very good private lesson where she learned a lot.

What a silly girl I am thought Tricia, but never mind; I can play with my favourite toy rabbit, Buzzy again. But it was not to be Tricia's night. The rabbit's battery had gone and the one thing Buzzy didn't do, was buzz! So, like the good girl she is, she fell into a deep contented sleep.

Chapter 2

Three Little Maids From School

This is going to be hard. Tina and I have agreed to go shopping in the middle of Manchester dressed with Georgina. I have never been out of the village before (except the hundred yards from the hotel). Inside the village I am starting to get to be known, which is good. By the way, I think this song sums up where us three girls currently are,

> Everything is a source of fun
> Nobody's safe, for we care for none
> Life is a joke that's just begun
> Three little maids from school

In which the girls go shopping, are introduced to the limpet, meet the horrid Sonia and have lots of fun. It seems our heroine may be growing up.

It was Saturday morning and the sun was shining again. The girls were very happy because Georgina had a pass to go into the big City with them, and they were all going in school uniform as well. They all loved their school. The girls met at a different shop where the ginger pop wasn't quite so good but Georgina knew the shop keeper who was called Sue. Then they moved onto the old girls common room because Tina and Tricia wanted to talk to the girls playing in the big hockey match the next day. There was something called a munch going on and the girls wondered what scrummy cakes and biscuits you could eat; but they were not old enough to go in. They did meet Rascal who had only recently left school. She was being lead round on a leash by her new owner, but looked very beautiful and was obviously very, very happy. The girls thought how jolly it would be if they were lead around on a leash when they grew up.

Eventually our intrepid three went into the big City in their school uniform. Tina in her short school dress, Tricia in her school blouse and trousers and Georgina in her pretty pink dress with marching pig-tails. They needed some new school knickers so needed to go to the school outfitters called Primark. The girls were amazed at the number and choice of school knickers available.

"Gosh", exclaimed Tricia

"Gosh" exclaimed Georgina

"Josh" exclaimed Tina

"Golly Gosh" laughed all three girls together,

but Tricia noticed that Tina had got a very red face. This was better even than the sweet shop they thought. As they were rummaging through trying to choose some for themselves a group of horrid boys turned up and started pointing and laughing at them. What the boys were doing in the girls part of the school outfitters they didn't know, but our brave girls carried on as if nothing had happened and Georgina and Tina in particular bought enough knickers to last them the term. Then the girls went to the cosmetic store. Tina and Tricia were now old enough to wear make-up at school and both girls enjoyed shopping for lipstick, blush and foundation. Georgina too bought some make-up which she was going to smuggle back into school when she could.

After all that shopping the girls were very thirsty and decided it was time for some ginger pop. Georgina was an extremely brave girl and went to a milk bar called Wetherspoons. Despite being younger, she was far braver than Tina and Tricia because Wetherspoons was a place where all the naughty boys and girls who had been expelled from school went. It was Tina's first time enjoying pop in the big City so maybe it wasn't too surprising that she wanted it to be fun. So Tina and Tricia walked around the corner and found a lovely café which served very yummy ginger pop. The girls then rushed back to school before the gates shut, made it just in time, and headed straight for the tuck shop to meet up with Georgina again.

They had got the taste and fancied lashings more ginger pop. There they met Crystal Chandelier, the oldest girl, at 75, in the school, although this was her final year, and her friend the limpet. The limpet was a strange boy who looked very young and frail but in fact was the complete opposite. He was called the limpet because if anything touched him, it was impossible for it to break free. The girls had also been warned about the limpet's chocolate fingers. Normally they loved anything sticky and creamy but apparently his chocolate fingers made you ill and tasted yucky. At least they knew. Poor Tina; they had barely sat down before she somehow got herself attached to the limpet. It took a good few minutes for her to break free. Tricia and Georgina were very surprised when a few moments later Tina got stuck to the limpet again. Tina did seem a bit more ready this time as she took a deep breath before it happened. When it happened a third time Tricia shook her head. "Tina must have had too many of those sweets which make you giggle last night", she thought .The girls said goodnight to Georgina, as it was that time again and went back to Tricia's dorm.

They were very happy when matron said that Tina could change in Tricia's room for Saturday was always busy in the big girls club and the girls wanted to look their best. Matron also said that it was alright for Tricia to stay with Tina on Sunday night. They were lucky girls! In fact Matron had a soft spot for them both. Though sometimes they were rather too high spirited they worked hard on their studies and were a credit to the school. The girls tried to get some sleep but were too excited so instead practiced putting on their new make-up and helped each other get dressed in their glad rags before going back to the tuck shop for one final ginger pop and then on to the big girls club.

They weren't however aware of the trouble ahead at the tuck shop. For there, looking at herself in the mirror, was Sonia. The girls tried to hide from her but to no avail. "Are they straight", Sonia said to them. Sonia was the leader of a gang of girls, the most horrid in the school. It was said that if a boy gave one of the gang a sweet which made you giggle, she would let the boy play with her. This is something our girls were not at all sure about. It was alright for teachers, but boys? Sonia also spent nearly all the time looking into the mirror; even longer than Tina, Tricia thought. In fact Sonia spent more time looking in the mirror than she did not looking in the mirror. The one problem if you spend all the time looking in the mirror is that you can't see behind you. Tina and Tricia were repeatedly asked if the seams of her stockings were straight. They always were, in fact they were the only part of her which could possibly be described as straight. The girls finally managed to break away from Sonia to go to the big girls club, but she seemed rather too interested in them. This was not good.

The big girls club was already filling nicely when Tina and Tricia arrived. They met loads and loads of friends, old and new and had a spiffing time. Then Tina met an old boy she had played with before when she had a lot of fun but ended up with her knees a little sore. He owned another big girls club in the West End of the biggest city and claims to have played with more than 3,000 girls (which would mean, on average, approximately one new girl per week if he started at the age of twelve). Tina wanted to play with him for one more time. Tricia didn't mind so kissed Tina goodbye and wished her oodles of fun.

There were two reasons Tricia didn't mind. Most important, Tina was her best chum and she wanted her to be happy; but also she had been doing private dancing lessons and was looking forward to practicing her moves on the lovely dance floor with mirrors all round (perfect for Sonia, Tricia thought). So Tricia went upstairs and was very pleased with the way she was dancing. The extra lessons and her practicing had paid off. She was joined on the dance floor by six big girls who had just left school. Tricia let them play with her and one-by-one each of the girls danced behind Tricia pretending to be a horrid boy while the others cheered. Tricia didn't mind that either. It was good fun finding out what it will be like when I'm a big girl, she thought. Then Tricia saw someone she thought she recognized, shuffling in front of her with eyes low. By the time it had registered the girl had gone and, despite searching the big girls club high and low, Tricia couldn't find her again. Tricia couldn't be absolutely certain but was fairly sure it was the girl, Joanne, whom she had helped get dressed on her first day at school. She so hoped that it was Joanne and was sure, if it was, that Joanne would be starting to feel happier at school. Tricia, exhausted, slumped into a soft sofa; it was very late for a girl her age. A boy slumped alongside her. "Mind if I sit here" he said. There were other sofa's available so Tricia was a little surprised he chose that one but since he was quite dishy (she giggled to herself) she let him. Before long the boy had one arm around Tricia's shoulder. When the boy snuggled further up to her she went all gooey inside, and when he started stroking her thigh under her dress, she simply melted. The boy wanted to play with her and she really wanted to let him. Then she remembered; she couldn't have anyone else in her dorm with her and there was no chance of her being allowed in the boys' school. "Oh no, no, no, you silly, silly girl".

Reluctantly, and sadly, Tricia went back to her dorm. She had also forgotten to get a battery so no Buzzy bee tonight either. "I have never known Buzzy so quiet", she mused. She changed into her baby-doll and suddenly her mood lightened. She had learnt so much today, she thought. She never wanted to leave school before, but now she is finding out how fun it is being a big girl, she is much happier. Then she realised what it was all about. She was growing up! Anyway, there is the big hockey match tomorrow. Jolly, jolly hockey sticks! And with a trace of a smile on her face; our by now young lady, fell quickly and silently into a deep, contented sleep.

Chapter 3

Happy Talk

I must be mad. During the week my other side entered me in a beauty contest. I've got no chance, I'm not even old enough. It will be fun trying though. It was another brill day apart from Sonia, who seemed to follow us everywhere. I also got a cab for the first time dressed to meet Tina at t-Girl Towers. I was a bit nervous but there was no problem. As I caught it in the village I suppose there wouldn't be. They must be very used to girls like me. By the way I do have a dream, and I'm starting to live it. I can't say I'm proud yet but I am determined.

> Talk about the boy sayin' to the girl:
> "Golly, baby, I'm a lucky cause."
> Talk about the girl sayin' to the boy:
> "You an' me is lucky to be us!"

Part 3 – The day of the big hockey match; in which Georgina is found in the closet, Tina may have been recruited and Tricia becomes a top model.

So the day of the big hockey match arrived and Tricia awoke, bleary eyed, after far too little sleep for a girl her age. First thing to do was to decamp to T-Girl Towers but getting hold of Tina was proving a problem. Tina must have had a jolly fun night, she thought. Eventually she managed and checked out of her dorm to a cab rank in school uniform for the first time. She picked up some money from Matron and got a lift to Tina's.

Poor Tina, her knees were sore again. Tricia wondered what game they were playing which kept making Tina's knees sore, but was too shy to ask. The girls were really looking forward to the big hockey match. "Rah, Rah, Rah" they shouted.

There was a special school bus to take them in because of the big hockey match. Tricia was very surprised when Tina hid her legs behind a rubbish bin in case the boys saw them. Normally, thought Tricia, the boys could see Tina's school knickers never mind her legs. But then she woke up. It was because her knees were so sore and red, she realised. I am a silly sausage sometimes and must get some more sleep, she thought to herself.

They met up with Georgina at the Tuck Shop. Georgina was too young for the big hockey match, but as chance would have it she met up with some older friends, Glenda and Mark, who agreed to look after her while it was on. Also at the tuck shop was Sonia again. "No, no, no" thought the girls. Sonia invited Tina out, but all they did was sit down showing their knickers and wave at all the passing cars. Tina came back puzzled but they had to get to the big hockey match.

Tina and Tricia cheered all the way through. Not only did their girls win by two goals to nil but it also meant they had won the whole competition. Even better; the girls from the horrid school at the other side of the City, where they wore sweat shirts and trousers lost eight one. "Ha ha ha" said Tina, "That'll teach them for lifting our skirts and laughing at our school knickers" "Ha, ha, ha" said Tricia, who wondered why Tina got special attention.

While Tricia and Tina were watching the big hockey match, Georgina wasn't seeing much at all. Somehow she had managed to lock herself in the wardrobe and it took Mark and Glenda a good hour to find her. They were very cross when they did and Georgina got a frightful spanking which made her cry. Poor Georgina, thought Tricia.

To celebrate the girls went back to school for more fizzy pop. To steer clear of Sonia they went to another tuck shop but it seemed Sonia could read their mind. She asked Tina to go down to the little girls room with her. Fortunately for Tina, the little girls room had a very big mirror which distracted Sonia, and, after telling her that her seams were straight seven times, Tina re-appeared and hugged Tricia tightly. The girls wondered if Sonia wanted to recruit Tina into her gang; but it seemed like they had got away with it, this time at least.

So Tina and Tricia went back to T-Girl Towers to spend a girls' night in. They listened to music and talked and talked; Tina on a chair, Tricia lying on the bed. To be fair they a did talk about school and the curriculum ahead, but mostly they talked about boys. Tricia realised that Tina was growing up just like her, in fact maybe even faster. While they were talking Tina looked down on Tricia lying on the bed.

"Trish, do you really want to end up like me. Look at the way you are lying, legs splayed apart, knickers on display. Its not very ladylike".

"But I love my panties. The trouble is I never get any chance to show them off, unless …."

"That can be arranged"

"How?"

"There are many ways". The voice of experience was indeed a voice of experience.

"You can use nature. Look for wind tunnels which can blow up your dress. When you bend over everyone can see your knickers if you are wearing a short skirt. And if you're standing next to someone you fancy you can accidently brush your skirt up".

"Oh, I see, I think. What about my bra? Sometimes I'd like to show off my bra too, some of them are so pretty".

"Well, you can unbutton your blouse a little. Or you can make sure your straps are showing through."

Tricia was learning such a lot in a short space of time and a long discussion followed about lingerie of all types. What the girls liked wearing what and what they didn't. To be truthful though there were hardly any items of lingerie the girls didn't like. Tricia was really enjoying the chat and eventually took it to likely the only possible conclusion.

"Tina, would you like to see my new baby-doll. It's ever so sexy".

"Have you got it with you?"

"Yes, it's in my handbag. It hardly takes up any room and I never know when I may need it".

"Well it is bedtime so I don't see why not".

After about five minutes Tricia had worked out (again) how the straps went and was looking resplendent in her flowery nightie with matching panties.

"There Tina, what do you think".

Tricia will never know because in the intervening time Tina had fallen asleep on the chair.

That didn't worry Tricia too much though. She started to walk up and down the bedroom modelling her nightwear. Arms on hips she wiggled her backside and practiced her pout. She imagined how wonderful it would be to be on a catwalk in beautiful clothes in front of lots of people. It wasn't too fanciful was it? After all, she does have the body of a super-model. Doesn't she?

Chapter 4

There's a Place for Us

No Georgina this weekend so just Tina and me. We decided to go into town again which was very brave without Georgina. I did enjoy although I got quite a lot of attention. I think I am finally getting used to it and know I have to. So the song, by the way, is meant to suggest that the place for people like us is maybe closer than we think. Although I suspect my thinking is maybe flawed. I am beginning to realise that Manchester is a wonderful, chilled, accepting City.

> There's a time for us,
> Some day a time for us,
> Time together with time spare,
> Time to learn, time to care,

In which there is sadly no Georgina, Tina has another haircut, Tricia (Trinny) almost has her hair cut and they are allowed out from school again (hoorah!).

Georgina was on an exchange trip so wouldn't be around for a few days which left just Tina and Tricia to have fun together. Jolly good girls to a T. Matron had finally decided that Tricia was well enough to share a dorm; originally it was going to be for four people but for some reason it later transpired that it was only for two. That was a pity as we shall see, but the good news for the girls was that to get Tricia used to sharing again, Tina was allowed to stay for the first couple of nights.

So Tricia decamped in her new dorm and met up with Tina. Luckily there was a tuck shop downstairs so, having packed away their clothes like good girls, they went downstairs to enjoy some fizzy pop. There they met up with Terry who was grazing for the night.

"Baa", bleated Terry.

The girls looked at each other. What do you do when someone baa's at you they though. Eventually, and a little unwisely, Tina went "baa" back and both girls giggled.

"You know I'm Welsh boyo", said Terry, "baa".

"We couldn't tell actually", said Tricia. "Baa sounds the same in most accents". The girls looked at each other and knew it was time for a hasty exit.

"Baa baa" they said

"Baa" said Terry; he seemed happy enough.

And the girls ran off to their favourite tuck shop as quickly as their legs could carry them; which wasn't easy in such high-heels.

When they arrived they were very glad to see a lot of their chums. Everyone seemed to be coming in together. Mark and Glenda, Josh; and Paula who we haven't yet met. Paula is a peer of Tina and Tricia and is jolly good friends with both them. "Baa", said Paula, and all the girls went into fits of giggles. The girls could only admire Paula's beautiful breasts and hoped to have some like hers when they grew up.

Now Tina, vain girl that she was, wanted yet another new hairstyle; so our brave girls yet again had to run the gauntlet in the big City. Matron was very kind, and smiling, gave them a pass. She knew they were growing up and wanted to encourage them. Tina was still very nervous about stepping out of school so it was a good job Tricia was with her. So Tricia held her hand as they walked out of the school gates; their first task being to buy Tina some (almost) new school uniform.

They decide to try the second-hand school outfitters as the girls had spent most of their money on fizzy pop. Tricia had never been here before but it was good fun! Tricia bought a school blouse which said "American Airline Hostess" on it. Tina bought a bright yellow mini-skirt and then spent an hour looking for something to match.

Tricia went out for some fresh air and while she was standing there five horrid girls from the bad school on the other of the City walked past. The closest one looked at Tricia and giggled. "Look at that silly girl in her school uniform on a Saturday" she said. One by one the other girls looked back at Tricia, but, and as you know, Tricia is a very brave girl. So she waved to all them. Tricia thinks they were giggling rather too much though.

Tina knew of another second-hand school outfitters which was supposedly up-market. Tricia, who was fast becoming Trinny – and desperately missing Susanah - wasn't so sure. The clothes looked exactly the same but Tina bought a lovely new school dress which she promises she will wear the next time the girls meet. Where was Susanah!

So to the hairdressers for Tina's new haircut. Tricia spent most of the time outside, enjoying watching girls and boys watching a girl or a boy. Tina came out looking delightful; with a fuller darker style. Trinny thought it suited her.

So, back to the tuck shop and back to their friends. Tina's new hair got a resounding (how English can I be?) yes except from Paula who didn't recognise her at all The girls also met up with Habib and the Prodder. Habib was bright, intelligent and witty. Three things which couldn't describe the Prodder. Unfortunately Tricia was the perfect target for the Prodder because, which she didn't realise, there was a small gap between her buttons which was showing off her tummy button. Prod went Prodders finger into the gap again and again and again......and again.

To try to distract him Tina took out her bright yellow mini-skirt and bemoaned the fact that nothing would go with it.

"Green would be good", said Habib

"You'd look like a canary", said the Prodder

"Cheep"; said Tricia, and they all giggled.

Then Prodder found a loose thread on the hem of Tricia's dress and tried to unravel it. Prodder wanted to reveal Tricia's deepest secrets; but our brave girl wasn't ready yet. Josh arrived and with Habib managed to get rid of the Prodder and protect Tricia's innocence. But for how long?

The girls had to go. Josh arranged an extra lesson with Tina and Habib was worried about his partner. Was she really going to leave him? The girls went back to Tricia's dorm and had a lie down before glamming themselves up for Saturday night at the big girls club.

What could possibly happen?

Diddlydiddlydiddlydiddlydee

Chapter 5

Two Ladies

All, please be aware that this is theraputic for me as I have failed in my attempt to become a beauty queen. But I know that is the right decision - I need more time and more exposure (the next few days bring some) and some burlesque lessons which I have hopefully arranged for Tuesday. Now, in the real "Wizard of Oz" the twister comes at the start of the film, so this is about right for the book. Oh, and by the way, I couldn't find a song about four in a bed so this will have to do.

> We switch partners daily To play as he please,
> Twosie beats onsie, but nothing beats threes.
> I sleep in the middle, I'm left, And I'm right.
> But there's room on the bottom If you drop in some night!

Our girls have a jolly fun time!

It started off a fairly quiet, normal night in the big girls club. Tricia was doing her dancing queen act upstairs (rather well actually) while Tina was chatting up the boys downstairs. Occasionally they would meet in the middle for some ginger pop and to discuss options. By the end of the evening there appeared to be two boys who were interested in our brave and sexy girls; Pete and Steve.

"I know", said Tina, "lets go back to Tricia's dorm and we can play Twister"

"Yummy", said Tricia, "I used to love playing Twister when I was a little girl. That sounds fun"

So the intrepid foursome did indeed return back to Tricia's dorm and fortunately it was so late at night that matron was asleep.

Tricia's first thought on entering her room was, how were they going to play Twister when she didn't have a twister mat or one of those funny spinner things? When everybody starting taking their clothes off Tricia became really confused. Tina took Tricia aside,

"This is a type of Twister big girls like us play", she said.

"Gosh", said Tricia and immediately removed her sexy black dress, "can I wear my pretty baby-doll?"

"If you like" said the boys, "it will give us a challenge"

"Not a very big challenge", said Tina

"But I haven't got a mat or one of those funny spinner things" said Tricia.

"I suppose we'll have to use the bed and our imagination", said Tina.

"Of course", said Tricia, "what a silly goose I am". Tricia was trying to sound far older than her years.

However for the next four hours she could certainly have been described as a goose, as for the silly bit – I'll leave you to make up your own mind. There were arms and legs and bodies everywhere. Boy with girl, girl with boy, boy with boy, girl with girl, oh the positions they managed to find. Gosh, thought Tricia, I'll be really good at the young girls Twister now! The game was well refereed by Steve who would occasionally shout "move over" and they would all change places. Eventually, but only for an hour, the game stopped and the four fell asleep exhausted.

Tricia's eyes opened very slowly. It was like they were stuck together with glue. She looked next to her and could see Pete's eyes struggling to open just like hers. On her other side she could hear gentle snoring. Pete murmured something incomprehensible then took a deep breath and tried again.

"Oh Trish, I'm absolutely exhausted. Could you make me a milky coffee to wake me up?"

"Milky Coffee? What do you think I am, a cow? All we've got are these horrible sachet things that are pretty much impossible to open, even with my long nails. And when you finally manage it the milk spills everywhere so there was no point in the first place". Tricia clearly wasn't at her best.

"Ok Trish, just do the best you can. And I wouldn't describe you as a cow at all, more a sexy bitch".

"Thanks, and I'll take that as a compliment though I'm not sure why".

"It was meant as a compliment hen. Come and give me a cuddle".

And there we must leave our intrepid foursome. The weekend started off with a sheep and geese, cows, dogs and hens have also been touched upon. The book is beginning to resemble a farmyard!

Chapter 6

Que Sera Sera

Now I've swapped the next two chapters of the story since it's my story and I can do what I like! It also works better so you'll have to wait for the slushy bit.

You may realise by now that I am an English girl so my morals are based on the Empire and a stiff upper lip; yes lip. This is instilled into children at posh English schools like mine by using the arts and in particular by using poetry written at the height of England's power and in particular by using Rudyard Kipling. His most famous poem, 'If', describes what I need to understand at the moment (I'm not sure about being a man my son though) and particularly the following two lines:

> If you can meet with Triumph and Disaster
> And treat those two imposters just the same

So we'll start with disaster; it's a shorter chapter than triumph anyway. Oh, and by the way, I also need to understand the following: .....

> Que Sera, Sera,
> Whatever will be, will be
> The future's not ours, to see
> Que Sera, Sera

DISASTER – in which our heroine's first attempt to be head girl fails.

Now our young girl was either very brave, very stupid or both; she was told that in her last discussion group. Though young for her age, she was jolly keen to become the head girl of the school. She wasn't even a prefect yet but she entered the competition nevertheless. What was worse was that the naïve young madam thought she had a chance of getting to the finals. She entered her application form in the nick of time. It read as follows:

~~~~~~

Miss Sparkle 2008 Contestant Entry Form

NB. Please provide as much information as possible as this is all that the independent judging panel will have to go on when deciding if you should be selected as a finalist. Any false or misleading information could result in disqualification.

Name Tricia Dale

Are you TV, TS etc. etc.

Age 50

Height/Weight 5ft 10in – 9.5st

Eye/Hair Colour Auburn/ hazel

Where are you from? Manchester

Occupation Schoolgirl

Describe yourself in three words? Open, Caring, Committed

What are your Hobbies/Interests & do you have any interesting skills?

You know my main interests; but I also like cricket and baseball, classical music (especially Opera) and literature. Oh, and real ale, red wine, port and cheese. I can't get enough cheese. I am currently learning Burlesque and am taking private courses in Sheffield. I have been given exercises to strengthen my legs and improve my posture which will enable me to dance in very high stilettos. I think I am now ready for my next lesson. Fabulous!

I can bowl an un-pickable googly, which is difficult in a bra and I'm told I do a particularly interesting version of "Wild Thing" by the Troggs.

Have you had any surgery (if yes please provide details)?

When I was younger I had a lump removed from my neck.

How do you think your friends would describe you?

Fun to be with, sometimes very serious but sometimes ridiculously silly. It keeps people on their toes! They will know that I care deeply about them and that it is important to me that they are happy. They will trust me and they will know I'm there if they have problems; or more likely "that slapper over there".

What are you best qualities & why?

I am open, honest, fair and approachable but I am most proud of my enthusiasm. I try in all walks of life, At work, at play, with my children, everything is important to me. In short, I care. I have found that is the best way to be loved. I smile because I know that rubs off on other people. Actually my best quality is that I have the body of a supermodel (no boobs included) because people are then naturally attracted to me.

If there was one thing that you could change about yourself (other than gender related changes) what would it be?

I can change anything about myself – except; I can't change the past. I'd like to be younger and go through this all over again. Actually I'd love to be younger and go through this all again.

If you could have three wishes what would they be?

Either:

-   A proper education for all in the world. I'm sure that's more important than anything else.

- No negative discrimination on any grounds (hence no wars and no hate)

- The elimination of poverty and greed.

Or

- To play the part of Sally Bowles on Broadway

- A designer handbag costing at least £3000 with matching shoes

- To be Victoria Beckham for a night; as long as the kids are with her Mum.

Is there anything that makes you stand out in the crowd?

My intelligence, my body and the fact that I am a leader. Chicken legs. My six inch stilettos, now I can stand in them.

Why do you want to be Miss Sparkle 2008?

After years suppressing what is inside me I have finally come out and am loving every minute of it. However I regret the wasted years when I denied who I was. So there are two reasons I would like to be Miss Sparkle; firstly to continue the path I am on by being able to openly express myself to whoever and in different ways; but also to help other transgendered people not fall into the same trap I did. I believe Miss Sparkle would provide an ideal vehicle to enable me to do this. Also I love showing off and would just adore the photo-shoot opportunities, the frocks, the make-overs, the style, the glamour.... I just can't wait!

Is there any additional information that you would you like to provide in support of your entry?

It has been only nine months since I made the decision to deal with my gender issues. I have moved a vast distance since then and am very proud of the person I am becoming. It has not been easy as I have to juggle with family life and work for the moment. Maybe this Sparkle is a bit too early for me but I do want to push myself to the limit (and have fun!). But, what the heck, and after all; Life is a Cabaret, old chum, AND I LOVE A CABARET!

~~~~~~

She also attached two photos. One of her looking dead sexy (well she thought so anyway) posing outside the tuck shop. The other of her on a freezing day in the playground. In the latter she thought she looked enigmatic; in fact she looked more like a car mechanic. It was this photo which was to prove her downfall.

Now, what everybody knows is that you can't become head girl on words alone. Tricia, being so young, was unaware of this. What of course she should have done was put on her best school uniform, had a makeover from the girls studying fashion and beauty in the top year, and visited the school photographer for a proper head and shoulders picture. A picture which could paint a thousand words. Well she didn't so she is not yet ready to be head girl. But she is still young and there is plenty more time yet. Chin up girl!!

Chapter 7

When You Wish Upon a Star

And the bell rings for the end of term. If this were a play, all the naughty boys would go to the bike sheds for a sneaky fag while the scenery got moved about. It is not a play but that has given me an idea (dangerous). The trouble is I'm no good at dialogue which is a bit of a handicap.

This was the most amazing experience of my life so far. Where it will lead who knows but it took me days to come back to earth. I think I am getting to the end of my rainbow, but have a way to go yet by the way.

> When you wish upon a star
> Makes no difference who you are
> Anything your heart desires
> Will come to you

TRIUMPH - In which our heroine learns to fly solo.

It was a big day in young Tricia's life. She had earlier asked Matron for a pass to go out of school, on her own and Matron said yes! Matron actually thought that girls grew up rather too quickly these days, but as we know she liked Tricia's spunk. She felt Tricia was just about ready and she was such a good girl too.

So Tricia, dressed in her best school uniform, made up to perfection (who's kidding who) entered the tuck shop a little nervously to prepare herself for the big expedition. There she found Josh which was a bit of a surprise. Josh was supposed to be at T-Girl Towers giving Tina an extra-curriculum lesson. Tricia, being her best friend, warned Tina via text. Just another fizzy pop said Josh when Tina called him. When Tricia started her momentous walk Josh was still there. Poor Tina, thought Tricia, I suppose she's learning just how hard it is to be a big girl.

She also met her old school chum Habib. She wasn't sure about Habib. He was a bit Shirley Bassey and a bit Tom Jones. He was also a bit Albert Einstein which is why Tricia liked him so much. He was on the precipice too as he was going out with a big girl who had just left school. They had had an argument. Would she come back? Would she not? Would Habib be happy? Would he not? Tricia left this predicament at the tuck shop. After all, there's only so much a young girl can do, isn't there?

It was 15:00 on Monday 26th May (Bank Holiday Monday) 2008 when our brave girl walked out of the school gates, on her own for the first time and into the sunshine. She looked as good as she could but she wasn't fooling anyone. She was a very young girl in a big big world. Bravely she went to the great big shopping centre in the middle of the third biggest City in England. All of the girls who have left the school told her it was amazing. Tricia couldn't believe it. It was fantastic! Shop after shop with beautiful clothes everywhere. She loved it!

Into the first shop she strode where she saw a lovely sundress. She tried it on; it fit but it wasn't quite her so she took it back. She learned that the second floor was best as it contained all the boutiques. She was quite good at shopping and knew very quickly if she liked something or not. In one shop she found some dead sexy white jeans. She thought she had dropped a size so asked to try them on. A look of surprise but again no problem; although she didn't know she needed to take two other items of clothing in with her. Fortunately they were provided by the shop assistant. She struggled to get into them but when she managed it she loved them. They fit her perfectly and clung to her every contour. Yes, she had dropped a size. She was now a size 8 (UK) size 4 (US), lucky girl! She had to buy them. She found a khaki jump-suit in another shop. Again she tried it on and it fitted so she bought that too. Tired she went to Nero's to have a cappuccino and, while drinking it, touched up her make-up in front of everybody.

She wanted to carry on shopping but had a predicament. She also wanted a wee but didn't have the right change for the Ladies and daren't use the Gents. The only thing to do was to go back to the Tuck Shop. The shops were starting to close anyway. But Tricia was on an absolute high, ignoring the occasional comments of "look there's a schoolgirl in her school uniform on a bank holiday" she could hear as she clip clopped her was back to the school gates.

"Yay, yay, yay", thought Tricia and paused.

"Golly gosh, I'm a big girl now, I have passed the test. I can use the back of the tuck shop. All that beer and wine; all those cigarettes and drugs available to me, super duper!" She was such a good girl though; and for now could be found way up high on the other side of the rainbow"

P.S. When she got back to the tuck shop, Josh had gone for his lesson with Tina and Habib's girlfriend had indeed come back. So it was a good day for all!

Chapter 8

One Hand, One Heart

Where troubles melt like lemondrops
Away above the chimney tops
That's where you'll find me

Someone told me on chat that troubles can't melt like lemondrops, so I thought about it and they do. When I go on holiday I take my troubles with me. Are the kids enjoying themselves? How are they getting on back at work? What's the money situation? When I go Manchester I'm so focused on being Tricia that literally everything else disappears.

This is the start of the three most amazing days of my entire life. Hugely emotional, I don't think I have ever laughed or cried so much. I am extremely lucky to have found a wonderful friend in Tina. It is so much easier and you learn so much more when you share each other's experience. We are so close we are beginning to be called sisters, and that is how it feels. By the way, the song could be about me and the constant boy/girl struggle but in fact is for Antonia and how I felt during our meeting, I think she'll approve and yes, I know I have already used West Side Story but its about as good as they get and Manchester is on the west side of England. So it's relevant, isn't it? And I think Natalie Wood is so pretty!

Make of our hands one hand,
Make of our hearts one heart,
Make of our vows one last vow:
Only death will part us now.

In which our girls are re-united, Tina strikes it lucky (or so she thinks) and Tricia meets a working girl

The backstage boys worked hard to prepare the scene before Tricia's arrival. The tuck shop would soon become a pub called The Irish pub which the girls would simply refer to as Paddys. The big girls club was to become a night club called Napoleons which the girls would refer to as Naps. The playground would become the campus. Yes, Tricia had finished school and was travelling up for her first day as a college student. The very good news for her was that Tina was joining her. They had arranged to meet at Tricia's digs, The New Union, at 18:00 that evening. "Golly gosh", thought Tricia, possibly for the last time, "I'm so excited!"

Tricia arrived at around 15:00 and checked in. She made herself hairless then had a shower. She hung up her skirts and dresses and neatly folded her t-shirts. Then slowly, carefully but with relish dressed and made-herself up. She was to remain dressed for the duration of her stay. What to wear? She was fed up lugging her suitcase around but now, when she looked at the array of choices she had, she realised it was worth it. She wanted to show off her (chicken) legs and wanted to try something new, so opted for her green khaki jump suit. Then for the best bit, oh how she loved doing this! As she put on her wig and applied her lipstick in the mirror she thought she could see Lara Croft looking back at her. She was mistaken but she didn't look half bad.

My how the girls hugged when they met each other again and how they talked. They were sitting outside drinking, the sun was shining, when they bumped into Sally, or more precisely Sally bumped into them. Sally, a genuine girl, was going through a difficult time. Suffice it to say that she hated men, but quite liked t-Girls because they were kind and gentle. They talked and in time the sun went down and Sally's legs were cold. "That's ok", said Tricia, resourceful girl that she was "you can borrow a pair of my tights, my room is only upstairs and Tina has to drop her stuff off anyway". So the girls went up to drop off Tina's clothes and Tricia shoved a pair of new tights in her handbag. When they returned downstairs however, Sally was nowhere to be found.

So back to Paddys for the first time in a while. Inside, Tricia was quite proud of herself for she had once read somewhere that a spare pair of tights was one of the most popular possessions a woman kept in her bag. She thought she was becoming a lady ha-ha-ha-ha. When they arrived Josh was there (surprised?) but Habib not, Habib had not got a pass which worried Tricia. So the girls and Josh had a chat.

The Irish pub is an old fashioned English pub, probably in its prime in the 40's and 50's. You could easily imagine the scene then in the smoke filled single bar. Sadly smoking is no longer allowed inside English pubs but, the girls found, the best way to meet people was to have a cigarette in the small smoking area outside. Music of the 50's and 60's is played at an acceptable level, easy to talk over but also possible to listen to. They even play "Over the Rainbow" sometimes. The girls like to sit in the corner where they can watch the guys coming in. Chic it is not, but it is clean, friendly and serves excellent food with good beer. It is an honest pub. It is also probably the most famous gay pub in Manchester.

The girls had a good gossip and got to know each other again before going back to Tricia's to change for the night. They wanted an easy first night so not too much to drink and to leave early. Tricia wore her pretty blue dress; most un-Tricia like she thought but she loved wearing it. Tina was onto a promise she said. She was waiting for a call from Harvey. Back to Paddys for one final pint then onto Naps.

Napoleons looks a small unimposing building from the outside but reveals its charms if you manage to get through the bouncers on the door. Tricia was once refused entry after having had far too much ginger pop for her own good. There is a downstairs bar where you can talk quietly, a middle bar with video screens strategically placed playing music and luxurious settees where you can lounge. Tricia has been known to 'pull' on these settees more than once. The upstairs bar is the home to the mirrored dance floor. There is a large smoking area outside, and like Paddy's it is another area useful for chatting and picking up guys. Tricia's backside has been pinched on more than one occasion out there. Chic it is not, but at its best it is vibrant, noisy and fun. It is also probably the most famous transgendered nightclub in Manchester.

Tricia and Tina worked as a team with Tina covering the ground floor and Tricia the top floor. Occasionally they would meet in the middle or in the smoking area and compare notes to ensure they were both aware of all the available talent. This particular night Naps was quiet, but not that quiet that Tina couldn't pull and at about 2:00 in the morning she took her guy back to T-Girl Towers. Tricia was dancing with a girl and suggested, since it was late, they went back to Tricia's room. Antonia agreed.

There then followed the most exhilarating few hours in Tricia's young life. It turned out that Antonia used to be a violin player in a concert orchestra. She gave it all up to become a transsexual prostitute. She originally came from Russia but has lived in England most of her life. None of that matters. What matters is that she is a beautiful, intelligent, loving, caring, giving person. They talked for hour after hour; they laughed, they cried, they went deep inside each other, they talked shop, they kissed, they hugged, they smoked (Tricia's first time) and they drank. "Sometimes", said Antonia, "it's nice not to sleep with a man". Tricia felt so proud. At about 6:00 Tricia led Antonia out of her apartment. They kissed and cuddled each other one final time and vowed to meet again. "Wow", thought Tricia, "college is such fun and I haven't even been here a day yet. I think I'm going to love it!".

With that school disappeared over the horizon.

Tricia and Antonia have arranged to meet again in two weeks time. A bit of a dispute over Mahler!

Chapter 9

The Sun has got Her Hat on

Let's lighten up a bit; but the weekend was like that. One minute intense, the next hilarious.

The day happened pretty much as written. I have elaborated the telephone conversations (though we did have a laugh on similar lines afterwards) but the texts were exactly as sent. I copied them from my phone. As you can probably gather I was in a bit of a euphoric mood.

Oh and a famous TV reality series had just started in the UK. I'll leave you to guess what it is!

My male side will likely never appear in the story but will occasionally slip in by accident. – the quote near the end is from his favourite album when he was growing up. It is about living in a parallel universe and this is exactly how I a feel right now. There is the universe I am living here (and really living here), in Manchester, and the universe at home/work. They are absolutely totally different lives. So, and by the way, how jolly English!

The sun has got her hat on
Hip-hip-hip-hooray!
The sun has got her hat on,
She's coming out today.

In which Tricia takes the opportunity to go solo again while Tina is having one of those days you'd rather forget. It was Friday 13th after all.

Friday 13th June 2008. Communications from Tricia to Tina:

10:00 Text

Big sister diary day nine. Tricia learns about what big girls do for a living from a violin playing ex concert musician. Might as well get paid for it hon! Will give you a bell about eleven

11:10 Phone

Hi hon -

Yes I'll be quick, whose coming round? -

Not another admirer, you've only just seen one out the door haven't you. Was it a good night? - .

Long and slim, shaped a bit like a trowel, sounds interesting –

yes can imagine it could hurt –

every position under the sun, but you weren't under the sun were you? –

sorry I am silly, forty minutes to get comfy, suppose that's called foreplay, you did well hon, how long did he last? -

Only three minutes. Not sure he's worth it., was it a good three minutes though –

oh, flat, sorry, that figures -

Stay out of Paddy's, whatever for, your beginning to sound like my Mother –

I know we've got a busy weekend but at the moment you seem rather busier than me, Mum! Who is he, Harvey? –

Alan, from Liverpool, can't have seen your picture then ha-ha –

But have you seen his? It could be shaped like the leaning tower of Pisa, or a polo mint, imagine that, all the pain and none of the pl...-

Only teasing you darling -

You might be out later –

ok I'll text, don't want to disturb your fun hon. Don't do anything I wouldn't do. As if -

hugs hon, byeee

12:30 Text

Big sister diary day nine. In Paddys writing about disaster. Sorry Mum

12:50 Text

Big sister diary day nine pint two. In Paddys writing about triumph. Pulled if I want, I don't; gross. Very sorry Mum.

13:20 Text

Big sister diary day nine pint three. In Paddys writing about triumph. Just noticed …

The sun has got his hat on

Hip hip hip hooray

The sun has got his hat on

Is Tina coming out today

Very very sorry Mum

13:50 Text

Big sister diary day nine pint four: In Paddys still writing about triumph.

The pub is full of t-Girls

Hip hip hip hooray

The pub is full of t-Girls

And no-one here is gay!

Very, very, very sorry Mum

14:30 Text

Hi hon. And the lamb lies down on broadway. Here I go!

Da da da da da da da da da da da

Will phone at 3

14:50 Text

Big sister diary day seven coffee one.

Everybody's happy

Hip hip hip hooray

Everybody's happy

because Tricia's out to play.

15:45 Phone

Hi hon, I'm sitting in Starbucks in the Arndale sipping coffee -.

Yes wonderful, no trouble at all, people know and a few are shocked when they get close but its great fun. –

Wearing my sexy white jeans, they're drop dead gorgeous!. -

Yes, I'm beginning to enjoy being noticed –

Been in a few shops but not seen anything yet, anyway how did your Liverpudlian get on –

still there, crikey he must have some stamina –

Sorry hon, reception here isn't good, every time he was about to come the what phone beeped?

well I did say I was going to text you –

Every twenty minutes is a bit excessive I suppose, but how was I to know it was going to take him twenty minutes, the last one only lasted three -

Keep your voice down, I'm in the middle of town, anyway why didn't you turn your phone off? -

Calm down, I suppose it is impossible to move when you're in that position -

That's ok, I didn't get much sleep last night either. Suggest we get a couple of hours and meet up later. I'll go to sleep about six —

meet nine, fine, rhyme ha-ha -

ok Mum I'll shut up -

bye hon love you loads.

17:30 Text

Big sister diary day nine pint five.

When I was just a little girl I asked my Mother what would I be. You would be proud of me Mum, Honest! About to go to sleep. Night, night. Your loving daughter xx.

Chapter 10

Your Tiny Hand is Frozen

Ok, just to annoy Tina lets go a bit up market for the by the way this time. It was quite a quiet evening actually. I do occasionally need quite evenings as I am a bit old to go clubbing every night. I have noticed I am far quicker at getting ready now. I have a make-up routine which I follow religiously. I also think I'm beginning to look and act in a more feminine way. But then that may be the pink fog.

> Speak, tell me who you are.
> Please do!
>
> SÃ¬. Mi chiamano TriciÃ¬,.........

In which the girls have a fun night together, though there is a dispute over a rabbit. They meet a character from a picture show, and Tina's worst nightmare comes true.

Tina woke Tricia at eight. At least I had a couple of hours, Tricia thought. She quickly got herself ready, sparkly gold top, denim mini and patterned tights, to meet Tina at Paddys for nine. Tricia is now comfortably capable of getting ready in an hour.

"How was he", said Tricia as they hugged.

"Yummy", said Tina, "and he wants more"

"We're college girls now, we don't use words like yummy", replied Tricia.

"Your turning into my Mother", said Tina with a smile on her face.

"Has Harvey rung yet?".

"No, I'm surprised at that".

"I don't believe he exists".

"He does!".

"He's just a figment of your imagination".

"In fact he's a rabbit", added Tricia.

"He is not a figment of my imagination and he is not a rabbit. He's hairy not furry", replied Tina sternly.

"Yummy", said Tricia

"He wants a threesome"

"Yummy, yummy, yummy" said Tricia, "Lets go for a smoke".

Outside the girls were being eyed up and down in a familiar manner by a tall man.

"You two look dead sexy, are you sisters?" said the man

"No", replied the girls in unison.

"I dress sometimes, but not like you, you are very brave"

"How do you mean?" asked Tina.

"I like Rocky Horror and sometimes go round the pubs in heavy make-up in my clothes", said Frank-n-furtive

"What do people think?" asked Tricia.

"They think it's a laugh, not as serious as you girls"

The girls laughed.

"Have you seen Harvey?" said Tricia.

"Whose Harvey?" replied Frank-n-furtive.

"A rabbit" said Tricia.

"He is not a rabbit" said Tina, angrily.

"He is a hairy rabbit" explained Tricia.

"Are you two sure your not sisters" said Frank-n-furtive.

"Certain" said the girls

And they decided to move on, back to Tricia's lodgings for a drink. It was very quiet but they did find the weirdest thing. A cubicle with two toilets. So Tricia and Tina could continue to gossip while doing their business. It was quite good fun actually.

Then onto the AX bar and Tina picked up the key to the changing room. This was where girls visiting for the day could get changed. The lighting was superb and Tricia and Tina took many pictures of each other adjusting their make-up and dancing to the music going on in the bar. They were so happy together.

So onto Naps and the pair promised themselves an early night as they had plans for the morning. The usual tactics were employed and there was a fair bit of talent around, but as we know by now, they are such good girls.

They went out for a smoke where they met some theatrical people. If there's one thing Tina doesn't like its theatrical people. She is into heavy rock not arty-farty stuff as she calls it. So she kept quiet while Tricia discussed the great musicals with Rhyanne. To their left a make-up lesson was about to start from an Aussie guy who worked for MAC. Tricia and Rhyanne tossed their make-up into the ring. The Aussie was quite impressed with what they had, but it was not as good as MAC apparently. Tricia was quite pleased with that.

As the make-up artist took some mascara from Rhyanne he said "your little hand is frozen".

"Actually", said Tricia, "its your tiny hand is frozen. Bet you don't know who wrote that?"

"Was it Steps?"

Tricia and Rhyanne shook their heads in despair.

Tina had had enough culture and suggested they went back. Tricia was tired too and agreed. They had a chat with a glass of wine for a while before Tina dropped off. She was lying diagonally across the bed. If Tricia was to get any sleep that night she had to turn her straight. Some things, thought Tricia, are beyond even me.

Chapter 11

Oh What a Beautiful Morning

You need to be both very brave and very aware to dress like I do when going around town. Though I am getting better I am still easily read, although most people are too busy in their day-to-day lives.

Undoubtedly it is dangerous out there in straight City although, ironically, I seem to get more grief from the stag and hen parties in the Village than I do in the Arndale. Still it was a lovely, sunny Sunday and Sunday, for some reason, feels far more chilled and easier than Saturday or Friday night.

> Oh what a beautiful morning,
> Oh what a beautiful day,
> I've got a wonderful feeling,
> Everything's going my way.

In which the young ladies travel far, make rash promises and meet up with Pete again.

"Cock-a-doodle-do" said Tina as she woke up at least three hours later than the laziest hen in the world.

"Cock-a-doodle-what?" said Tricia, "this is the first morning this week you haven't had any cock-a-doodle-do"

"Maybe that's why I feel so good, let's hit town early, whose getting ready first"

"You seem full of the joys of spring so you go", Tricia was barely awake.

Tricia had almost hummed up to the part where Mimi was dying in Act 4 of La Boheme by Puccini when Tina announced she was ready to face the world.

"Your turn", she said

"I thought this was going to be an early morning raid" said Tricia who promptly got herself moving.

While Tricia was getting ready, Tina was poring over a map of Manchester like an Army General.

"Whatever are you doing?" asked Tricia, putting on her foundation.

"Trish, whatever you do, look after yourself girl. It's a jungle out there!" said Tina, "and I'm trying to avoid ambushes of any kind".

"No your not Tina", replied Tricia, "You're trying to avoid people of any kind". Tricia was well aware that it actually is safest when there are lots of people around and also well aware that Tina would be well aware soon. She smiled to herself.

"Anyway, has Harvey phoned yet?"

"No, he still hasn't"

"He is an imaginary rabbit isn't he?"

"Shut it!, I love you really"

So, zigzagging their way through tracks strewn with weeds, unused by civilisation for hundreds of years, the girls finally hit the big city. "Ouch" said the big city. Now General Tina had a real problem. She looked left. People. She looked right. People. She looked straight ahead. People; but straight ahead there were slightly fewer people. "Let's be brave Trish" she said and for possibly the first time in her young life, Tina went straight. Tricia bravely followed smiling to herself again.

First stop Primark to top up on panties and stockings. Tricia also found a lovely red top. It had a picture of a pretty girl just like Tricia (ha-ha) on it with a speech bubble coming out of her mouth. Four hearts were at the top of the speech bubble followed by:

"I just love those shoes"

"I have to have a pair"

Next on to Tina's favourite charity shop. Tricia had a quick look round but didn't see anything she wanted so went out for a smoke and to watch people watching her. Half a pack of cigarettes later a triumphant Tina emerged with a bag full of clothes, the content of which will become apparent later, but probably not here. "Its great shopping in the morning, people are so chilled" said Tina who was starting to chill herself. Indeed she was so relaxed that the girls decided to trek further into the City. Farther than they'd ever gone before.

Now it's not commonly known but when girls like these are walking through town they sing little tunes in their head. I think we can guess what Tricia was singing, after all it was a beautiful morning. Tricia was intrigued to find out what Tina was singing. It was a song by Nazareth:

> *Born under the wrong sign*
> *Trouble is my middle name*
> *Born under the wrong sign*

Tricia seemed to be doing a lot of head shaking now she was a college girl. But at least they were going to the Northern Quarter; the cultural heart of the City.

There they found a nice little bar and were quietly sitting outside watching people watching them when they bumped into Alan. Alan was intrigued by the girls although he was quite disparaging about the way Tricia had powdered her nose and about Tina's dress sense which he described as "eighties throwback". Tricia thought that Tina would secretly be pleased with that description.

It was a long way back to the campus, about a 30 minute walk. Tina was still in charge of navigation and still steered clear of crowds. They stopped to buy some cigarettes and an umbrella. Inside the campus they decided to have a drink outside by the canal. Unknown to them there was a stag party going on in the bar next door. 23 guys and two pretty girls. What chance did they have? One of the guys wandered across and asked them to join the party, but the girls played hard to get. "We've just been shopping and were very tired, can we have a moment to ourselves" said Tricia. The guy agreed but asked the girls to promise they would join them later. Foolishly the girls agreed.

Sometimes however life works in your favour. The guys in the stag party were that drunk that they forgot about the promise and eventually moved off down the road. Lucky girls! The guys had however taken a number of pictures of our belles which they have no doubt hung on their bedroom walls to give them something to dream about when they go to sleep. No doubt!

The girls went back to Tricia's dorm to get ready for Naps. Tricia decides to wear her very slinky black dress. Tina dressed like a Bay City Roller. In Naps they met Zara and Michelle amongst others who seem to have a similar love/hate relationship as our sisters. They also meet Pete again, roll back a few chapters, and give him a promise. Pete stays with the girls until nearly closing time. Michelle describes them as a 'ménage à trois' which was particularly apt, considering they took Pete back to Tricia's dorm to give him the time of his life.

What actually happened we will never know because I ran out of paper but I think it can be assumed that a good time was had by all.

Re-stocked because I needed it to write this it was a sad day for Tricia as she had to leave. Dressed in mufti (Tricia) and looking resplendent (Tina) they went to Paddy's for their final goodbyes. There they met Tom, A very keen Liverpool Football supporter who also apparently was almost the size of a twelve inch ruler when happy. He was great fun to talk to and a lot had happened in his life. He may well appear later. But as Trish and Tina were tearfully saying their goodbyes, Tina's phone rang.

It was Harvey. Tina's face lit up. He would be round in the evening. Or at least Tina hopes so.

Chapter 12

Singin' in the Rain

When I come back from Manchester I am hugely emotional. I cry (good), I think of music and poetry and the book and how I can write up what happened. I am going through that now, as I write.

When I go to Manchester it takes time for Trish to kick in completely, but Iain gives her that. Iain wants Tricia to have all the fun in the world. So, Sparkle weekend, the biggest transgender celebration in England and its in Manchester YAY. By the way it was rainy and wet but I suppose you can't have a rainbow without rain. Some bits in this chapter are very English but you're all on the Internet for goodness sake so look them up and have fun reading; as much as Iain did writing.

> I'm singing in the rain
> Just singing in the rain
> What a glorious feelin'
> I'm happy again

In which the two girls share some texts, discover Tina's surname, meet a felon, sing and get very wet

"She's coming home, she's coming home; Tricia's coming home". Tricia views Manchester as her home. It was where she was born, in 1995 actually (she knows because of the Windows Operating System sadly) and where she has been bred since, although there was a long gap in between. She is more than happy to support Manchester United (Tina approves) and would quite like a not-so-quiet night in with Andrew Flintoff, though Freddie and Rachel may think otherwise. Despite what she says, Manchester is also a

City of culture. It is a prosperous, vibrant City with tolerant, lovely people. It also has a gay village that's the best in England. "Manchester-la-la-la-la, Manchester la-la-la-la"

Tina's mobile was on the blink, or it may have been her signal. "Don't send me texts" she texted. Then it was working again

"Testes testes" was sent to Tricia

"Leave them alone!" was the reply. Tricia had more of an idea than Tina where they had been.

It was Thursday evening and the rain was lashing down. That's the worst thing about Manchester, the rain lashes down quite often. The girls had swapped a couple of other texts.

"What do you think about Tina Travain"? texted Tina Travain

"I'd go with Tina Tresvain" texted Tricia Dale

Eventually Tina worked out it was French, like the letters she uses almost every day of her life.

"I think Tricia Trollope" texted Tina Tresvain; not knowing that Tricia Trollope had already been rejected much earlier in the young girl's life. It was discussed by her first, very strict schoolmarm. It was agreed that, like everybody else, Tricia's parents should name her. Her Father was called Patrick, hence Tricia, her Mother's stage name was Margaret Dale. So Tricia Dale. After that meeting with the schoolmarm Tricia couldn't sit down for two days. Why hadn't she learned her abc?

So what do you do on a rainy in Manchester. Well, you go to Paddy's where, if there is a transgender fest going on, you will meet up with other like-minded people. There they bump into (it isn't hard but very pleasant) the ample chested Paula who is talking to a guy. She wishes to palm him off and sees a couple of likely candidates.

"This is Burglar Bill" said Paula

"You must be Rod Stewart" said Burglar Bill

"Ha ha ha ha ha" laughed Tricia

"And you must be Mick Jagger" said Burglar Bill

Tricia shut up.

So onwards and to the New Union where there is a karaoke going on. It is still raining hard but inside the weather is cloudy. Paula sings "Angels" by Robbie Williams. Rather well thought Tina and Tricia. Tricia sings "Wild Thing" by the Troggs. That was different think Paula, Tina and Burglar Bill who is stroking Tricia's hand (?) and looking into her bloodshot eyes with lust.

Finally to Naps which is quiet apart from a lot of t-Girls. The dance floor isn't open which annoys the girls. At about two o'clock Tina announces she is going back to T-Girl Towers. On her arm is not just her handbag but also Burglar Bill. Tricia smiles to herself, gets another drink and waits to see if anything develops. It doesn't so she goes back to her hotel, happy and ready for sleep and action the following day.

Chapter 13

You'll Never Walk Alone

Let's get inside my head for a while. Its important for all of us, I think. This chapter is an amalgam of the number of different times I shopped in the City. I now feel very relaxed about doing it but still get a great rush.

Oh, and by the way, Tara is my dance teacher. She is absolutely gorgeous and I love her to death! She is also in love with musicals. Like me she saw this coming, as should you, from a mile off. But what's this? I am a Manchester United not a Liverpool fan!

> Walk on, walk on with hope in your heart
> And you'll never walk alone,
> You'll never, ever walk alone.

Walkies with Tricia.

Tricia thinks deeply about what to wear; not deeply enough as we shall see. Check tea-dress, white jeans or short skirt with leggings. She decides on her white jeans with her "These shoes look fab I have to have a pair" red top. Twenty minutes later after much jumping and grinding she has somehow managed to pour into her jeans and is happily sitting at the mirror doing her make-up. Jewellery, wig, lippy and she is ready. She checks her handbag; keys, purse, camera and tissues are already there. She adds her little cosmetics bag filled with the essentials, her hair brush and her cigarettes and lighter and zips it up. White jacket on, handbag over shoulder, final check in the mirror, sexy bitch, then the door clicks shut and Tricia is free.

Be confident girl, I say to myself as I walk through the corridor and get into the lift. I wonder if anyone will join me, they don't, and I get out, pass reception with a smile, get a smile back, and out into Manchester. Left, let's go to Primark because I need some make-up brushes and sponges and some tights. A young girl walks past, she doesn't notice. An elderly man walks past. He doesn't notice. Going good Trish but there are three young guys heading your way. Run, hide? No be confident. Stride, remember what Tara has told you. Back straight, pencil behind the shoulder blades, head high. Heel, toe, slightly cross your legs. Good girl. They're passed you and you passed; well at least they didn't recognise me.

Getting busier now as I approach Piccadilly Gardens. Left, then right, over the tram lines and I am in the open in the middle of the City. Yay this is brilliant! Very young girl doesn't recognise me. Older one a few steps further on does, but gives me a lovely smile. I smile back. Through the doors and into Primark. I know this shop well but still get lost. I finally track down the sponges and brushes. £2 for three of each; definitely a bargain. Two pairs of patterned tights, I love patterned tights. Those girls are watching me. I look at them and smile, they smile back. Those two seem amused, but then I suppose its not often you see a t-Girl browsing the skirt rail. Need a new black belt to replace the one which broke yesterday. That's nice and only £3. To the check-out. Queue not too bad. Three girls and a bloke; who is going to have the pleasure of serving me. She's a pretty girl, another nice smile and out of Primark onto the Arndale Centre. Really busy now. Up the escalators because the second floor has all the girly shops. Vestry, no nothing in there; Dot P, no try West One sometimes you can find .... wow look at that slinky red dress. Any in my size, Yay size 12. "Yes, I'm fine, just browsing but I think … can I try it on?"

Now a lesson for all aspiring girls out there. If you are going shopping don't put your sexy white jeans which take twenty minutes to put on, on. Beads of sweat are bouncing off the floor of the changing room like the raindrops yesterday as I finally manage to peel them off. But it was worth it. The dress is just gorgeous. Dead slinky like my black one and fits perfectly. She'll more than do and is under £30. I go and pay. "Yes, I'm out all weekend, it wonderful. Will wear it tonight, yes, thank you, you have a good night too, bye". Brill, sorted so outfit is slinky red dress, gold flats, white coat and handbag.

Lets go downstairs and try Peacocks, you can often get a bargain there.

Wow, black cotton dress, short, definitely Tricia, under £20 and its mine ….. £14.99, my size. But there is no way I'm going through the rigmarole of getting my jeans off and on again. So ask girl. Yes, it is refundable if it doesn't fit. Let's go for it. Bra for my red dress, 38C, yes, that's pretty I'll get that one. Look at those panties, 3 for a fiver. I know I've got loads but a girl can never have enough panties. Go on Trish, you deserve them. Black jacket. Hmm that will go with slinky red dress and my white jacket needs a rest. Try it on girl you're dressed as a woman for goodness sake! Fits well. Yes I must have it. Check-out girl smiles nicely at me.

I hate this, fumbling around in my purse . Why are my hands shaking so much; I am not nervous. Is it the beer or is it the rush? I suspect its a bit of both. Pay by card girl its easier. "Thank you, and I will enjoy my day". Have I really spent that much? Ouch, sorry Iain. Its gone twelve already and I've agreed to meet Tina. Good morning's work though!

And our brave young lady clip clops out of the Arndale Centre and to Piccadilly Gardens hardly creating a stir at all. She gets noticed by a few, but only a very few people. She calls Tina who isn't even dressed yet, so has not started on her make-up, so is going to be at the very least an hour. Tricia goes into Nero's in Piccadilly Gardens and buys a coffee. She takes it outside and drinks it slowly. She is very, very, happy. She is herself.

I turn into the campus, to the gay village I know and love. I relax and drop my guard. I am spotted by a car waiting at the lights.

"Beep beep"

"Beep beep"

"Beep beep"

And other cars join in. I smile to myself as I cross the road and wiggle through the car park and into the village. I so love being Tricia.

Chapter 14

The Pearl Fishers

A lovely day for Tina and I, we had fun and there was more to come, but that will have to wait until the next chapter. I think what this proves is that Tina and I can spend a day around Manchester just the same as any other normal girl. I though have become far more confident than Tina but that is because I spend so much time in town. It's almost becoming second nature dressing as a girl. But then that is precisely what I want.

By the way, this is one of my favourite songs of all time. It shakes me to the core (and will annoy Tina ha-ha).

> It is her, the goddess,
> who comes to unite us this day!
> Yes, let us share the same fate,
> let us be united until death!

The Girls go Fishing

The girls readied their bait for the trip ahead.

Tina chose the hippy look; flared blue jeans, gypsy blouse and black shrug and her favourite pink and white long socks.

Tricia chose her new black dress from Peacock's, patterned black tights and ankle boots.

Yes, they were going fishing. Not only that, but Tina has agreed and was ready to go to one of the largest fishing areas in the country, Arnpool.

The Arndale Centre is massive. It consists of three floors. The ground floor has mostly menswear shops but you can get girly stuff there; in fact Quiz, Tricia's favourite shop, is on the ground floor. Up the escalators and there are girly shops all around you. There is also a market on the first floor where can get specialist stuff like tattoos and wigs. All the High Street stores can be found here (New Look, Next, Top Shop, Dot P etc) as well as independent fashion retailers. The third floor is the food hall, cheap and tacky and dotted round the centre are plastic coffee houses. Needless to say it gets very busy, but for girls like Tina and Tricia, its paradise.

In the downpour on Friday something very bizarre happened. Tina's right boot began talking to her.

"Help" it said.

Tina looked down, puzzled.

"My inside used to be warm and smelly. Now its cold and wet"

Tina looked down again, aghast.

"And while I've got YOUR attention I would like some of my own. I do not like the short skirts and stockings you wear. It takes the attention away from me"

Tricia covered her mouth with her hand and giggled to herself.

Now some girls are stockings girls and some girls are tights girls. Tina is definitely in the former camp. Her belief is that a flash of flesh between her very short skirt and her sexy stocking tops attracts the men. This is one of the reasons it takes her so long to get ready. Tricia, on the other hand, is more practical. Stockings are far too much trouble and, like socks, one always gets lost in the wash. Where do they all go? Is there a Planet sock and a Planet stocking?

Tricia shudders as she remembers her first experience with stockings. She spent an age trying to get them clipped into her suspended belt. Much like pouring into her white jeans she got hot, sweaty and delayed; so went out with make-up all over the place and hair a mess. She was only out for ten minutes when she needed the Ladies. Like the good girl she is she took down her skirt, then tried to take down her panties. They wouldn't budge! As all girls know you put your panties on over your stockings. Tricia didn't. Unclipping her suspenders was easy. Doing them up again was a different matter.

The poor girl was under enough pressure as it was, but girls kept knocking on the door and asking how long she was going to be. She heard them discussing whether she had a man in there with her (she wished, he could have helped getting her stockings back on) but she bravely ignored all this to concentrate on the job in hand. Finally she managed it, opened the door and tried to keep her calm while walking past a queue of irate girls jumping up and down and crossing their legs. The queue for the Ladies was considerably longer than the queue for the bar.

Whilst Trish was daydreaming, Tina and her right boot were having a furious row.

"Cobblers" said Tina, "we'll have to go to the cobblers"

"Cobblers?" said the boot, "I can see them from here"

"Where?" said Tina

"Above me", said the boot "there always there"

"Not my cobblers" said Tina, "The cobblers"

"What's The cobblers" said the boot

"Somewhere I can shut you up, you old boot" said Tina

"Now, now" said the boot.

The cobbler did his best and glued the sole together again. He didn't hold much hope of it lasting though.

"I need some new boots" announced Tina

"I see a charity shop coming, I'll buy forty Bensons then" said Tricia

"No, they haven't got any. I always look for boots"

"You always look for everything in the charity shop" Tricia shrugged her shoulders

"I suppose the only option is to go to the Arndale then"

To Tricia's amazement Tina agreed. So, for the want of a sole the girls would go fishing in the morning.

After twenty minutes meandering around Tina's favourite 'look after yourself' route, Tricia felt she had to say something.

"Why can't we be like other girls and just walk up the road and turn left, OUCH!". She had just been stung by a nettle as the path disintegrated into a tiny track.

"Because I need time to psyche myself up" said Tina, chuckling "Here, have some dock leaves"

"But this is ridiculous" said an annoyed Tricia as she applied the dock leaves to her left bottom cheek. She wished she had worn her sexy white jeans!

Eventually they reached civilization again. "I'm in charge now because I know where we are going". Tricia breathed a sigh of relief.

"Big breaths hon, and look confident"

"There not as big as yours darling, but I only because I don't use chicken fillets" said Tina

"What are you talking about?"

"Your breasts silly" Tina paused

" Ha ha chicken fillets to go with your chicken legs"

"Can we not discuss my breasts, or even my legs, when we're in the middle of Manchester with hundreds of people ear-wigging?"

"Keep your voice down Trish, those girls heard, look at them giggling". Tina paused,

"Maybe we should put corn on the shopping list"

"Shut up, think about your song"

"What song?"

"The song that's in your head when you walk around the middle of Manchester attracting scorn, silly"

"Corn?"

"No scorn"

"Willow, tit willow, tit willow"

"Can you please leave my breasts alone?"

"Burglar Bill didn't yesterday"

"What do you mean?"

"He told me you let him have a good grope. He thought they were real, ha ha ha"

"I didn't notice, he must have had very light fingers"

"Liar!"

The girls turned right into TK-Max, the gateway to the Arndale and the discussion at last turned away from Tricia's breasts and onto more mundane things; like shoes, dresses and handbags. To their left they saw a rail of evening gowns. They couldn't resist. For a good fifteen minutes they picked dresses from the rails and held them against themselves asking each other for comments. Then they went to Tricia's favourite part of the shop; the cut-price designer handbags. Tricia could browse through these all morning. They were really enjoying themselves but this wasn't getting Tina's boots and Tricia wanted a new dress for Saturday night so, reluctantly they moved into the Arndale Centre itself.

First shop Shoezone. Tricia had warned Tina that it was the wrong time of year to buy boots, that she should wait until the autumn but Tina was adamant. There was a small selection of boots in the shop but nothing Tina liked. So they walked around the corner and into Peacocks. Tina immediately saw what she wanted, but they were not boots. They were silver wedges, quite high, and they would go with a lot of her wardrobe. The problem was she could find one her size, but not the other. She started to get angry. Silver wedges of various sizes (except size 7) were flung around the shop as she desperately tried to find the match. Tricia approached a shop assistant.

"Excuse me, can you help Cinderella over there. She's getting a bit irate"

The girl professionally approached Tina despite having to duck and weave to avoid being hit by a silver wedge.

"I'll get you a pair from the store room" she told Tina. While she was gone a triumphant cheer emerged from the corner of the shop.

"You just need a bit of patience" she told Tricia who was frantically trying to gather together and put back the sea of silver wedges on the shop floor.

"They've got some pretty panties in here, over there, I bought some yesterday" said Tricia who needed to buy some time to make a presentable display of silver wedges. By the time she had finished Tina had bought six pairs of panties and two silver platform shoes.

"Sorry", Tricia said to the shop assistant on their way out.

The shop assistant smiled.

"Time for a cigarette, where can we smoke", said Tina, happy with her purchases.

"We have to go outside" said Tricia

The girls walked out of the Arndale Centre and onto the steps leading to the Cathedral.

"Lets sit down over there, I'm tired" said Tricia

"I'm not sitting over there, there's hundreds of people" said Tina starting to get jittery again.

"Hon, we're in the middle of Manchester as it is, just relax"

Before the girls could start a squabble, they were approached by a funny looking man with a goatee beard.

"Excuse me (cough) young ladies"

The girls wondered whether the cough was for the young or the ladies or both.

"I am a follower of Hari Krishna, would you care to contribute to our cause.

Tina, who was still euphoric over her new shoes, fumbled in the purse and found £2.

"Then you are entitled to a gift (cough), young lady". The man reached inside his bag and presented Tina with a book entitled 'The journey of self-discovery'

"Have a lovely day (cough) girls"

They finished their cigarettes.

"I need a new dress, lets try Quiz, it's just round the corner", said Tricia

"I still need some boots" said Tina

The girls entered Quiz and Tina went straight to the shoe section. Tricia immediately saw exactly what she want. It was a beautiful sparkly gold dress. It was similar to her other broken sparkly gold dress, more about that later. She carefully worked her way through the rail, eventually finding one her size. YAY she thought.

"Nothing in here Trish, I'm going to look around the shoe shop next door".

"Ok Tina, I want to try this on, I'll be a few minutes".

Tricia was again allowed into a changing room. This time it was far easier to get dressed and undressed. The dress was gorgeous and Tricia knew she had to have it. It was so pretty she didn't want to take it off. Tina was prowling around inside the shop wondering why Tricia was taking so long (for a change). It was good she wasn't here yesterday, thought Tricia. She paid and two happy girls walked out of the shop well pleased with their morning's work.

Tricia's last sparkly gold dress was very flimsy and she managed to wear it out on its fifth outing. A strap broke while she was putting it on which she managed to fix using tit tape. Fortunately for her, she was dancing with half a dozen genuine girls at Naps when the second strap broke quickly followed by the tit tape giving way. An embarrassed Tricia was therefore stuck in the middle of the dance floor in just her underwear. The girls however rallied to her cause and with pins and tape they managed to make Tricia look presentable again. Well, they did the best they could.

"To the pub Trish" said Tina

"To the straight pub" said Tricia.

They got themselves a drink, went onto the balcony upstairs and inspected their haul.

Two shoes (silver wedges)

Six pairs of panties (various)

One sexy dress (sparkly gold)

One book called the journey of self discovery.

Not a great catch, but not bad for two inexperienced anglers.

Chapter 15

Windy City

Oh you pretty things, don't you know your driving your Mamas and Papas insane.

I didn't spend much time at Sparkle itself because I was more interested in doing my own thing. There are moves afoot to make this all more permanent. The trouble is that there were so many threads over the weekend that this is a bit disjointed. But then it all happened so, so what! It was great to be with so many t-Girls though; some of them even ventured around town. By the way, and I know I'm skirting around the issue, but this one's from Calamity Jane. Did I tell you I love Doris Day?

> I just blew in from the windy city
> The windy city is mighty pretty
> But they ain't got what we got, no sirree

In which Tricia's slinky red dress goes out for the first time, Tricia has a ballet lesson, and the girls meet loads and loads of people.

Tricia's sexy red dress made its debut the previous night. Leaving Tina asleep, she was eventually to wake up, it made a mistake crossing the road at eleven o'clock. The lights changed to green when it was half way across forcing it to walk down the middle of the street. Cars on both sides were beeping their horns furiously. Tricia realised that they were not beeping their horns because she looked like a man; with her slinky red dress and fishnet stockings in the middle of the night, they were beeping their horns because she looked like a prostitute. Tricia loved the attention and wiggled more provocatively, if that was at all possible.

She had previously sent her dance teacher a text for advice.

"Now I shout it from the highest hills, but how do I do a pliet?" she wrote.

Tara replied, "Hiya Calam hows life in the Windy City? Sorry sugar having a bad week. You need to turn your feet out and tilt your pelvis forward so that your spine straightens. Then bend your knees out so that they point in the same direction as your toes, and don't let your knees go further than your toes. Move your feet wider instead".

Tricia replied "Thanks Tara, I'll do my best. Windy City no good for wigs! Hugs Calam."

Tara replied "Ha ha how true x"

Tricia quite likes Calam. There is an element of truth in it. The subject is all about getting Tricia's back straight and improving her posture, Ballet lessons! What ever next?

So back to chronological order, which is the only order in the girls' lives, Tina and Tricia returned to Paddys where they met up with Janine and Emma. Emma is living full time, Janine is not. Janine travelled up to Manchester from Nottingham on the train dressed. It was the most frightening experience of her life as she made one fatal mistake. She forgot to bring anything to read so she had to spend the whole journey in the headlights, watching people watching her. She survived though, and did look good. Tricia has yet to do this although it doesn't frighten her any more. Her time will come.

While out having a smoke, the girls met Peta. Peta described the most frantic sexual period of her life. The time when she became, as she put it, a dump truck. Tina's ears pricked up or something. She was going through precisely that now. Peta said it lasted about six months but now she is far more choosy about whom she sleeps with. Tricia's ears pricked up, "ha ha there's mileage in that; Tina the dump truck ha ha" she thought.

The girls were obviously drinking far too much for there own good so decided to go for a curry. They had never been for a sit down meal dressed before so it was a first. The Ashoka looked shut from the outside as there were building works going on all around it. Inside though it was as warm and friendly as the waiter who served them. The girls had a long chat with him about, well, what it was like to be girls. He was charming and polite and the food was excellent. So if you're ever in Manchester look it up, it comes highly recommended.

Antonia (Silver Shadow) texted Trish "I am in AXS, meet me soon". So the girls met up again with Anonia who was with Tracey and was to remain with Tracey for the weekend. Who was who and what was what was never really established but they all had a good laugh anyway.

Suzy texted Trish "I am in the park at the first tent on your right". Trish said her goodbyes and went to have a chat with Suzy. Suzy works for the same Company as me. She has just had the operation and is struggling a bit at the moment. It does take time to recover, but Tricia could tell she would soon be fully fit. The Company they work for is very good with issues like this. Tricia has now told HR about herself and will be opening up further shortly. She is a brave girl!

It was about this time that Tina scrawled on Tricia's notepad. The one she uses to write all this up, that "Tricia becomes drunk as a newt". So we better stop here. There is much more to tell however. Sparkle weekend, girls everyone (even some in town) fun, fun, fun!

Chapter 16

Tomorrow Belongs to Me

The story covers a couple of days of my life which again were great fun, but I struggle to remember a lot which went on. I wonder why that is?

By the way, there are two reasons for the song. The most important for me being the realisation on the Sunday morning that pretty much everything is possible now. It is like being re-born, and I do think tomorrow might belong to me (Tricia). It was also nice to agree with Michelle that this is the best clip from any musical.

I also learned that I can only do so much. I am trying to run too fast when I am here. I must somehow slow down. I'm not sure how to do that yet because everything is so new and exciting. I'll have to think about it.

> The sun on the meadow is summery warm
> The stag in the forest runs free
> But gathered together to greet the storm
> Tomorrow belongs to me

In which the girls help the homeless, Jayne joins the fun, Tricia extends her welcome and they meet maid Michelle who leads Tricia into bad ways (I am such an unbiased storyteller)

Jayne was about to meet the girls. It was feverishly arranged during the week. Trish wasn't sure whether she would actually turn up but Jayne was there and, sort of, ready. She was very nervous as it was to be her debut. What would Tricia do next?

Well at least she had done her homework. She had brought loads of clothes for Jayne to choose from, Tina had brought a lot too, and shoes, make-up and spare wig. It was how to do the make-up that worried Tricia. She was only just getting reasonable at doing her own make-up but how was she going to apply it, and what should she apply, on somebody different?

Then, as so often in life, along came lady luck. Tricia was outside having a smoke downstairs, watching others watching her, when a young lady asked her for a cigarette. Debs was homeless, cold and wet so when Tricia offered her back to her room to warm up, she jumped at the chance. She loved Tricia's make-up and used it both on herself and on Jayne. Problem solved,

Jayne wore Tricia's gold flapper dress, gold flats, sequined white stole and gold handbag. She should have won a gold medal as she was still very nervous, but the girls saw her through it and got her to Paddys. Tricia was wearing sexy sparkly gold dress number two with white handbag and shoes and felt good. All four girls looked radiant. Debs had a few drinks with the girls in Paddys before saying her goodbyes.

So onto Naps; and dancing, and smoking, and talking, and drinking. Tricia thought Jayne did really well but didn't think Jayne ever really properly relaxed. Eventually she had to go back to her hotel. So Tina and Tricia went back with her to Tricia's and Jayne changed back again, both her clothes and into a different life. The girls hope Jayne enjoyed herself and had a memorable time.

In the morning Tricia hastily arranged another day and another night at the hotel. She was just enjoying herself too much. Leaving Tina asleep yet again, off she went around town. It is now like a drug for her. She adores doing it and loves showing people exactly what she is. There were loads of t-Girls out. One took a picture of her in Piccadilly Gardens. It was sunny, it was fun, and it was the first time Tricia realised she could do anything Iain could do. No; no song, they do it together. She bought some girly stuff, including a new black jacket and passed Tina, dressed in mufti, on her way back to the hotel. "Paddys" said Tina

"Paddys" said Tricia, "see you in ten minutes, new clothes to try on".

Fifty minutes, a change of clothes and two irate phone calls from Tina later, Tricia appeared in Paddy's.

"What kept you, I'm on my own here dressed as a bloke" said Tina,

"Complete vanity, go and change back and look gorgeous like me",

"I can't, I've got work tomorrow, love your new outfit though",

"Oh hon, you're so sweet. Am I forgiven then?",

"Of course",

"Will you give me a kiss then?",

"Is that just because I'm dressed as a bloke?",

"It seems to me you feel safer in here dressed as a girl than as a bloke. What were those phone calls about?"

"Yes I do. Girls like us get protected by blokes like us",

"Not sure about your logic hon" Tricia paused,

"But you are really sweet, that means you would protect me" Tricia paused again,

"Protect my honour" Tricia paused again, for a even longer this time.

"But I may not want my honour protecting"

"How do you mean?"

"Well, if some young studmuffin suddenly started ravishing me, the last thing I'd want is your protection!"

"Some young studmuffin, who are you kidding? Ha ha ha ha"

The girls had no idea where this was taking them but fortunately for us all they were never to find out. Maid Michelle joined them at the table, though you couldn't actually tell it was Maid Michelle as she was wearing t-shirt and jeans. The girls got on really well; Michelle and Tricia in particular who shared the same interests and tastes; even as far as agreeing on what the greatest clip from any film of all time was. Now I wonder what that could be? Actually the only clip Tricia thinks can compete is the first time you see Harry Lime in the Third Man.

Tina had to go back to T-Girl Towers to prepare for the work the next day, leaving Tricia and Michelle to explore the back streets of Manchester looking for varied and different pubs and pints. At about 17:00 Michelle had to leave to get her train. Tricia staggered, by far the worse for wear, back to her hotel. On her way home she received a text from Antonia (Silver Shadow).

"Hi honey we are still in Manchesta tonite. U? Your dress was FAB last night !!! love u, A-a".

Tricia crashed on top of the bed with a smile on her face. There she was to remain until just after midnight when she woke up, still fully dressed, with a start. Its 00:30 must go to Naps, must go to Naps she thought, need a cigarette first though. She went all the way back down the stairs of the hotel to the smoking area outside and lit up and thought again. No she mustn't. Its Sunday night, Naps will be quiet and she is still shattered. She must text Silver Shadow to apologise. Go back to bed girl, this time put your nightie on. Although you act like an eighteen year old girl you know the truth.

Eighteen? My hasn't she grown up fast.

Chapter 17

What a Wonderful World

So I thought about it. I desperately need some quiet time, some time simply to relax and consider my life. It's not easy because I now have so many friends who all want to talk to me. But I must be strong and resist, or find another pub where I can just grab an hour to be alone and think. So for this chapter, just chill.

> I see trees of green and red roses too
> I watch them bloom for me and you
> And I think to myself, oh what a wonderful world
> I think to myself, ooh what a wonderful world

Peace and Quiet

Its Friday lunchtime and Paddys is quite. Tricia has to change hotels so has a couple of idle hours on her hands and, with her heavy suitcase stuffed full of beautiful clothes, can't really do much. So she just chills, has a couple of beers, and is totally relaxed. She is dressed of course, pink top, sexy white jeans (no shopping for a while). She looks divine and she doesn't have a care in the world.

Tonight, with Tina, she is to see the real professionals which she is looking forward to. Than back to Paddys and Naps. Whatever will happen to her? Who knows, and that is fun, fun, fun. There needs to be a balance though. The time Tricia is spending now, quietly, is very important. I know that and Tricia is beginning to learn it. It is simply not possible to run around at one hundred miles an hour all the time.

She has to check into posh hotel in an hour but that no longer concerns her, despite what it says on my credit card. Then she is going to dump her bags, hang up her wig and dresses, have a shower, change and go shopping in the big City. She needs another pair of jeans; black she thinks and a denim dress. It doesn't matter if she can't find them, the search will be fun (actually she didn't and the search was fun).

She goes to the ladies. Like the good girl she is pulls down her panties to sit down. On the front are the words http://www.signin........ On the back are the words ......and poke me. Tricia sometimes wonders whether its worth bothering with knickers at all. She thinks sometimes they get a bit too much in the way. But she loves wearing them, so she will.

She touches up her make-up; recognises that her nails need re-doing before tonight. Tonight is sparkly gold dress number 2 night. Tonight she is going to compete with the professionals. She isn't going to win but that doesn't matter. It's the taking part that counts. She is mildly annoyed that her sexy white jeans won't fit properly and completely over her ankle boots, but understands that she has chicken legs and she has to live with it.

She goes back into the bar. She notices the rain lashing down again outside and is pleased that she had the sense to put her girly pink umbrella in her handbag. The Eva Cassidy version of Wonderful World comes on the juke-box. Tricia sits down, listens and thinks to herself… "yes, it is a wonderful world"

Ohh yeah

Bye Tricia, enjoy yourself!

Chapter 18

There's No Business like Show Business

I'm beginning to realise the importance of a stage. Maybe it was going to the Ladyboy's that triggered it. Tina and I got great applause when we went on stage there for our photos. I think of the dance floor at Naps. That is in a way a stage and is becoming very important to me. I am on stage when sitting at the bar with Georgina and Tina. There is no doubt that the customers are watching us and eyeing us. Then I thought even deeper. As a trandgendered person I am potentially on stage at all times, especially in town.

But then aren't we all?

There's no business like show business
like no business I know
Everything about it is appealing,
everything that traffic will allow
Nowhere could you get that happy feeling
when you are stealing that extra bow

In which Tricia can't understand Mark, the girls become ladyboys and Tricia struggles to walk

An English summer? Is there such a thing any more. All weekend Tricia had to carry both girly umbrella and sunglasses with her. She's amazed her handbag stood up to it. The weather was a bit like Tina, thought Tricia, it never knew what to do.

On Thursday night she had a long and deep chat with Mark. Tina was

68

nairing so wouldn't be out until Friday. Though, as you know, that isn't strictly true. Tricia had just one task to perform. To book two tickets for 'The Ladyboys of Bangkok" for Friday night. How appropriate thought Tricia. She achieved the task and the girls were put right at the front, next to the stage, GULP.

Now Mark is a lapsed t-girl. Tricia doesn't understand at all; but then there are a lot of things Tricia doesn't understand, particularly to do with nails. How, for example, when you are right handed, do you put nail varnish on your right finger nails without getting it all over your skin is one thing she doesn't understand. How can anybody possibly be capable of doing a French manicure, is another. Tricia knows she has a lot to learn, but is keen and eager to do so. It now only takes her five minutes to do the clasp on a necklace at least.

How can you be a lapsed? Either you love being one, like Tina and Tricia, or you don't. Mark tried to explain but Tricia just couldn't get it. She loved the 45 minutes (only) it now took her to get ready to go out. She loved putting on her jewellery, doing her make-up, styling her wig; that was all part of the fun. And Tricia loves fun! Mark never did convince Tricia, but then did Tricia convince Mark, or anyone else come to that. Tricia doesn't care. She is who she is.

"Hiya Gal", Tricia met Tina in Paddys at 8:30 on Friday night.

"Two pints and we go to the Ladyboys"

"Two pints Trish, we've got to be there for nine!"

"Sounds about right Tina, and its your round"

"I'm not round Trish, I'm straight!"

"Ha ha ha ha ha"

The girls were back together and straight away were enjoying themselves.

They were put on a table with six genuine girls. Tricia immediately got talking to Caroline, and Tina to Lynne. The girls really loved having some real ladyboys on their table. The girls really loved having some real girls on their table. It was fun, fun, fun all round, or all straight or whatever.

In the interval there was the opportunity for Tina and Tricia to have their picture taken on stage. We know that our brave girls never miss such opportunities. Lead by their table there were huge cheers and whistles from the audience as they walked onto the stage. And they looked so pretty! Sparkly gold dress number two works for Tricia.

The table got more raucous as the night wore on but all the girls, genuine or not, had a great time. They went together back to Paddys after the show and carried on talking and drinking. The genuine girls eventually had to go home but another meeting is being arranged.

Onto Naps and the usual routine. Tina downstairs, Tricia up. Meet in the middle for a smoke and an update. Tricia's ballet had improved and she was getting reasonably good at pliets, but Tara had given her another task, one which was to prove much more difficult. To walk with her toes slightly turned out. The dance floor at Naps, with mirrors all around, was the perfect place to try it out. Tricia found it impossible; she was by nature pigeon toed! It totally threw her balance. She tried to look cool as she bumped into the umpteenth person but failed miserably. She didn't know that Tina was watching.

"Ha-ha-ha your drunk again, its hard to disguise that fact if you've got chicken legs" said Tina

"I'm not drunk, I'm practicing my walk" replied Tricia, bouncing into a couple on her right.

"Walk? Its a dance floor for goodness sake"

"My dance instructor has instructed me to turn my toes out when I walk" said Tricia, still walking up and down, "And its not easy".

"What sort of dance teacher is she?" said Tina. "You're bumping into everybody, there are people in the corners afraid to move in case they are mown over. You are a safety hazard – in fact you are like a dodgem car!"

The tannoy behind the bar then added more pressure. "If anybody has any crash helmets can they please bring them up to the dance floor, quickly!" it announced.

"Don't you dare question my dance teacher, she is simply lovely and knows what she is doing" said Tricia who, at that precise moment, bumped into four girls with very high heels, knocking them to the floor instantly.

"Strike!" shouted Tina "Ha-ha-ha you're not a dodgem car you're a bowling ball. Lets go and have a smoke, I'll roll you down the stairs".

Tina tugged Tricia from off the dance floor. The all clear alert was sounded at the bar. The dance floor filled again and the people in the corners felt free to move. Tina and Tricia had a long chat. "Wait until it's not so busy before you try your walk again", said Tina. "And I'm still not sure about your dance teacher".

"I am", said Tricia, "don't you ever say anything against her. She is with me every minute of the day, every step that I take".

The girls later met Lady Morgana who asked Tricia to write a sonnet for her. That will be fun, thought Tricia, not realising how difficult it was actually going to be. And what is happening in Frankfurt in September? There are still plenty of different things going on in Tricia's life but they are all fun. Now, what are the rules of a sonnet?

Chapter 19

How do you solve a Problem like Tricia

The difficulty I have is that I am too wild, too random and at times almost uncontrollable. I have been told that, for my own good, I need to take on some more responsibility. People don't want to change me too much, because then you lose what is inside me but I just need to tone it all down a bit. By the way, this is what they sing to me.

> Oh how do you solve a problem like Tricia?
> How do you hold a moon beam in your hand?

In which Tricia moves into T-Girl Towers and explores the area, Tina has main course and afters with Harvey and Tricia acts very, very, responsibly for a girl of her age

Tricia has made a decision, or at least it was made for her. She is moving in with Tina at weekends. This has been agreed with her family. The thought of being dressed and being herself all weekend fills her with joy; but there is much to do. It is this which may help Tricia. She needs to take on more responsibility if she is to grow as a person.

Tina works away from T-Girl Towers during the week so stays with her parents. This has meant that nothing much has been done at the flat so it is a bit of a mess at the moment. First the girls need to sort out some keys for Tricia, then Tricia needs to get the electricity connected.

Then there is Tricia's bedroom. This will need to be converted to look much more girly. Tricia is going to have real fun doing this as she is going to get it all sorted dressed. Going to DIY shops, picking wardrobes and mirrors etc all dressed as Tricia; wonderful. She stayed there last weekend. The girls cleared a lot of space in the bedroom (well Tina did mostly) and Tina made a temporary wardrobe using some old wood lying about and a coffin. Tricia has never slept with a coffin before; but she's still living. The bed was very comfy but it was only a single bed. This will need changing quickly as she is sure to bring someone back with her before very long.

On Saturday afternoon Tina got a surprise. Out of the blue, her doorbell chimed. It was Harvey and he was to become the first test for the girls. Tricia decided to stay in her room and read but it wasn't long before Harvey came in stark naked flashing his impressively large manhood. He wanted Tricia to join them but Tina hadn't agreed so Tricia declined. Instead she went out to buy some milk. She didn't want to intrude or invade upon Tina's space. To put it bluntly, Tricia didn't want to queer Tina's pitch! She also felt that if she was to stay here at weekends she ought to get to know the neighbourhood. They might enjoy having another t-Girl amongst them.

Now, there are plenty of ways out of Tina's front door. If you turn right and cross the road (where the girls wait for Taxis dressed as hookers) and keep walking, pretty soon you come to the posh area and the closest shop which sells milk. Tricia bought the milk, noticed there was a bar next door, so went in and ordered a drink. The bar was modern and plastic with airport music coming out of the speakers. It was totally soulless inside so Tricia decided to sit outside. A sunny day in Manchester? What ever next. She sat down and in full view of everybody slowly sipped her drink. It was clear to her that nothing exciting was going to happen; the bar was simply too lifeless. A disappointed young lady drank up and went back to T-Girl Towers where she was let in by a smiling Harvey on his way out.

The girls made themselves a coffee and sat on Tina's bed discussing what a perfect fit Harvey was. Half-an-hour later Tina's doorbell chimed once more. It was Harvey again. He had come back for a second helping. What would Tricia do now?

Now, there are plenty of ways out of Tina's front door. If you turn left and keep walking, pretty soon you come to the dodgy area where the shops are boarded up. Tricia kept walking, passed some children playing in the street and carried on. Shortly she heard some tiny footsteps behind her and turned round to see a little girl of about six or seven looking at her with interest.

"Excuse me", said the girl.

"Yes", said the t_Girl.

"You're not a real girl are you" said the girl.

Tricia smiled and winked.

"Yes, but don't tell anyone, ssssshhh"

Tricia put her perfectly manicured finger to her lips.

The little girl rushed back to her friends. As Tricia carried on down the street she heard a voice, shouting.

"I've told someone!"

Tricia had decided she was going to have a drink in the first pub she came to, brave girl, and she could see one in the distance. As she got closer it looked like it was closed since it was all locked up. As she got closer still though, she noticed that people were drinking inside. Very strange. She tried to open the door but it was indeed locked. She was about to give up when the door opened from the inside and Tricia was beckoned in by the landlady.

"You can never be too careful around here but you look safe enough" she said.

"I'll let you know that I'm extremely vicious with my handbag" Tricia replied.

"Don't worry sweetie, your safe in here with me, what are you drinking?"

The landlady locked the door again.

Apart from being like Fort Knox, it was an old traditional Manchester pub. There were a few men playing darts on the other side of the bar and a few more watching some intolerably dreary game show on the television perched high in the corner. It was the type of pub which probably hadn't seen a woman for twenty years or more. It still hadn't. Tricia however did feel safe in there and received some lovely smiles from the men. She drunk up and the landlady let her out.

"Come back again, honey," she said "but not too late at night"

The children had been called in for their tea but it was a happy if a little disturbed Tricia who made her way back to t-Girl Towers. It must be a very, very dodgy place if you have to lock the pub doors, she thought. She was again let in by a smiling Harvey on his way out.

"Georgina's texted," said Tina, "we've got one hour to get to Paddys. Do you know what you're wearing tonight. Tricia did, she always thinks things out beforehand. She was also pleased with herself. Moving in with Tina was a good idea. She was aware of how responsible she had been that afternoon. Unfortunately that responsibility was not to last very long at all.

Chapter 20

Summertime

By the way, the sun was shining in Manchesta, YAY!

> Summertime,
> And the livin' is easy
> Fish are jumpin'
> And Tricia is high

Where Tricia goes into a space she can't remember or forget and is very, very, irresponsible. She was however ecstatic.

Tricia had lots of friends around her. Crystal Chandelier and the Limpet were there, Mark and Glenda were there as of course was Tina and a lovely young girl they had just met called Aba. So she was in safe hands.

Easy Trish, easy. Just melt away. Its fun and its different. It's very, very different. Easy does it girl.

Chapter 21

Ladies who Lunch

This completes a totally mad weekend where I did a lot of things I shouldn't. I can't say I'm particularly proud of myself but was lead astray (believe that and you'll believe anything). It was great to meet up with Antonia again, by the way, hence the song. It was also really good to meet up with Georgina again, however briefly.

> Perhaps a piece of Mahler's.
> I'll drink to that.
> And one for Mahler!

In which Tricia reads her sonnet, Georgina returns to town, as does Antonia and Tricia is irresponsible again!

Tina picked Tricia up from Paddy's, both under-dressed after a hard days work and took her to T-Girl Towers. Tricia had previously got her mind into gear on the train coming down. It used to take her the best part of a day, now a couple of hours will do. She was writing the book and listening to Cabaret on her headphones. Back at their flat the girls chatted as they got ready for the evening. Tricia recited the sonnet she had written for Lady Morgana. It is called 'A Love Shared'

I kneel down at my Goddess's throne,
Head lowered, my tongue caresses her feet
Slowly I descend into the zone
The space where they both long to meet

I rise; I pass her well and peaks
I inhale deeply, she looks divine
I very gently kiss her cheeks
I realise it will soon be time

Her pouting lips betray a grin
As all of my resistance dies
She motions me, time to begin
I gracefully lie between her thighs

As the crop lashes down from high up above
They were as one, sharing their love

Tricia hoped to meet Lady Morgana again over the weekend, but there was no rush. She was quite pleased with her first effort because a sonnet is not an easy thing to write. The girls dressed quietly for the Friday night out, but sexily. Tricia wore her black dress, Tina her tartan skirt. The weather was warm so there were plenty of legs in evidence. Maybe they didn't look too much like prostitutes as they waited for the cab to take them back to Paddys, and to Georgina who was back in England with some news.

Despite her best efforts to land a job as a papergirl, she ended up second in command of an engineering company in San Marino with a brief to turn the country round. Poor Georgina, but you know what they say. "Look after your Pennies and the pounds will take care of themselves". Georgina will naturally dress like a schoolboy in her new role.

Onto Naps where the girls bump into Habib and Amanda. They are pleased that everything is going extremely well between them. Then Josh turns up and Trish and Tina decide to take him back home with them. Tricia was used as the fluff girl before warming up herself in her new bed for the first time. Very comfortable is was too. She managed to get to sleep despite all the noise emanating from Tina's room.

The next day the girls walked in to Paddys through the canals. Tricia wrote a poem about walking through canals and locks but it is not sure why she did so. Tina made an unfortunate fashion howler, wearing white socks with her black stilettos. All the girls could hear were chants of "white socks, white socks as they were walking. Maybe the chapter should have been Chicago (think baseball) but the song had already been chosen. Unfortunately Tina was not Anna Kornikova and neither was her outfit. Trinny tried to warn her but to no avail. So they get to Paddys and begin to realise just strong, for a twelve year old girl, Georgina's mind is.

"Just take those ridiculous things off" she said. And Tina did. Tricia realised that she needed to be more assertive.

The girls, back together, wondered around Canal Street where they met up with Aba. Aba was a very young, very attractive genuine girl with some demons in the closet. She didn't know what she was meant to be. Tricia felt she just needed some time to sort herself out; but there was no denying what a lovely girl she was. She was interested in our girls' lifestyle but didn't pry too much. Tricia hopes they meet up again and expects Aba to have a very successful and happy life.

Georgina had to leave to go to to San Marino at this point, so the girls said their goodbyes and Tina, Tricia and Aba went back to Paddys where you already know what happened. Oh Tricia, how could you? Tricia found it amazing though.

Trish was woken up (she did eventually get back to her bed) by a text from Antonia.

"Hi honey sorry I've not been in touch lately. Hope you r well? Not sure if u r in Manchesta today bit I am. Fancy a lunch? Xx"

Tricia, though ready herself, expected Tina would be about another hour. She had only just decided what to wear and informed Antonia of that fact. She was sitting outside on the balcony of T-Girl Towers when she received another text.

"See me outside pub Mahler, I mean Via, lol"

Eventually, and after much cajoling, Tina was ready and the girls took the cab to meet Antonia.

Antonia looked absolutely stunning sitting outside Via Fosse in the sunshine. She certainly had a body to die for. The talk quickly got round to her profession and why she is called Silver Shadow. The girls now understand.

"What I sell is not sex" said Antonia, "but love". Then the talked turned to how stoned Tricia was the previous evening and to drugs in general. Antonia was already on the look-out. As Tina went inside to buy the next round, behind them, coming down Canal Street, was a two-man band collecting for charity. As Antonia and Tricia tossed their coins into the bucket, Trish recognized the tune being played. It was 'Can't buy me love' by the Beatles. We now know for sure that this isn't true.

So finally, well after lunchtime in fact, the girls grabbed a bite to eat. Well Tina and Antonia did in any case. Tricia didn't want any food stopping her drinking which was now in full flow. They took Antonia to Paddy's but the girls felt that Antonia wasn't over-impressed with the fifties style décor. It wasn't really Antonia's cup of tea, or wine, or vodka come to that.

Antonia discussed some of the tools of her trade. Her £800 handbag; her absolutely gorgeous travel bag. She put on her hooker lipstick and boy, did it make a difference. She was very, very high maintenance. She also got chatting to very strange black man who disappeared for a while but returned, with exactly what Antonia wanted.

Now, where do naughty girls go when they don't want anyone to see what they are doing. Why, the changing room of course. They borrowed the key from the bar at Via using the ruse that Antonia hadn't seen it before, went downstairs and locked themselves in. They were very careful. They left the changing room exactly as they had found it. There was not a speck of dust to be found anywhere. Oh Tricia, how could you do it again? Twice in two days. So much for your new found responsibility.

The girls, now pretty high, went back to T-Girl Towers where they talked some more before falling asleep, holding each others hands, on Tina's bed. What a mad weekend! But no Lady Morgana!

Chapter 22

Every Time we say Goodbye I Cry a Little

This is the probably the hardest chapter of all to write. But then I'm also a Father of twins so its hard the other way too.

> There's no love song finer
> But how strange
> The change from major to minor
> Every time we say goodbye

Leaving

The Company mobile phone warbles and it's the most difficult time of all for Tricia. Its 7:00 a.m. on Monday morning and she has to change back to a male professional and be in work for ten. She still has make-up and nail varnish on from last night. She is in her nightie but wishes to remain as Tricia as long as she can. She sighs, gets out of bed, and puts on her pink dressing gown.

There is no electricity in T-Girl Towers so her first job is to boil up some water on the camper gas stove. She puts a big pan on. Some for her coffee and some for her to wash in. She relieves herself in her accustomed manner, sitting down (ha-ha who's kidding who) and she gets her girly pill ready to take with her coffee. At this stage the gas cylinder may have exploded, but as we know Tricia can sort these things out?

She makes her coffee and leaves it to cool. She removes her make-up using cotton buds and make-up remover. She then puts the remains of the hot water into the sink and thoroughly washes her hands and face. She brushes her teeth, packs up her sponge bag and puts it in her holdall. She does not shave. She wants to look manly ha-ha and look like an office worker. It gets harder every time. One day she is sure she will leave Manchester as Tricia.

Next she sorts out which clothes she needs to take back with her to wash. No electricity so no washing machine in T-Girl Towers. She packs those then makes sure all her dresses are properly hung in her coffin and her make-up and jewellery are correctly stored away where they should be. She doesn't forget her nails so on with the nail-varnish remover. There will still be some traces left (as they were painted red) but Tricia doesn't mind. It will remind her during the week. She smells her wrists. She can still smell her perfume. She smiles.

Now's the time Tricia, time to go!

She puts on her drab.

He looks at himself in Tina's full length mirror. I can't convince anyone he thinks and soon he won't. He'll just about do for now though. Check no jewellery, which will shortly change, lock the door, down the lift and out (or back in the closet). Goodbye Manchester, goodbye Tricia, but he will make the most of a bad job.

He walks to the station using the streets, not the canals; don't think too hard – have to be him, not her. At the station he has fifteen minutes to wait for a train. He has a cigarette outside the station. He loves that girls outfit. Where did she get it? Would it suit Trish? Wow look at that handbag, bet that cost a bomb. He goes into the station and buys a cappuccino. The train pulls in. He is lucky, he finds a seat. He gets out his girly pink mp3 player and puts on Rachmaninov. He opens his diary, this diary, to start on this chapter. The one you are reading now. What happened at the weekend? Where are her notes?

The train pulls out and Manchester is about to become Tricia-less. Is it better for it? He thinks. Probably not, but it will still be there when Tricia returns in only 104 hours and 30 minutes times He bets it will still be raining.

The wretched mobile phone wakes up again. At least its tune reminds him of happy things, actually of cricket.

"Hi Iain, Are you ok for a meeting at eleven". Iain? Whose Iain? Oh yes he remembers now.

"Think so, won't be in until ten though, will let you know for sure then".

From the timeless, open, friendly, free world Tricia has come, Iain has joined the rat race. He is about to lead a life of deadlines, blame, avoidance of responsibility, greed, finance, politics and stress. A world ruled by time and that wretched Company mobile phone. Never mind. He'll survive, and he needs to earn some money to fund all the gorgeous dresses and make-up.

Tricia is happy, Iain is happy for Tricia, Tricia is lucky, very lucky. Thank you Iain.

Chapter 23

Tricia

"Hiya Tricia"

"Hello Trish"

"You been a good girl Trish?"

"Tricia, you back again"

"Tricia, what are you drinking?" (I wish)

"Trish, is Tina out tonight?"

"Tricia, you up for it tonight" (I wish again)

"Tricia, lovely to see you again"

"Hi Trish, love that outfit"

"Tricia, are you going to stay sober this time"

"Trish, you got a spare fag"

"Trish, your looking good"

"Tricia, how much did you have yesterday"

I am now known around the village and that is brilliant. Not only to I get to dress for two or three days a week but I am also constantly called Tricia or Trish. It all helps me become her. It makes it easier to chant:

"I am Tricia Dale"

"I am Tricia Dale"

I so enjoyed the weekend. I really felt like a woman with Alex. The reaction to what happened later will be interesting though. I've been told there will initially be lot of gossip and micky taking but that will eventually die down. I do put Iain through difficult times.

> Tricia . . .
> The most beautiful sound I ever heard:
> Tricia, Tricia, Tricia, Tricia . . .
> All the beautiful sounds of the world in a single word . .

In which a lot of Tricia's body gets invaded.

Tina met Tricia in Paddys, took her back to T-Girl Towers and gave her the key fob. Tina had to work the following day so Tricia had to go solo that night. Thursday night, quiet night, so Tricia put on her patterned tea dress and black tights. She likes that outfit. She's such a conservative girl. Tina dropped her back at Paddys where she had a chat with Mark before bumping into Alex.

Alex likes to talk but Tricia was more than happy with that after working all day and travelling down. Tricia actually is a very good listener. Eventually the bell sounded announcing closing time and Alex asked Tricia if he could come back. Tricia said yes and they walked the canals hand in hand under the moonlight.

Back at T-Girl Towers Alex asked Tricia whether she still had her school uniform. She did, but not with her unfortunately. Alex then asked whether Tricia had a secretary's outfit. Did she just! Tricia quickly changed into red blouse and sexy black pencil skirt with stockings and suspenders.

Had Tricia been a naughty girl? Had she just! And about three minutes later the sexy black pencil skirt was around her ankles, as were her panties. How could she have been so silly? Why had she forgotten to post the letter? How could she have known it was going to cost her boss money?

And the rugged Northern Mill Owner pulled the poor defenceless girl across his solid thighs. Her backside twitched as she prepared herself for what was to happen. And his hand came down and she gave a little cry. Both of pain and of delight. She wasn't finished with, even after that though. The strong Mancunian entrepreneur lifted her like a rag doll and positioned her on the bed. He was very rough with her but she now realised; the rougher the better. Shortly afterwards they were lying in bed; him snoring gently, her with her head on his chest thinking. That was lovely.

Tricia got up at around 10 in the morning, made Alex a coffee and took her time getting dressed. Well it wasn't just getting dressed! In fact it took her so long to get ready that they didn't leave the flat until 12:30. She was getting as bad as Tina. They walked back to Paddys through the canals and met Tom. On the television was the opening ceremony of the Olympic Games which was very impressive. Tricia only had one thing on her mind though and no, it wasn't that!

She left Paddys at half three and walked into town, to where she thought she could get what she needed. She could. She made an appointment for 16:50. Her head was in a bit of a whirl though so she went shopping and bought herself a coffee to clear it. She returned at the appointed time and was told to sit down on the chair. She was also told that it would be fine and it wouldn't hurt.

She shut her eyes. She heard one thud, then another and indeed it didn't hurt. Next she was covered with two wax strips which were abruptly pulled off. That didn't hurt either. Then the lady expertly tweezered around where the wax strips were. This was easy. But what would be the reaction? Particularly at work. Tricia would worry about that later. For now she proudly walked out of the salon with two feminine studs in each ear and her eyebrows shaped. It was time to go back to Paddys to meet Tina.

Chapter 24

Wouldn't it be Lovely

The new, slightly more responsible me, needed to do something with my room at T-Girl Towers. On the plus side I had a bed (single), a chair (with the stuffing coming out), a coffin for my clothes, a sideboard for my make-up. On the minus side that was all I had. And in the flat we had no electricity, no hot water and a camper gas stove that blew up your face when you changed the gas. As with clothes shopping I decided to prep first. So, by the way, this is an obvious choice.

All I want is a room somewhere,
Far away from the cold night air.
With one enormous chair,
Aow, wouldn't it be loverly?

In which Tricia meets Tina's new boyfriend (for five minutes), looks for paint and plans her room

Tina's new boyfriend, Nick phoned. It was Saturday morning.

"We've got to look for paint for Tricia" said Tina.

"That's ok, mind if I come along too", said Nick.

"We can try Homebase and if not there then go to the Trafford Centre"

"It's a deal", said Tina

Tricia was glad people were organizing her life rather that the other way round for a change.

Eventually they got into the car, picked up Nick and stopped at Homebase. Guess what, the rain was lashing down again. Tricia got some ideas. Lilac she thinks and realises she probably needs Ikea for the furniture. She'll have fun putting that lot together. She is utterly hopeless at things like that. She supposes she'll have to find a man to do it for her. She thinks she will be able to.

Into the Trafford Centre and shops and sales galore. Poor Nick, but the girls were in their element. They went into shop after shop trying to save money; checking things out for each other. It was clear that the Trafford Centre had never seen t-Girls before. They went into Wilkos to check paint prices. Wilko's seemed the cheapest around; how suitable. Tricia is fairly sure she knows what she wants but just needs to mull it over for a while. It transpires that Nick is not allowed in Wilkos as he had an altercation with one of the members of staff. That has to be well weird. Barred from a pub yes, but barred from a shop???

Anyway, opposite Wilko's was a real discovery for the girls. A sensational boutique. With help from the enthusiastic shop assistants, Tina managed to spend two months wages. Tricia bought a pretty pink top and a dead sexy yellow dress to match the dead sexy purple dress Tina had bought. They were going to dress as twins during Pride weekend which was just around the corner. Poor Nick; he was stuck with two young ladies in the dress shop of their dreams. So he took his revenge.

"I know a good pub only a minute away from here", he said.

"Goody", said Tricia not knowing the area.

"Are you sure?" said Tina, knowing the area well.

They walked past a gang of youths who whistled and jeered at them and into a pub protected by a guard-dog. Tina had a cigarette outside. Tricia went in; after all, she had been in a pub with a locked door before. Tina eventually came in and bought herself a drink. A guy wandered across to them and mentioned that they weren't really welcome there. Not nastily at all, but they were a bit too much for people to handle. He later withdrew the remark but the girls took the hint. They walked back into the Trafford Centre past the leering youths.

"There's the pimp and his two bitches" Laughter and catcalls.

"Life can only get better", said Tina

"Life is fun", said Tricia

They went back to Paddys and met up with Tom who was going to paint Tricia's room for her. Tina took Tricia outside.

"I've ditched Nick", she said

"How can you possibly go out with someone whose been banned from Wilkos?"

"Don't blame you hon", said Tricia.

"But you've been out with much worse I reckon", Tricia was on the attack.

"What do you mean?" said Tina

"Like burglar Bill", said Tricia

"Who, Alex" said Tina

"Damn. I must stay sober in future", said Tricia knowing there was no chance,

Chapter 25

Endgame

My walk and my deportment are so important to me at the moment. My make-up is getting better, my looks are getting better but I let myself down because I stoop a little. Tina keeps shouting "straight" at me for me to straighten my back. This is in fact holding me back which is why I need to concentrate on it. Oh, and by the way, this one's from Chess.

> Nothing could be worse
> Than self-denial
> Having to rehearse
> To endless trial

In which Tricia designs her room , its Marlon's birthday, there is some good news and some bad news, the girls join a hen party and Tricia makes a discovery.

Tricia has to think about her bedroom. The good new is that she has. The bad news is that its time for action. She has a budget, she has a coffin, she has a single bed but that's about it at the moment. The first step is to get the electricity on.

Tricia believes in P,D,I,M which stands for Plan, Design, Implement, Manage. She has done the plan bit and is now onto design,

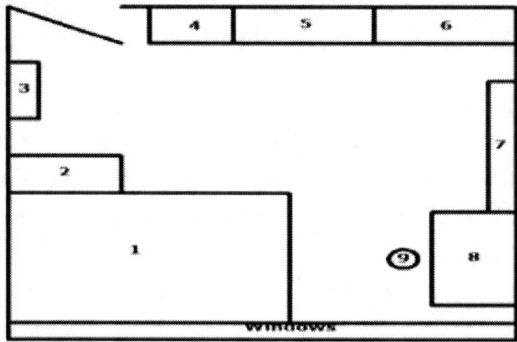

She needs two full length wardrobes for all her dresses (numbers 5 and 6), a four shelf unit for all her undies (number 4), a dressing table with drawers and a make-up mirror (number 8) for all her cosmetics, cleansers and jewellery. With a stool (number 9). A shelf unit (number 7), She's not quite sure why yet but she'll think of something. A double bed (number 1) because she doesn't intend playing with buzzy bee all the time. A bedside table (number 2), preferably with a drawer where she can put her lube and condoms. A full length mirror (number 3) because she likes looking at herself, vain cow that she is. Curtains carpets and paint. First she needs paint because Tom is going to do it for her.

She is thinking lilac for the walls and red for the ceiling. But then she thinks again. Maybe red for the walls so her room will resemble a brothel. No, definitely lilac and she needs to think how it will all work with Tina's room and the rest of the flat, which comes later. As no doubt will all the people who share Tricia's double bed with her. Grape ceiling. There, she's decided.

The girls were ready for an afternoon's socializing. Tina is a hippy again, she likes hippy stuff and looks good in it. Trish looks seductive in her black dress. They maybe don't look too much like prostitutes as they wait for a cab to take them to Paddys; and in truth, do not create much of a stir.

A couple of cabs go by, the girls can't see if there is anybody in them (apart from the drivers) but it annoys Tina. Tricia is fairly chilled about it, she just loves being out there. Actually she prefers walking. She gets more exposure that way and its only about half-an-hour along the towpath of the canal. It's a nice walk and gives her time to herself, to think and to plan. Anyway, the third cab stops for them and takes them outside clone-zone where its just a short walk to Paddys. We need a map.

At the bar are Mark and Tom. Tom is going to paint Tricia's room for her so she needs to keep him sweet. But sweet is Tricia's middle name. He is unimpressed about the lack of electricity in the flat and doesn't think Tricia will sort it out. She will though. He suggests Tricia buys nothing until the room is painted, but as we know Tricia has a plan. Clear out absolutely everything she can next weekend then Tom can get working.

Sadly for Mark, his Father recently passed away and he is left dealing with the estate. It's a funny old world. Tricia learned earlier that very day that her eldest daughter is pregnant; so she is going to be a grandmother ha-ha. Later in the week she learned that a friend she confides in also suffered a loss on the same day in the shape of her eldest son. Tricia feels very sorry for her, that must be devastating as he was only 19. How do these things all join up? Are they connected or are they as random as Tricia herself?

Marlon came from the smoking shelter. "It's my birthday, are you girls going to buy me a drink?" Typical Marlon he's always after something. Marlon was twenty. Tina and Tricia wish they were still twenty although they act like it (Tricia 20 already, what is going on?) They do however celebrate Marlon's birthday with a glass of sambuca, lovely.

The girls decide to move on to Canal Street and Tina notices a hen party and, being the shy person she is, decides to sit next to them. Tina is getting more confident by the day. The hen party are pleased to see the two girls, particularly Melissa who talks to Tricia and Kellie who talks to Tina. It is agreed that if Tina wishes to have breasts, the best thing to do is to have implants and that Tricia should carry on doing what she is i.e. taking her tablets, as she doesn't yet know for sure whether she is TV or TS. The girls pose for some pictures with the hen party who go on their way happy.

Off to Naps where Tricia gets to meet Donna and Donna. Donna one is the other way altogether, girl wanting to be boy; and she's doing a very good job of it although she finds it draining and frustrating. Donna two is her girlfriend, very pretty, very sexy. Donna one is lucky boy thinks Tricia.

Onto the dance floor and Tricia makes a discovery.

"Tina, I think I know what the problem is" said Tricia

"Well at least your not knocking everybody over" said Tina

"Its my left leg, I broke it once skiing. Look my right foot opens out perfectly, as Tara told me. My left foot really struggles though.

"So that's why your dancing from corner to corner in a perfectly predictable manner"

"Yes, and nobody's cowering in the corner now"

"No, they're now cowering on the sides", said Tina jokingly. "I think I'll call you the bishop"

"You know I'm not a bishop Tina, I'm a dancing Queen!"

"No your not Trish, you're a pawn remember".

"Maybe I should concentrate on being a knight for now as it will be an improvement and that will please Tara.

Tricia did improve as the night wore on and, in fact, by the end of the evening did have a rather good night.

Chapter 26

Secret Love

The nicest way to get to the village from t-Girl Towers is to walk along the canal paths. I love doing this; it gives me time to think. About half way there is a bar called Duke's where I often stop and have a beer.

By the way, and about time! If you get the chance to watch Calamity Jane, look at the different way Doris Day rides the horse, in the countryside and in the town. Seems familiar to me, though I can't ride horses!

> Now I shout it from the highest hills
> Even told the golden daffodils
> At last my heart's an open door
> And my secret love's no secret anymore

Arrival

I walk along canals and locks
I watch a young girl feed the ducks
The sun is high, the breeze is strong
This is a place where I belong

I buy a beer, I feel so calm
I'm looking pretty, I'm feeling fine
Dressed to kill and made-up too
Now what does Tricia want to do?

Buy some shoes or buy a dress
She's waited too long to impress

94

Fifty years to be here
Celebrate with another beer?

To the boutiques she will go
Her vulnerability will be on show
But boys and girls, its fine to talk
That t-girl there walks the walk

She struts her stuff, she feels so proud
She needs to scream, to shout out loud
I am Tricia, I am she
I am who I want to be.

Chapter 27

Lili Marlene

I am definitely nearly there. I am so much more confident (maybe too confident) walking around town. I now am looking for people to make comments and enjoying them. Story this time is of Tina — you've read enough of me - who was compared to Marlene Dietrich. It's amazing what a few beers can do. It reminds me of a story.

A man who was sitting in the pub one evening drinking pint after pint of beer kept looking into his shirt pocket after each pint.

"Why do you keep looking in your pocket", said the guy opposite.

"Are, well you see; in there is a picture of my wife and when she looks attractive enough I know its time to go home"

By the way and for Tina.

> You wait where that lantern softly gleams
> Your sweet face seems to haunt my dreams
> My Lili of the lamplight
> My own Lili Marlene

In which the girls are accused of being thieves, Tina get likened to a film star, they meet up with Megan and Becky for the first time and Tricia gets lost.

Tina did the usual on Friday night. The girls were about to go home and she hadn't yet pulled so she went up to the first guy she could find and chatted him up. He was called Martin. The three shared a cab back to

T-Girl Towers. In the cab Martin says to the girls "You're not going to rob me are you?" then he asks them to share the cab fare. Share the cab fare? What's that all about? Martin is about to be given his wicked way with Tina and she has to share the cab fare. Who is the prostitute there then for goodness sake?

It was quite ironic when the following day in the smoking shelter at Paddy's Tina made a pithy remark and commented,

"God, I sound like a prostitute"

"No your not Tina, your just a tart" was Tricia's immediate response.

It was during that time when someone, whose glasses were full of beer said to Tina,

"You know who remind me of?" the question was loaded; both girls' ears pricked up.

"No", said Tina

"Marlene Dietrich, that's who"

Tricia's beer spluttered out of her mouth into the smoking shelter and all over everyone.

"Marlene Dietrich?"

"Marlene Dietrich?"

"She has elegance, class, beauty, style, intelligence, wit and can sing. Tina sings' Born on the wrong side badly'", Tricia was being a little harsh.

Tina simply smiled contentedly to herself.

"I'll have to look her up on the Internet, Trish"

"Think you'd better leave" said Tricia to Harry, the perpetrator of the remark "You're causing ructions"

They were also talking to a couple. Megan, originally from Oz so she knows about cricket, and Becky from Manchester via USA, so she knows about musicals. It was a match made in heaven for Megan, Becky and Tricia. Tina will learn soon thought Tricia but they all had a great time and a load of beer in any case. Megan and Becky eventually had to leave, because Megan is a chef and needed to chop things with a steady hand in the morning. That got Tricia wondering whether she should go along as well. Not yet she thought, I am no where near ready for that and, in any case, I am far too happy where I am at the moment.

The girls, that's Tricia and Tina, argue about three things:

1. Music; Tricia likes classical, opera, musicals, romantic, melodic, Pink Floyd and Peter Gabriel. Tina likes Hawkwind, Pink Floyd and Peter Gabriel so there is some common ground.

2. Travel. We already know that Tricia likes walking along the canal. Tina always prefers to take a taxi which, after all, is only £5 from T-Girl Towers (£6 after 8 p.m.)

3. Food and when to eat. Tina is a northerner (from Manchester) so likes her meals at given times. Tricia however eats when she feels like it but prefers to drink, and eating gets in the way.

It was Tricia's predilection for drink that nearly proved her downfall that night. They continued drinking in Paddy's and then went on to Naps where she had even more. Tricia drunk so much in fact that Tina had to intervene and kindly put her on a cab back giving the driver instructions. Unfortunately the driver got lost and asked Tricia the way. No chance! Not only was Tricia drunk but she also only knew three routes back; one using the canal was not much use to a cab driver, and they were off the other two. So she used what little she had left of her brain. She knew the cab cost £6 so she waited until the clock moved on to £6 then she told the driver to let her off. She must be close.

So there was Tricia, in miniscule white dress and glossy tights at 2:30 in the morning in the outskirts of Manchester, lost. She could have been in Moss Side for all she knew. She decided to go for it. She turned left, clutching her handbag for dear life, because she thought she recognized something. She passed a crowd of youths across the other side of the street. They started catcalling and whistling. They didn't know the truth however. They thought she was a prostitute not a t-girl. Tricia quickly pulled herself together. The only chance was to get another taxi, but where was she going to? Where on earth was T-Girl Towers? She flagged a taxi down and thought hard.

"Do you know the big roundabout where Mancunian way joins Deansgate?" she asked

"I think I know where you mean"

"Well tell me when you are close and I will look for landmarks. There is an old church."

"Ok, I think we'll find it" the cab driver was nice, Tricia was lucky.

"Ok, were nearly there, tell me if you recognize anything" he said.

"Yes, there's the church, pull up on the left, thank you, thank you, can I give you a big hug?"

"Sorry darling, I'm straight"

He could have got a lot more than a hug if he knew what Tricia knew. That we are all born bisexual and its society that changes us, but never mind, the cab fare was only £6 so she must have gone in a triangle!

She was a lucky, lucky girl!

She knows!

Chapter 28

I Feel Pretty

This one just had to happen. So without further ado, and by the way:

> I feel pretty, oh, so pretty,
> I feel pretty and witty and bright!
> And I pity
> Any girl who isn't me tonight.

Make-up make-up never do it again. If you do you get the cane - yes please!

Having washed, shaved, cleaned her teeth and dressed, she props her mirror on her pillow and lies on the bed. She doesn't yet have a dressing table though sometimes she can use Tina's. First she puts on her foundation. She has had her foundation the whole time and it is still only half used. Mind it did cost her £60. It is thick and creamy. With a sponge she covers her face and neck. It is the start.

Now for the powder. She has a big brush to put that on with. She can either go brown by using the centre of her press or natural by using the edge. She doesn't suppose it matters much. She is quite pragmatic. She knows that however long she takes tucking her jeans into her boots at home, as soon as she takes one step outside they will flap out. So she mixes the powder; she will be a Mediterranean girl again today. She waits a while for the powder to settle.

While she is waiting she touches up her finger nails with pink polish. She is not very good at this, particularly on her right hand because she is right handed. She somehow manages only getting a little on her skin which she removes using a pad and remover. She waits a moment for the nail varnish to dry blowing slightly on her nails.

Next is concealer. Most of the products she used are from Lancome including Renergie Lift Concealer SPF20. Lancome is expensive but it thick, creamy and luscious and is lovely to put on. It has the hardest job in the world. With all the beer she drinks it might as well give up; but it doesn't. She uses her finger tips to try to cover the bags under her eyes and her laughter lines. It sort of works.

Then the eyes. She doesn't want to emphasize them too much as she has a spot on her left eyelid. She keeps meaning to have it cut off but never finds the time to get to the doctor. Life is too hectic. The hardest part of all is the eyeliner. She has tried so many but has finally found one which works. It is liquid and this one is from Max Factor. It is called Masterpiece Glide & Define eyeliner. The problem now is that it goes on too easily so she puts too much on and it smudges everywhere. She has to take it off and start again. It doesn't help that she has drunk far too much the night before and that her hands are shaking like she is in an earthquake. This time however she manages it, just, and her Japanese eyes are defined.

Time for her mascara. She is much better at this. She uses CILS design Pro again by Lancombe. She paid a lot for it but it is worth it. It is so black and thick that it doubles the length of her previously unacceptable lashes. She puts on two coats. While waiting for it to dry she puts on her blush. It is supposed to cover where you naturally blush but she hasn't blushed for a year. How can you possibly get embarrassed when you do what she does? She got advice from a MAC consultant to put two stripe of blush down her cheeks (after all she fights like a tiger). It seems to work for her though so that's what she does. The mascara has by now dried so back to her eyes. She doesn't wish to over-emphasize them so keeps it simple. A light, almost natural shade above the lids which slightly accentuates her now shaped eyebrows. Darker on the lids themselves because she wants people to see she is wearing eye shadow when she blinks. She thinks that is dead sexy.

Next comes jewellery and perfume before the big flourish. She has studs in her ears which she has to keep turning, well for a few more weeks yet, so no worries about earrings. She likes her bangles, on this occasion ethnic and they will go with her ethnic necklace; she is a fashionable girl after all. Three rings which seem to go on easily but are a nightmare to get off. Then perfume (Victoria Beckham's Intimately range) on both wrists and elbows (in the evening she will spray some on her ear lobes as well).

So, to the final and best bit. First some lip plumper which, given a couple of minutes, will make her lips full and easy to paint. While she is waiting for the limp plumper to work she fluffs out and re-brushes her wig then puts it on. She now needs Tina's full length mirror to straighten it and style it with her hands. She loves this bit. The wig can settle in all sorts of different positions and she needs to be imaginative about how she finally styles it. Wig done, its time for the lippy which she paints on using a small sponge tipped brush. Subsequent applications will be straight from the tube but it helps to get it just right at the start. In the evening she might add lip gloss but not now. She is ready, she feels sexy, she feels gorgeous, she looks and smells Tricia. One cigarette to let everything settle, one final look in Tina's big mirror, jacket on then she is out into the big wide wild world. What happens next she doesn't know? That is why it's such fun being Tricia.

Chapter 29

Hallelujah

I had a problem here. I agreed with Megan and Becky that we would choose a Leonard Cohen song as we all adore Leonard Cohen; but the rules of my particular game are that the song must come from a film, musical or show. This was Pride weekend and the village was buzzing. I had a great time, but I don't think Iain approved!

So, by the way, a bit of bondage. This one's from Shrek! (Pity it wasn't from Lion King)

> She tied you
> To a kitchen chair
> She broke your throne, and she cut your hair
> And from your lips she drew the Hallelujah

Pride Weekend.

It is Pride. Are we proud? Is Tricia proud? Tricia is proud. She has gone a huge distance in a short space of time and is still (just about) controlling it all. Having just done Sparkle, for transgendered people, this really is the big one. The biggest GBLT fest in the country. The village will not be Tricia's any more. It will be shared with over a thousand people. There are three stages, there are acts, there is music, there is poetry, there is comedy, there are exhibitions. There will be no stag or hen parties to disturb Tricia this weekend. Its £17 just to drink at her local. I sense something is wrong.

Never mind. She has her ticket and is intrigued to find what its all about. It is her first time. She is a Pride virgin. Soon she will lose her virginity again. Will it be fun? She worries a little as she walks through the village in drab early Friday evening on her way to T-Girl Towers. She notices the fast food vans already selling burgers and chips. Tricia doesn't do chips. Tricia likes to keep nice and slim so chips are out. She has to go through a gate, which later on will be protected by security guards She keeps walking. The way out of the village by the canal is blocked up so she has to do the first bit at street level. A quick beer at Dukes as her shoulder is getting sore carrying her bag and then onto Tina's, onto dressing, onto fun. The key fob works and lets her in. Into the lift, up eight floors, left into her room and breathe in.

On her battered sideboard she can see her wig, her make-up, her shoes, her handbags, her jewellery and her boobs. In her coffin she can see all her lovely dresses. In her drawers are her skirts and tops and her underwear. On her table, neatly folded, are her two pairs of jeans. One white, one denim. She is back in heaven.

"Hi Trish, good week?" Tina arrived but the girls didn't say much to each other as they got ready.. They were too busy choosing their clothes and concentrating on their make-up. Tricia had already worked out what she was going to wear. It was a Bank holiday weekend so she needed clothes for three and a half days. Wow, she thought, that's half a week dressed, Yay! Her wardrobe was to be as follows:

Friday Night:	Slinky black dress, black fishnets, white jacket, white handbag, gold flats
Saturday Day:	Jeans with purple top, black jacket, black handbag, white open toe sandals
Saturday Night:	Dead sexy yellow dress, bare legs, white jacket, white handbag, white shoes
Sunday Day:	Denim jump suit, clear tights, black handbag, black jacket, black ankle boots
Sunday Night:	Sparkly gold dress number two, glossy tights, white jacket, white handbag, gold flats
Monday Day:	Yellow top, white skinny jeans, black handbag, black jacket, black ankle boots

Monday Night: Slinky red dress, black fishnets, white jacket, white handbag, gold flats

So a pattern was emerging but this was right. Her ankle boots are solid and good for walking. Her flats are good for dancing. Her black handbag can (and does) hold the kitchen sink, her white handbag has limited space. So she is developing one set of outfits for daytime and one for evenings.

As the girls approached the village, Tricia noticed it was like a prison. They had to queue to convert their £17 tickets into yellow wrist bands. Then they were frisked as opposed to frisky and their handbags checked before they were allowed inside their own village. There were eight gates. Eight entry and exit points guarded by security. There was no other way in. The village was packed. There were people milling around everywhere.

Straight to Paddys to meet up with Megan and Becky. Becky had found a whip which she didn't know what do with (Megan had some ideas) because it wasn't hers. Tina got a text from Marjorie. "I've left a whip at Paddys, can you find it me?" Problem solved. They left the whip behind the bar for Marjorie to pick up later.

Everything about the village seemed different. There weren't even many t-girls in either Paddys or Naps. The atmosphere was less chilled, more raucous. Not necessarily a bad thing, but different. Many of the people Tina and Tricia had got to know over the last year weren't there; either because they baulked at the £17 ticket (a day ticket was £10) or they weren't particularly fond of Pride itself. The road (all 30 meters of it) to Naps was packed, but not as packed as it was to be the following night. Naps itself was full but didn't seem so full of predators, touching or pinching Tricia's backside, casually holding her hand. The girls enjoyed themselves anyway. It was good meeting new and different people from all over the country. That night they were good girls; but aren't they always? They went home reasonably early. But what is reasonable and what is early? There was the big procession tomorrow and they wanted to see if they could blag there way onto a float.

They weren't early enough. The girls got up late so couldn't get to the procession in time. Tricia hopes she will be a bit more alert when it comes to the church. She stuck with her white gear, Tina wore black, so they contrasted nicely. Tonight Tricia was going to wear her dead sexy Chinese yellow dress and was looking forward to it. Taxi in and beer in. A few pints and they split up to look at the exhibitions. Tricia was impressed with the number of whips on display and realised where Marjorie had got hers but she didn't purchase any.

Then she went to the edge of the village to watch the procession she wanted to take part in. There was a huge crowd jostling for space as it approached. One unfortunate girl slipped over in the melee and got her necklace caught in Tricia's big toenail. Not a pretty sight, not a pretty toenail! At least Tricia had put some nail varnish on in the morning while she was waiting for Tina.

Tricia was due back at Paddy's at 16:30 to meet Tina but got there earlier. Silly girl, it was obvious that Tina would be late. She was amazed to find that the bar area was virtually empty but that the queue for the ladies was stretched right through the pub and almost out into the street. This was a problem because it was the major reason why Tricia had got there early. She is however a resourceful girl. The queue for the gents was much smaller so she joined that instead; after all, it wasn't exactly foreign territory. Sometimes it's good to have a choice.

Tina arrived announcing that there was parade of drag queens at New York, New York so the girls wandered down to see. They wondered whether should join in but decided against it. They were t-Girls not drag queens. To confirm that that fact, as Tricia walked away afterwards someone passing her made the comment "now that is a real transvestite". She felt so proud.

After a few more lively beers and livelier chat the girls went home. Tricia wanted to walk the canals as she needed some air and some space. Tina wanted the cab but then she decided she wanted something to eat so Tricia walked anyway. While they had been drinking a small shower had hit Manchester leaving the cobblestones on the canal towpath slippery. Tricia, practicing her walk and her attitude, went over causing scar on her knee and breaking her sunglasses (£2 from Primark). It was only later that she noticed something much worse had happened. Her right nipple had come away from her boob. Lucky it was caught in her bra. Never mind she thought, I can buy some superglue tomorrow. Some things are easy to mend.

"Ha, ha, ha" said Tina later, "told you should have got a cab".

Saturday night and the village was heaving. They watched a few bands then went to Paddies. Megan and Becky had done too much on Friday night and were still nursing their hangovers. Paddies was an oasis of calm compared to the mayhem outside. A few pints in there and then onto Naps. The atmosphere was very, very different. While Tricia was trying to find a square metre on the dance floor, Tina bumped into Michelle and Zoey. They decided to move onto Spirit. Tricia gave up, there simply wasn't enough room and went to join them at Spirit. It took her twenty five minutes to get the hundred yards between the two nightclubs. Everybody wanted to kiss her; everybody wanted to have their picture taken with her. After all, she did look dead glam in her sexy yellow Chinese dress.

The following morning Tricia went shopping, agreeing to meet Tina later. She put on her new denim jumpsuit. The trousers were so short they barely covered her backside. She went bare legged wearing her white strappy sandals. She walked along the canal then went up the stairs at Oxford Road to enter the village. Her walk was really improving. The first guy who passed banged his head with his fists. From afar she looked sexy as hell; but up close? She got many, many comments that day, many unprintable, but she loved the attention, it was what she needed.

Back at Paddy's to meet Tina, the village was still packed. She noticed a sign on the Gents. It said "Men only – NO LADIES"

"Am I allowed in then? Tricia said to Lee behind the bar.

"I think so" Lee replied

"Then it should say, people with balls only allowed" said Tricia, "that would cover it".

"No we don't" said Steve, overhearing the conversation.

She met Tina, had a few more beers, had a wander round the village then back to change into slinky red dress and fishnets. They were meeting up with Megan and Becky to see Proms in the Park which tuned out to be disappointing. It should be called 'Film music in the Park' thought Tricia; and modern film music at that. An early night, but what's early, because everybody was tired out.

Monday, the last day of Pride, a bank holiday.. Tricia walked into the village, Tina has departed to prepare for a mornings strimming the following day.

Practicing her walk just before entering security gate seven, she slips again as her heel slides across the pavement. This time it wasn't wet. This time there was no physical damage but plenty of the mental type as a crowd of people laughed at her. She dusted herself down, laughed back, and entered the village, with a very red face, through security gate six.

She was dressed much more soberly this time and wanted one last hike around Manchester to see what reaction she would get. She brought her third empty glass back to Lee behind the bar.

"That's it" she said "Tricia is ready for Manchester",

"But is Manchester ready for Tricia?" asked Lee,

"It will be", Tricia paused "in about fifty years".

She hardly caused a ripple; was it her missing nipple? She remembered to get some glue.

Back to the village where she met Megan and Becky and they watched a hilarious concert by Frisky and Mannish. Well worth going to see if they are in your area. They parody songs in a gay way and are very, very, professional and very, very funny. Back in Paddy's and Tricia gets a surprise.

"I've forgotten, I've got something for you" said Steve

"Ooooh how exciting" said Tricia

She was passed a small thin parcel. She quickly realised. It was not for her at all, it was the whip which Becky found on Friday.

"No Steve its not for me"

"You're Tricia aren't you?"

"Yes but this isn't for me. I'll tell you who it is for in a minute.

She opened her tiny notepad where she writes the notes for the book. It was for Marjorie so she wrote Marjorie on the parcel and gave it back to Steve.

Ultimately Marjorie was to pick it up so was to be happy. Even more ultimately, Tricia supposed, she was to be very, very happy; if a little sore. Tricia was jealous.

Finally they walked into the park for the Candlelight Vigil. This was in remembrance of all the people in the world who have died of Aids. Megan was not looking forward to it as she knew some friends who suffered because of it. Sadly the vigil was much like the rest of Pride.; cheap and commercial. The speeches and the rallying calls should happen elsewhere. This should have been a peaceful, conservative affair. It wasn't. The three were disappointed. After holding their candles up for a minute the fireworks started. Pride was over for another year.

Hallelujah.

Bang!

Chapter 30

And this is my Beloved

Whatever you do in life, you can't get away from your roots, but I have learned that you can add to them.

By the way the words are from Kismet, the music is by Borodin from Prince Igor, (Ovlur's theme); and is beautiful. My Mother once received a standing ovation singing the song. My Father conducted the orchestra. I was ten and cried with pride. We buried my Father to the music. That was the day I became free, though that was no fault of his.

Strange spice from the south
Honey through the comb sifting
Imagine these in one eager mouth
And this is my beloved

Being Tricia

Tricia is proud of herself. Of course when she's walking around she gets some remarks and caustic comments, but she will always look people in the eye and comment back. She is open, she is honest, she is herself and has absolutely nothing to hide. She loves being the person she has become. She is not frightened about what is around the corner but thinks it fun (and she likes fun) that she doesn't know what it will be.

Other people are proud of Tricia too. How can she possibly have the nerve to do what she does? Her Mother is proud of her. She sent this card on her birthday:

Today loving wishes
and thoughts come to mind
For a son who was born to be
one of a kind,
Making his way
with a mind of his own,
Making a difference
and making it known
That he has his own hopes
and dreams to pursue -
Which is why, Son,
these wishes are special,
like you.

Other genuine girls are proud of her. She can see it in their eyes when she walks around Manchester dressed, as she normally does, in a slightly provocative manner. Sometimes however she likes to dress tartily because she wants people to stare, to look at her. Although she occasionally wants to be the centre of attention she can back off if necessary. She is pleased about that. She also notices that some other people are frightened of her. They will make space for her. They will not want to engage in conversation with her but if she manages to get over the initial hurdle then they have fun. Is this Tricia's fault or is it theirs?

Tricia can get into a zone I can't. She is in it now as I write this. There is a huge flood of thoughts and influences hitting her.; so many she can hardly cope. Her past, my past; references to her love of music, literature poetry; my love of music, literature, poetry engulf her. She is in a zone where she is totally relaxed, chilled and can take this all in. She does not have to worry about children, work, money; she can appreciate everything that is good about life. She hasn't a care in the world and is totally happy. It is being yourself that's important, not hiding away, not being frightened of anything. Tricia loves this space.

But there's even more to it. She adores the whole thing. Getting up in the morning, putting on her pretty pink dressing gown and deciding what to wear; washing, shaving, putting on her outfit; slowly applying her make-up; the jewellery, the perfume, the lip plumper; then finally and best of all putting on and styling her wig and then her lippy. She takes her time because she so enjoys doing it although she can do it quickly if necessary. Then there is the satisfaction of seeing her reflection in the mirror.

Walking in along the towpath, preparing her next venture into the big City. What does she need? What does she want? What should she look for? She reads magazines and newspapers for fashion hints and make-up tips. She loves that too. Even I turn to the woman's section of the paper first, then the sport, then the news. After all, you can't do much about the news, its already happened.

The fact she can now go anywhere as Tricia also makes her happy. She has been to the cinema, the theatre, restaurants, bars, cafes, pubs and of course the shops. There are plenty more places she would like to go to but there's no rush. Tricia doesn't do time. She has yet to do public transport but that will happen shortly. She would like to go to Liverpool for a day trip; to see how it has changed since my University days. To get further back into her roots, my roots. Maybe that will happen next month as Tina is pondering her finances at the moment and is likely to be out less often.

Tricia doesn't like or believe in labels but has heard of something that makes her feel comfortable while talking to others. She is not just a crossdresser, she is much more than that. She is not a transvestite, she is more than that. She is not a transsexual, she is less than that, for now anyway. She is a t-girl quite simply. That pretty much defines her and is not really a label. Above all though; she is Tricia, she is she; she is who she wants to be. Happy!

Chapter 31

I Could have Danced all Night

This weekend was dominated by one thing. I had been preparing a trip to Liverpool all week. This was going to be major. It would require me to get on a train, dressed and made-up for fifty minutes. I wanted to pick up stuff from my roots. Go to the University where I studied 32 years ago. Try to find the pubs I drank in, the house I lived in and walk through the City. Iain hasn't been back for 25 years and I of course have never been there at all. Let's hope that I'm brave enough because it is bound to be fun, and I like fun! By the way, I nearly forgot, dancing produces attitude. I'm likely going to need a lot of that.

> I could have danced all night!
> I could have danced all night!
> And still have begged for more.

In which Tricia plans, meets up with some old friends and some new, Tina scores at least twice and Tricia builds up her confidence.

Tricia wasn't going to Manchester at all she was going to catch up with things at home. Something however was nagging at the back of her mind. She wanted to go back to Liverpool; she wanted to visit her past. She wanted Tricia to see her background. She worked really hard on Tuesday, Wednesday and Thursday so she could go back. She so loves Manchester. So she planned. This is her itinerary..

Friday – Chill into the weekend in slinky black dress. Paddy's and Naps.

Saturday – Paddy's then New York, New York for Liverpool v Manchester

United then book to get her eyebrows waxed then shopping for black jeans and purple blouse (to go with the autumn jacket she bought last week). Then back to change into slinky red dress then maybe Proms in the Park with Megan and Becky then back to Naps.

Sunday – Tina will be leaving early so she is on her own. First Paddy's to build up confidence and spirit. Then, at 13:45 the big challenge. To catch a train to Liverpool, to her roots. Tricia on public transport aaaaaarrrrrggggggghhhh!

She met Tina, Mark, Josh etc in drab. She was later to see them in slinky black dress and fishnets (Tricia that is). Becky and her sister Joy popped into the pub and the four girls had a good gossip. Megan was still ill but they were hoping to go to Proms in the Park in Salford the following night. That intrigued Tricia. She would think some more about it and maybe go herself. She didn't promise anything though.

Onto Naps. Tricia had the Merseyside very firmly on her mind. Tina had something else; something North not West of Manchester. Something Scottish. Tina pulled and brought back a Billy Connolly impersonator. No, this is true; he goes around Northern pubs in scruffy clothes posing for pictures with the punters. Och eye the noo, would you believe it?

Tricia meanwhile was pounding the dance floor, marching up and down, practicing her walk, getting her attitude up. She spent hour after hour on the dance floor not leaving until three. She marched back to T-Girl Towers through the streets of Manchester. She had attitude. She had confidence. She was Tricia.

The following morning the girls got up late and took a taxi into the village. Tricia wore her t-shirt with a girl just like her on it (?) and her purple skirt with patterned tights. She likes that outfit. Everything seems to merge into one. A quick pint in Paddys then to New York, New York for the football. Manchester United lose to Liverpool 2-1. Tricia doesn't mind too much. It may make the scousers more accepting of her tomorrow. She also found a place where she could practice her march. There is a big mirror on the way to the toilets in New York, New York. She excuses herself about twelve times in the ninety minutes of the match. "This beer's going right through me", she says to Tina.

A few more in Paddys and Tricia says excuse me again. This time for around an hour. Firstly she books her beautician for an eyebrow shaping session at 16:30. Then shopping for a purple blouse and black jeans. She doesn't have much luck. All the purple blouses she sees are too fussy. Most un-Tricia like. Eventually she finds some black jeans in T-K Max for £15 so quickly buys them. She desperately needs the ladies so has to march back to Paddy's as quickly as she can. She squats for an awfully long time, something she was to do on many occasions over the weekend.

One quick pint then back to the beautician's. She hears some very good news. Only two more weeks and she can start wearing earrings properly. Two more weeks with her studs in then she can wear the hooped gold earrings which have been lying on her battered sideboard for a month being admired. Tricia returned to Paddy's but she knew Tina had gone. She had instructions to wake her up at eight o'clock using any means possible (it was now five). Oh well a quick pint and she will get back too. She texted Megan to decline the offer of proms in the park. She was wary about coming back in the tram in the dark and wanted to save herself for Liverpool. She was just finishing her drink when a huge Nigerian came to sit next to her and they started talking.

She got back to T-Girl Towers on the dot at eight. Well, a girl's got to eat. The timing was perfect as Tina had to get up to unbolt the door. They were out by nine. Tricia changed into slinky red dress but her fishnet hold-ups didn't hold up so she gave up and went bare legged showing off the scar where she had fallen over during Pride. Tina was after only one thing again so went to Naps early. She was to get it but Tricia doesn't know who with, and suspects neither does Tina. Tricia didn't even go to Naps. No Naps on Saturday night, amazing. With tomorrow and Liverpool on her mind she just marched home through the streets. Sometimes she can be so sensible, but other times? .....

Chapter 32

Officer Kruppke

This is a bit of a side issue. It should really be about tomorrow. It is me going west in another way and by the way, I'll borrow from Leonard Bernstein and West Side Story again. After all Manchester is in the West of England. Liverpool is in fact a few miles further West. Will I do it? Today was cum and tomorrow will come.

> My sister wears a moustache
> I wear a dress
> Goodness gracious, that's why I'm a mess

Liverpool gets sidetracked

She met him at the candy store, you get the picture. He was dark, very, very, dark. He was Nigerian. She wanted to continue to enjoy this candy store so she went on to another one, about two minutes away. He didn't drink so bought himself a small orange and her a sherbert. They cuddled and snogged until they were ready. They both knew what they wanted, they both knew it didn't have legs, but they were determined to enjoy it. Forget Liverpool for a while, forget plans and aspirations, this is about the here and now.

Unfortunately what follows has had to be censored. However Tricia has had her first stab at writing song lyrics. So here is a song by Dale and McCartney. Doesn't seem to have the same ring to it does it?

Friday evening at five o'clock as the sun goes down
Joyfully opening the office front door

116

The week is over; he wished he'd done more
He walks briskly down to the station clutching the things he needs
Dreaming sweet dreams of the rest of the day
He's done his job, now she can play
He, (he gave it most of his life)
Is leaving, (sacrificed most of his life)
Work (He needs a job so that Trish can get by)
He's leaving work after living a lie for so many years

Friday evening at half past six he is far away
Carefully turning the front door key
Stepping inside she is free
She (He gives her most of his life)
Is coming (Surrenders most of his life)
Home (He gives her everything money can buy)
She's coming home after no life at all
For so many years.
Hello

Tricia smiles as she shaves then puts on her lingerie
Rushing to meet the appointment she made
Meeting a man who she hopes won't fade
She strolls out of the apartment, showing her attitude
Brazenly made-up with short, tight dress
She is a girl who is out to impress
She (She only thinks of herself)
Is having, (No thoughts for anyone else)
Fun (Fun is just one thing that money can buy)
She's coming home after living a lie for so many years

Friday night and at twelve o'clock she is there with him
She looks so pretty and feminine
He sits beside her and plies her with gin
They go down under the arches holding each other close
How could he treat me so thoughtlessly?
How could he do this to me?
She's having fun,
Hello!

Chapter 33

It's a Lovely Day Today

Yes I did it and I loved it. At the end of next month I am going down to London to show my American friend, Monica, the sites and then bring her back to Manchester for some fun and games. I intend to do it all as Tricia. This was therefore an important dress rehearsal. By the way the sun was shining in Manchester, and in Liverpool, so miracles do happen.

> But if you've got something that must be done
> And it can only be done by one
> There is nothing more to say
> Except its a lovely day for saying 'Its a lovely day'

One Goes Mad in Liverpool! (Or is it two?)

The sun was shining and Tricia was up bright and early, well before eight. She had been well behaved the previous night after the previous evening with the big Nigerian. She didn't even go to Naps. Unheard of on a Saturday night. But today, Sunday, was the big day, the day she had been planning all week. Today she was going to become a scouse girl.

> *"Oh Maggie Maggie May*
> *She is back and here to stay,*
> *And Lime Street will be Lime Street as before"*

What to wear for this, her first time on a train? She must dress soberly, she must not seek attention. She is happy with that though. Sometimes she craves attention and sometimes not, and this she knows is a not. So checked purple blouse, new skinny black jeans bought yesterday at TK-Max, black cropped jacket and ankle boots. She was going to be walking today. She was going to be clip-clopping around Liverpool today.

There's even enough time for Tina to get ready so they can have a couple of beers at Paddy's to settle Tricia's nerves. She doesn't really feel nervous though, she feels excited. Tom is there so they talk about the football yesterday and in the week. Soon its 13:45 and Tricia has to say her goodbyes.

She has decided not to do or wear anything special, anything flash. Just be a normal girl (?) Buying a ticket, catching and alighting a train. The journey itself is fifty minutes. Fifty minutes sitting in a carriage with others. A sitting target. She decides to buy Glamour magazine for company. That's what most normal girls would do, wouldn't they?

She has bought her ticket and is now on the train. There is a nice guy sitting next to her who knows, but listens to his headphones. He asks Tricia to look after his equipment for him while he goes, presumably to look after his equipment. Tricia's mind flashes back to yesterday evening. She would like to go with him. While he's gone the ticket inspector comes round. He punches her ticket and hands it back. "Thanks luv", he says.

The lady on the seat opposite is applying her make-up. Tricia wants to do that, Tricia wants people to know what a girl she really is. She will start when the train is past Warrington. She has had no difficulties so far and has enjoyed the journey. She needs to relax and watch so she stops writing for a while.

The train approaches Warrington. She can't believe that she is sitting on a train, obviously a t-Girl (but a good t-Girl) and there are no issues. She does look good though, as good as she can so far, as good as it gets. She has spent all weekend building up the courage, confidence and attitude to do this.

> *"She struts her stuff, she feels so proud,*
> *She needs to scream, to shout out loud,*
> *I am Tricia, I am she,*
> *I am who I want to be"*

She knows there is lots more that can happen. She knows that Liverpool is rougher around the edges and less cosmopolitan than Manchester. She looks forward to it. If Tricia didn't do this, if she didn't care, there would be no point in my investing the money. But she does care. We both want it more than anything in the world. We both want to be free and be ourselves. We will!

Warrington. Now its time to check her make-up. It is good, it is good enough, it is just right for daytime. Not too glary but you know its there. She simply tops up on lipstick and mascara and dabs a little more perfume on. She wants to feel and smell Tricia, to be Tricia. She is!

The train pulls in at Liverpool Lime Street Station. She gets out and has her first big problem. Ladies or Gents? She can't go back to Paddy's, she is in Liverpool. For the first time in the straight world Tricia takes the Ladies option. She is good enough, she is sexy enough, she is confident enough, she does it. She shakes her head, why had she put herself through this, she could have easily gone on the train. But she is pleased with herself, even though cost her 30 pence. 30 pence to spend a Penny, what is the world coming to? She had had four pints earlier at Paddy's and one on the train, so she probably got value for money. Next find one of the two pubs I used to drink in. She had to walk through the University campus to do this. I vaguely remembered where they were. Turn left and up the hill. On the way up she passes a pub with some lovely blues being played live. Look for the new cathedral.

"In our Liverpool homes"
"In our Liverpool homes"
"We speak with an accent exceedingly rare"
"Meet under a statue exceedingly bare"
"And if you want a cathedral we've got one to spare"

I think of my first two years at University. At the halls of residence near Sefton Park. Too far for Tricia to go today. There were Folk nights every Monday in the bar. I wouldn't sing when they asked for house singers. I bet Tricia would though. Life would be different is Tricia was in me as much then. She was in me but she was frightened. She isn't now.

Or

"You look in the dustbin for something to eat"

"You find a dead rat and you think it's a treat"
"In your Liverpool slums"
"In your Liverpool slums"

And worse to follow. I think of my final year in the house of Windsor Street. We used to sunbathe on the toilet roof. When we had a bath the condensation would drop on you from the ceiling of the bathroom. To describe it at a slum was probably generous. But it was my house.

The Cambridge, where she used to eat at lunchtimes as well as drink was no more. I remembered Sandy from behind the bar, he is probably no more too. The Caledonia, where I drank in the evenings, was open however. But there was no real ale for Tricia. There was satellite TV on showing the Everton game. The pub was full of Everton supporters but they all smiled at Tricia. Tricia was not a threat. She got her picture taken. They are good in Scouseland.

She walks out, walks to see if she can find the house she ended her University life in. Past the gothic cathedral (must nicer than the "Mersey Funnel or the wigwam" as it is locally known). She turns into Windsor Street. All has changed. There were seven pubs in Windsor Street, now there are only two. The seven pubs were always open. The two are shut and it's only around 16:00. It seems lighter, roomier, the road seems wider than when I remember it. In fact that is true of all Liverpool now. It does seem brighter. Maybe that is progress. She thinks she finds my old house but she's not 100% sure. Everything is so different.

She walks back. She needs the ladies again. She looks for Ye Cracke which is supposedly where John Lennon and Paul McCartney drank but can't find it. She finds the Grapes instead. Another place she used to drink. She buys a beer then back on the toilet, what is it with her and toilets this weekend? She goes outside and has a cigarette with her beer. She takes some flak from three guys who realise immediately what she is. She gives it back. It was not spiteful and it was amusing. The Scousers are known for their humour.

She walks into the City centre itself. The first thing she notices is that its almost identical to Manchester. The same shops, the same pedestrian area, the same everywhere. Surely we must fight this she thinks. She walks down to the pier head. Where she found the suburbs quite impressive, she sees the centre as a bit plastic. She's not sure she likes it. This isn't progress, this is rampant commercialism.

She gets to the pier head, the farthest west she can go before the sea. It is only then that she notices the air is different in Liverpool from Manchester, but it is. She has some banter with some stewards directing the traffic.

"You're a tranny aren't you?"

"No, but you're scousers, we all have our crosses to bare"

"You're nothing but a two bob tart"

"Ha ha, you couldn't afford me on Liverpool wages; at least you've got a job I suppose"

Tricia thinks. Two bob, that's a lot? And her mind goes all Nigerian. Actually he bought her a beer, so she goes for £2.50. She's not sure if that makes her comments justifiable though. Tricia turns to face them and laughs. They laugh back. It was a bit of fun. Laughter can diffuse any situation.

She had another beer in a plastic pub in a plastic glass next to the station while waiting for her train to take her back to Manchester. If she completes the journey she completes everything. She will we all know. Two young girls take pictures of her on the train. They ask and she says yes, providing they take one with Tricia's camera. Tricia is aware that as the day has gone on she has got worse in presenting herself. This is partly due to alcohol consumed and partly due to tiredness after all the walking. But she doesn't care. She is happy. She duly arrived back in Manchester at just after seven, safe, sound and exhilarated. Just a few pints in Paddy's then an early night. She still had much to do back home,

Tricia had changed a lot but there was still much more to see. She wanted to walk around her faculty, she wanted to visit the halls of residence. She still has some more of her roots to discover. She will be back though. She now knows she can do it whenever she wants. She likes Liverpool; in general.

Chapter 34

The Ugly Duckling

To get to the other side of the rainbow you not only have to have a dream, you not only need to wish it come true with all your might, but you also need to keep going, despite others trying to blow you off course. You need to work, work, work as hard as you can on it and have the confidence you can reach it. This is particularly true if you dream the type of dreams I do. Dreams which other people don't understand. I think I am getting close to the end of my rainbow.

But where is it?

> I'm not such an ugly duckling
> No feathers all stubby and brown
> For in fact these birds in so many words said
> The best in town, the best, the best, the best in town

A Fairy Story, how very apt.

Once upon a time, a long, long time ago, in a land about 200 miles away called London, a young princess, though she didn't know that then, woke up; though she didn't completely wake up for a long, long time.

She had been dreaming beautiful dreams. Of pretty fairy tale dresses made of silk; of figure hugging skirts and blouses; of sassy handbags and clutches in white, pink, black, red, silver and gold; of boots and shoes with wedges and heels or simply flat; of figure shaping skinny jeans and boot leg jeans; of Barbie pink nail varnish; of mascara, eye-liner, eye shadow, blusher, compact, brushes and sponges and luscious red lipstick so thick it oozed onto her pouting lips; of stockings of tights and of ankle socks; of panties, bra's, slips, camisoles and nighties; of earrings, necklaces, broaches, hair clips, bracelets and rings

She had been dreaming of shopping in the most fabulous shops which sell all those wonderful things; of drinking in the finest pubs and bars; of eating gourmet food in the best restaurants (though she didn't know about curry then); of listening live to the most beautiful music ever played; of driving in the largest cars imaginable; of watching the most challenging plays ever written; of handsome princes and beautiful princesses just like her and of dancing through the night.

Then, 40 years later, a handsome prince must have kissed her while she was dreaming because ...

Once upon a time, not so very long ago at all in a land called Manchester, an elderly Queen (who knew precisely what she was) woke up and got out of bed. She took off her nightie, put on, her underwear, her blouse, her pencil skirt, her boots. Then she put on foundation, compact, concealer, eye-liner, mascara, blush, eye shadow, lip plumper, lippy, then perfume; then her necklace, bangles and rings. Finally she put on her wig, loaded her handbag and put on her black jacket She left the house and headed for the shops through the canals and locks. She bought a beautiful pink dress and some blouses. She visited her local pub and met another aging Queen just like her. They had some wine and some beer then went to the finest Indian restaurant for something to eat.

They got into a cab to go to the theatre. There they meet up with a wonderful prince and princess just like her and enjoyed a stunning play which shocked them all. They got a taxi back to the pub before going on to the nightclub where she danced all night. She was a dancing Queen in Neverland. She had a smile on her face.

And she lived happily ever after (I think).

Chapter 35

Dancing Queen

Liverpool has certainly changed me. This weekend I was so much more confidant and my attitude was so much better. It was a tremendous weekend. I now walk around without a care in the world. It is now almost natural for me to go dressed and made-up. Friday night is the key. It is the dance floor at Naps where I build my attitude for the weekend ahead.

By the way, from Abba the Musical and Abba the Movie. Bit out of sync I know, but then aren't I? Anyway, its what I feel life's like!

> You are the dancing queen, young and sweet, only seventeen
> Dancing queen, feel the beat from the tambourine
> You can dance, you can jive, having the time of your life
> See that girl, watch that scene, dig in the dancing queen

Happy birthday dear Megan the film star who freaks, the girls discuss safety, watch a play and Trish develops even more attitude

The one thing Tricia learnt from her trip to Liverpool is that it is all about attitude and confidence. To be confident however, you need the attitude. She was going to further develop it this weekend. This weekend was to be seminal (careful how you read that) in her development.

Friday was Megan's birthday She and Becky had been to see the BBC perform Swan Lake but came back to the village afterwards and saw Tina and Tricia walking away from Paddy's for a change. To be fair though, they had been in there a couple of hours. Megan had also made her debut in front of the cameras. She was asked her opinion of the credit crunch. "What is the credit crunch?" asked Tricia who was far too wrapped up in her own little life to know about such things. Megan performed admirably but they were not to find out whether her footage was to be included.

A few beers in the pubs on Canal Street and then on to Naps. A normal Friday night in other words. They discussed the fact that a man had been badly hurt by thugs and was lucky to still be alive. He went to a fancy dress party as Lois Lane, his mate went as Superman. Of course the full details of the story weren't reported so it wasn't known whether he provoked the incident.

"Superman wasn't much help then" said Tina.

"Why on earth would a man want to dress up as a girl in any case? I don't understand." said Tricia. Yet safety was certainly a major concern for the girls. Tricia's rule is to stay with the crowds wherever possible and try not to be in a straight place late at night. This weekend it was inevitable that she would be, but then it was a very safe straight place indeed.

In Naps Tricia pounded the dance floor yet again. Up and down, up and down she marched, glaring at anyone who got in her way. She was psyching herself up, developing her attitude and with it her confidence. Meanwhile Megan and Tina discovered that they shared the same size feet. They were both size 7, so they swapped footwear. Megan totally freaked wearing Tina's boots. She burst into tears and was totally uncontrollable until Becky and Tina took them off. She just couldn't do girly. Rumour has it that she was once forced to wear a dress for a family event but rumour isn't always accurate.

The major event on Saturday was the play. Yes, our brave young girls were going to the Lowry to watch 'Miracle'. They agreed to meet Becky outside the theatre at 18:30. Well eventually arranged because Becky wasn't up until three in the afternoon after the previous night of excess. Poor Megan had to go to work at 11:00 and on a bicycle with a slow puncture at that. Nothing could puncture Megan's joi-de-vivre though.

Needless to say Tina was running late and Tricia needed all her patience to get her moving.

"Its time." said Tina, "It goes too quickly".

"Have you ever thought" said Tricia, "that it may not be time's fault; it may sometimes be Tina going too slowly".

Even so they got to the Lowry at 18:27.

Tina wore a fairly slutty (that is meant as a compliment) black mini dress and boots to the play. Tricia wore a just above the knee pencil skirt and cotton blouse with her ankle boots. She didn't want to look tarty. As they walked to the lift, Tina bumped into Tricia's heel.

"Foul, yellow card" shouted Tricia, "that was a tackle from behind".

It's a good job, she thought, that I spent fifteen minutes ensuring my tackle was behind. This skirt is very, very, tight.

The sun was shining though it was to get nippy later, so they decided to have a beer outside the Lowry bar in the open air. Becky joined them and they took some pictures and drank some beer.

"Tricia is what you might call a surrealist photographer" said Tina.

"What do you mean?" said Becky

"Here we go" said Tricia.

"All the pictures she takes are blurred because she shakes so much".

"Show Becky".

Tina handed Tricia her camera.

"That's not fair, you're putting me under far too much pressure, I'm bound to shake now".

Tricia concentrated with all her might, though there's not much might left in her now. She took a deep breath and gently squeezed the shutter.

"Crikey Trish, that wasn't bad" said Tina.

"Nothing wrong there" said Becky.

"There's some funny words on the screen" said Tricia, "I can't read them because I haven't got my glasses on".

She passed the camera to Tina

"Ha, ha, ha, ha, it says 'camera shake, the picture may be blurred', ha ha ha ha"

Tricia cursed silently.

Megan wobbled round the corner on her bike. She had ten minutes before the performance started so plenty of time for a quick beer. At this point it all got a bit hectic as they needed to order beers for the interval as well but they made it just in time.

The play itself was first class. It was about a guy who could cure people with terminal diseases by sodomizing them. There were only three people in the cast. Ben, 'The Miracle' himself, his psychiatrist and a Catholic Priest. The Catholic Priest viewed him as the new messiah but he renounced God and Jesus. A great theological debate ensued but it later transpired that the priest was suffering from an interminable disease and wished to be sodomized. So gay sex was validated. At the end of the play the psychiatrist broke down in tears, pleading for Ben to save her seven year old son who was also suffering from a terminal disease. This really got everybody thinking. How far do you go?

Megan had another shift at six in the morning so they went their separate ways. Tina and Trish did what they normally do; back to Paddy's then onto Naps. Did Tina pull? Of course she did. Did Tricia pull? Did she care? But she walked back to T-Girl Towers with attitude. Now that did matter.

Chapter 36

Underneath the Arches

I think I am breaking free; I feel so normal dressing now. It is still as exciting to me as it always was but now all the apprehension and nerves have gone. I want to keep pushing myself further, to do more and more things, to experience myself.

By the way there are plenty of ways of having fun! and this one just had to be done. It's by Flanagan and Allen. I'm an English girl and this is an English song.

Underneath the arches
I dream my dreams away,
Underneath the arches
on cobble stones I lay,

The difference between a t-girl and a transvestite

Tina and Tricia dress for different reasons. Tina's motivation is purely to attract men so she will use any technique she can to appear tarty. Tricia's main concern is that women accept her and think she looks good. A nice comment from a girl or woman gives her immense pleasure. She also likes to attract men, hence the short skirts and dresses, but doesn't over-do it. Tricia is starting to wear less and less make-up; Tina more.

Tina is like a predator as far as men are concerned; a hunter gatherer. It's a weird contrast. If any man shows any interest in her whatsoever she's on to him in a flash. Tricia can take it or leave it. She does get men coming onto her but doesn't mind if it doesn't happen. She also doesn't judge Tina. They both do what they do for one reason only. To have fun.

As well as developing her confidence and attitude, Tricia is also trying to develop a pout. Even during the week when in drab she is practicing pursing her lips together. It came out forcibly that she was doing in right in Paddys on Friday night. The girls met Jane, a lovely lesbian.

"Want me to go into bloke mode", she said.

She immediately widened her mouth and started talking in a mock cockney accent. Tricia commented on the wide mouth and Jane agreed. She had been practicing the opposite from Tricia for years. She kissed both girls goodbye.

"Bleeding heck Trish, she puts it on with a trowel; I've got gloss or something horrendous all over my cheeks, yuck".

After hour after hour on the dance floor Tricia struck lucky. She met Tim, or Handy Andy as she was to name him, since his hands couldn't leave her body alone. He wanted action, he wanted it now. Tricia was happy as it was at least two in the morning and all the marching up and down had made her tired. But where? She couldn't go to the Rembrandt like last week again, and she was certainly not risking being thrown out of Naps, and there are security cameras everywhere in the village. Tricia thought hard. Where is her favourite place to walk? Why the canal of course. What does the canal have? Why bridges and arches of course. So like a million horny tarts before her she took Handy Andy under the canal bridge. Some people even walked past while they were in the act so he grasped her tightly to himself and snogged, even then he couldn't stop his hand caressing her backside. Wow! The things one can get up to on a canal.

When she woke up Tricia noticed she has received a text the previous night. It was from Tina. It said: 'Bad bloke. Need you down here as my boyfriend'. The fact that Tricia was dressed as a woman; the fact that Tricia's phone was in her handbag which was in the corner of the dance floor which was playing very loud music seemed to pass Tina by. There was no way on earth Tricia was going to receive that message. "The scary thing" said Tina when they were discussing it, "is that I was actually quite turned on by the fear; I quite enjoyed completely giving control away". Tina, careful girl.

In Tricia's little diary where she makes notes she noticed Tina had put 'Bog rolls'. She could only assume Tina had put it on the wrong list.

It was Saturday lunchtime and Tricia was ready, and like most Saturday lunchtimes Tina was not. Tricia went for some milk and cigarettes and a lunchtime pint to give Tina some space and time. It was a glorious sunny day in Manchester. It was a glorious sunny day in Manchester. Tricia thoroughly enjoyed reading the paper on a table outside the pub with no atmosphere, tanning her chicken legs. All was peaceful and quiet. Even better, walking back to T-Girl Towers a guy wolf-whistled her from behind. Her first ever natural (not ironic) wolf-whistle. She was delighted.

The girls decided to go back to the Stretford Centre. There were some essentials they needed to pick up and there was also a certain boutique they both loved. They needed toilet rolls (you knew that) candles, batteries and wine glasses.

They got:

Tina – 1 skirt, 2 dresses, 3 tops, blue eye shadow, white stockings, body spray, powder, boots (again), eye liner, mascara.

Tricia – 1 dress, 1 blouse, 1 top.

Other - Toilet roll, candles, ouzo, 2 bottles white wine, port, milk.

Forgot – batteries and wine glasses

Only 50% success rate but that was good considering they spent more than forty five minutes in the boutique. Tina spent the rent money again.

On Sunday Tricia woke up bright and early at 09:00. The sun was still shining in Manchester. The sun was still shining in Manchester. She really needed a couple more hours sleep and would normally have put her head back down on the pillow. Not this time though. She knew what she wanted. She wanted to go out into Manchester. She wanted to put on her make-up. She wanted to dress up. She wanted to be Tricia. There was no fear, there was no doubt. Liverpool had changed her, dancing had changed her, she had so much more confidence, she had so much more attitude.

She walked in through the canals. She shopped for around two hours. She even went to the Ladies in the Arndale. She only bought a pair of sunglasses but that didn't matter. She browsed and browsed through the wonderful clothes on display in the shops. She was happy, she was free, she was Tricia, she was who she wanted to be. She had a coffee before meeting Tina in New York, New York where they watched Manchester United draw with Chelsea. Then to Paddy's and a lot of beer (Tricia) and wine (Tina). Then a curry then home for an early night. Work tomorrow. Tricia enjoyed her day immensely though; she was herself.

She really thinks she is She now.

Chapter 37

Handbags and Gladrags

I will have to extend the rules of the songs to include ones from TV (appropriate as that's what most people call me although I'm a t-girl). This is the signature tune to the Office, and I'm shortly to become a Grandad (?)

I do so love my handbags though!

> So what becomes of you my love
> When they have finally stripped you of
> The handbags and the gladrags
> That your poor old Grandad had to sweat to buy you

Tricia's Handbag

Tricia adores handbags. She loves the colours, she loves the straps, she loves their smell, initially of leather but after they are worn in of her perfume and her make-up. She loves playing with her handbag; one minute on one shoulder, one minute on the other, cradling it on her elbow, carrying it in her hand. She loves unzipping it to get out her purse or her make-up and she loves the way she keeps them meticulously clean. She looks back to her past. She treats her handbags with the same reverence as I treated my football boots.

Tricia adores buying handbags. She likes cut price designer ones and there are a number of shops who do them. She will spend an age trying them on; over her right shoulder, over her left shoulder, on her elbow, holding them low, holding them like a clutch; looking in the mirror at how she portrays herself, gauging how they feel on her arm, working out how much of her stuff they could contain.

So far Tricia has six handbags. Her two favourites are her black leather one with gold straps which can contain the kitchen sink and her white one with a gold patches which can almost contain the kitchen sink. She has another black handbag with a leopard skin bow. It is dead tarty and not at all Tricia (maybe she should give it to Tina ha-ha) which she bought in a mad moment. She also has a navy handbag, a gold clutch and a pink clutch. These are really evening bags and Tricia rarely carries them. Now she's bought a slinky pink dress though the pink one may come out of retirement.

It is therefore best to concentrate on the handbags she carries all the time, her black and white bags. She has developed a wardrobe which works with both bags. Black jacket, black boots, black bag. White jacket, gold flats, white bag. Daytime, black bag, because she needs everything with her. Nighttime, white bag, because she needs nearly everything with her and she likes to dance in her gold flats. She may change the rules sometimes but she is allowed to. After all she is a lady (?).

When she comes back to T-Girl Towers to change or first thing in the morning, she will empty the bag she last used and put everything on her bed. She will wash and shave, dress or re-dress and make-up her face. Her make-up bag is white with pink flowers and contains her essentials which are: nail varnish, concealer, eye-liner, mascara, blush, and blusher brush, eye shadow, eye liner, lip plumper, lipstick, lip liner, lip gloss and lip brush. She can just about squeeze in a small mirror, just in case. She has worked out that when she is out (and she certainly is that) the one thing she needs to top up on is the one thing she can't find and it's normally lipstick. She places her make-up bag in the bottom of her handbag because it is bulky and easily visible.

Next she put in her powder and her powder brush. If it is hot (is she hot?) she will quite often re-powder but most times (in England) she doesn't need to. She will then spray on some perfume and put that in her bag. She normally sprays herself every four hours or so. She likes smelling of Tricia. After brushing her wig she puts her hairbrush in. Finally she puts in items that can merely be transferred from her other bag; tissues, phone, purse and keys. Both bags have a secret pocket where she puts her keys. She also checks that she has a condom in the secret pocket of both bags. She never knows when she might strike it lucky; and a girl needs to be safe. Then her glasses, she puts a pen in the glasses case with them and her tiny notebook. Finally, on an outside pocket, she puts in her cigarettes and lighter. If she is wearing a new outfit she will take a picture of herself (vain cow) then put in her camera.

No tights then, no room for tights. If she snares the ones she's wearing she goes bare legged and throws them away. No spare anything actually, once she is out, she is out and that's it. It works for her.

Her purse contains coins, notes, credit cards, a picture of Tricia when she first started and tickets for any event. She will ensure it is on the top of her handbag, easily visible, because it is the most likely thing to be used.

Tricia used to struggle with her black handbag. It has two straps not one so didn't fit easily over her shoulder and a side strap which fastens between the shoulder straps and then a zip. She often found it hard to open, particularly when she was walking, because all the straps got in the way. She now knows why ladies spend so long at the checkout. Now she has attitude she is better though. She will take as long as is needed to ensure that her purse is back where it should be and her handbag is properly zipped up. She doesn't want to be stolen from. Let's hope she never grows old (?)

Tricia used to struggle with her purse. If she doesn't open it correctly all the coins will spill out over the floor and she has to crawl around trying to find them; most unladylike. Tricia has attitude. She now takes her time to make sure her purse is in the right position before opening it. She also ensures her money is carefully put away before she closes it and places it in her handbag. She feels a bit like Tina, making everybody wait. But Tina hasn't got a purse and is forever emptying her bag to get to her loose change.

Tricia used to struggle with make-up, particularly eye-liner. She doesn't any more now she has attitude. About every hour she will go to the ladies, do what ladies do most times, in an appropriate position(?) and then check herself in the mirror. She will carefully top up anything that needs topping up, normally lippy or blush. This usually means the entire contents of her make-up strewn all over the toilet shelf as she can never get to what she wants in her make-up bag. She will however be courteous and wait her turn if other girls are in a rush.

She also has a little mirror which lights up when you open it in her make-up bad. This means she can check herself out whenever she wants, normally in a café, bar or even on the train. Sometimes she likes to show off to others about how girly she is by touching up her blush, lippy or mascara in front of them. After all, she is Tricia, she is she, she is who she wants to be.

Then there are the optional items to put into her handbag. The white bag would now be completely full so nothing more can fit in,. That is another reason why she mainly carries it at night. There is however just enough room in her black bag to add her girly pink umbrella (likely), her sunglasses (unlikely) or her girly pink umbrella and her sunglasses (also likely, it is Manchester after all).

If she wishes to do some serious writing she can also put in her black bag her reporter's notebook; as long as she lays it flat across the bottom of the bag. It won't fit in her white bag at all. Normally she just packs her tiny little memo pad which she uses to make one line notes about her life.

That's about it; that is Tricia's handbag. Oh, and Tricia quite likes glad-rags as well. But you probably knew that already.

Chapter 38

I enjoy being a Girl

On Saturday I went shopping in my black jeans and purple top and didn't create a stir at all. That isn't really what I want to portray and got me thinking. I've got decent legs, I should show them off. I should wear short dresses and skirts; not over-tarty like Tina but sexy. That will get me noticed, that will get some comments, that is good. Iain tried to fight with me, he doesn't like the limelight but I do. This was one battle Iain wasn't going to win. After all, "I am Tricia, I am she, I am who I want to be!

I had to nurse Tina this weekend as you will hear. In two weeks time she is going to walk in the Himalayas; not, needless to say as Tina.

Oh, and by the way, I think you know this already:

When I have a brand new hairdo
With my eyelashes all in curl,
I float as the clouds on air do,
I enjoy being a girl!

Tricia goes shopping (again)

Tina had done her back in. There are three places where she may have done it. She could have done it at work where she strims and makes metal, but she didn't. She could have done it on her bed having fun with a man, but she didn't. She could have done it in the Oxfam shop bending down to pick out a skirt from the rail, and she did. Tina didn't go out Saturday night, she was in agony. Tricia stayed in too and between them they shared a bottle of port. They were such good girls!

Tricia has been thinking; a dangerous state of affairs for a girl like her. She thinks she is getting above her station. Her station is probably Queensway on the Central Line, although she realises now that there is nothing central about Tricia. Tricia is a t-girl yes, but she's also a girly girl. She likes nothing more than being in the arms of someone (male or female) totally dominant, totally in control of her; looking as pretty as a picture, as submissive as possible. So what's with the jeans Trish? You are sending out the wrong message. You are trying to protect yourself and that is not what you stated you would do; you know that. It is fine for normal girls to wear jeans but you are a girly girl, a special girl, a t-girl.

Tina has done her back in so Tricia is helping nurse her better. Tricia should look like a nurse so is wearing her skimpy white cotton dress today. Tricia must show that she is not just a t-girl, that she is a girly girl. Tricia likes challenges so she makes one up. Tricia must go into at least six shops and pick out two more dresses. That will give her week of dresses to wear around town and she has some skirts as well. She will need them all shortly. So Tricia will not be wearing jeans for a while.

Tina has done her back in so Tricia is free to explore the shops of Manchester. The girly-girl dresses she is going to buy must come from at least one of the following six shops; Miss Selfridge, H & M, Next, Quiz, New Look or Top Shop. She must therefore go into at least one of these shops twice; once to check it out and once to purchase. She is going in her little white cotton dress, sheer tights, ankle boots, black jacket and handbag.

Tricia goes for a coffee in town before hitting Paddy's. She is turning a lot of heads. A lot of people commented (not to her directly) that they couldn't believe she was a bloke until they got up close. Most don't notice. It's the teenage boys and girls who take it all in. Tricia has very long slender legs (chicken legs, though quite shapely) and when she shows them off like today she attracts attention. She also has a very, very, slender figure. She could model clothes if it wasn't for her boat race. She is very willowy and quite tall (5 feet 10 inches) but not too tall. Many girls are taller, many girls are less attractive. Tricia received two wolf-whistles coming back from the coffee house. Tricia is dead sexy. Tricia turns men's heads. Tricia knows. Tricia loves the attention.

The trouble with getting a day-wear dress that Tricia wanted to be dead sexy in, is that it is autumn, and is therefore covering up weather. Dead sexy dresses are really for the summer. Tricia wanted two dresses to go with her new jacket. She did indeed go into all six shops. This meant that she had to go to the ladies in the Arndale again and this time she had to queue for about ten minutes. No worries though. She got recognized by some boys in Quiz, who thought she was very funny, but she gave them a wink and they ran off. Other than a brief period of about ten minutes, Tricia didn't get that much attention. Tricia was puzzled. She had been shopping for over an hour and a half. She thinks, like Liverpool, she was tiring so she made an extra effort, straightened her back a little more, and the comments stopped. As well as the six shops she also went into Peacocks and T-K Max. Eventually, in New Look, she found a short denim dress and knitted red woolen dress. Both were very short. Normal girls would probably wear them with jeans or thick black tights but Tricia isn't a normal girl, she's a girly, girl who likes to show off her legs, so she will wear them with clear tights. She spent ten minutes in the changing room trying them on. They fitted well.

Tricia now has eight changes of daytime clothes. Five dresses; white, black, check, denim and red wool, and three skirts; black denim, blue denim and purple with numerous t-shirts; two pink, two yellow, two blue, one green, one silver. She also has a black pencil skirt and three blouses. That is longer but is sexy so that's ok too, with dark stockings. For nighttimes Tricia has nine glam gowns; white, black, pink, gold, yellow, two red, blue, purple. Tricia is getting together quite a wardrobe.

Tricia needs all these clothes. Tricia needs to be ready. In a months time she is meeting Monica Ann (from Afghanistan via Houston, Texas). She will have Saturday, Sunday, Monday and Tuesday in Manchester. She will have Wednesday, Thursday and Friday in London with Monica Ann to show her the sights. She will have Saturday, Sunday, and Monday in Manchester with Monica Ann to show her other sites. Ten days dressed? I wonder if she'll make it. My guess is she probably will.

They are also going to Herefordshire or Wales to see Monica's roots but they're not precisely sure where yet and Tricia is going to learn a bit about Buddhism. So these are eventful times for our young heroine who is still thirsting for knowledge...... and a beer or two.

Chapter 39

Smile

I have to stay at home next weekend, for the first weekend in over three months. That will be hard. I wanted to go out on a high this weekend but as you know Tina did her back in on the Saturday so it ended up quieter than I hoped.

Eleven days without being me, ouch, so by the way and I never knew it was written by Charlie Chaplin!

But then there is the end of October to look forward to and ten days being me, so the sun will come through eventually!

> If you smile through your fear and sorrow
> Smile and maybe tomorrow
> You'll see the sun come shining through for you

Tina does her back in so Tricia struts her stuff alone.

Tricia is fast approaching her first birthday. The hugely ironic thing about this is that next weekend, when she should be celebrating; she has to stay at home and not come up here to Manchester. It will be very painful for her. It will be the first weekend for three months that Tricia can't be herself. But Tricia looks on the bright side of most things; as you know her glass is normally half full. I am going to use the weekend to fund her future. I am going to extend the mortgage so she can continue to enjoy her lifestyle. She will still be able to buy beautiful clothes and make-up and of course arm candy.

She had been practicing two things during the week; her pout and her smile. She wants to be able to change from vampish pout to happy beaming face in an instant. Tricia knows the importance of smiling particularly in her position (on her knees?). It does diffuse most situations in an instant. Tricia wants to concentrate on her mouth, to make it the centrepiece of her face, because she has a spot above her left eye. The hugely ironic thing about this is that when she smiles, she is aware needs to smile with her eyes as well as her lips. It is going to take Tricia a long time to get her pout and her smile right, but she is a patient girl who knows that patience and practice pay off in the end. That is how she improved her walk so much. What she could do with, she thinks to herself, is a style advisor.

Tricia also wanted a make-up advisor. On Saturday she tried to book a makeover for the following day but had no joy. The good news however is that they would happily do it, just not on a Sunday because they work a skeleton staff. This gives Tricia a problem. She needs to book a day in advance and can't get to the Manchester shops before Saturday at the earliest. Tricia knows to be patient however; she has worked out when it can be done and that will be ideal. At the end of the month she is going to be dressed for ten days including the first three in Manchester. She can book the make-over then for the Monday; perfect timing! She will feel brilliant being made over in the shop with others watching. She bets she won't want to take the make-up off.

Life is weird sometimes however. That evening she met Lynne a genuine girl who she has met before and who works with cosmetics. She told Lynne her problem and Lynne volunteered to do Tricia's eyes. Wow, what a difference! At first Tricia didn't like it but as the make-up settled down she thought it was amazing. It's a pity she didn't have the sense to get a picture but that can come later. Tricia and Lynne swapped mobile numbers and Tricia can phone if she ever wants any help. She now has a posture advisor (Tara) and a make-up adviser. She is starting to get a team behind her. She is happy about that. She is still sad about next weekend though.

Tina did her back in on Saturday but you know that already. Tricia, dressed for the first time in her new slinky pink frock was about to put proper hooped earrings in for the first time also when she heard a wailing noise come from Tina's room.

"Trish, I can't do it",

"First time I've heard you say that hun",

"Not that, it's my back; I can't get out of bed. Though I couldn't do that either".

"I keep telling you not to go to bed in the evening. It takes too long to get going again"

"No Trish, I really am in trouble".

Poor Tina really was in trouble. She couldn't move at all.

"I need the toilet," said Tina, "and I can't get out of bed".

It was then Tricia realised that Tina's ridiculous shopping habits sometimes worked.

"Look behind my bed, there's a walking stick"

"What on earth have you got a walking stick for? You can walk perfectly well without it".

"Well I can't now! anyway it was on special offer at Aldi"

Tricia pulled the bed gently from the wall with Tina occasionally crying out in pain.

"There, one walking stick, and I still don't believe it!"

"Can you help me up?"

Ten minutes later, looking like a nonagenarian in a pink micro skirt with a pink slashed top and knee high socks with flowers on, Tina was on her feet, bent double, clutching the walking stick for dear life.

"I can't leave you hun, let's open the port"

So Saturday night, the busiest night of the week is ruled out for Tricia. No next Saturday night either. Keep smiling girl. She did, and they had as fun an evening as they possibly could when you have no electricity, no heating, no live batteries in the CD player and no hot water.

So onto Sunday and as you know already Trish decided to go all girly in her nurses outfit. She needed to smile on Sunday too. She was accosted by a gang of teenage girls in Miss Selfridge.

"You're not a real girl are you?"

"What is a real girl?" smiled Tricia

"You're a man aren't you"

"Well, my body says I'm a man but my brain says I'm a girl so I don't know the answer". Tricia smiled again.

"We think you are very brave".

"I know I am very brave. Are you comfortable with me?"

"Yes, you seem nice, you seem different, but we don't know if it's right"

"What's right? Remember that if I can do this and be like this then you can do anything"

"Suppose so"

"Think about it"

"Do you have, you know, with men?"

"I am bisexual as you are also probably".

"Oh no we're not and you haven't answered our question"

"Actually I have, and the answer is yes"

"Oh"

"Oh?" Smile

"I'm not sure we could have, you know, with women".

"I think you probably could. Don't rule it out. Don't ever rule anything out.

"We're confused"

"That's ok, so am I. But think what you can do, who you can be if you accept who and what you are. Be confident, be proud, have the right attitude and you can go far.

"Do you think so?"

"I know so".

Trish smiled at the girls and they smiled back; then disappeared out of the shop, hopefully to think about what she had said. But who knows. Tricia knows she is still considered a freak.

She continued shopping, bought two dresses and then went to watch the football in a packed straight pub. No worries. Tricia is confident, Tricia is brave, Tricia has attitude and Tricia smiles a lot. Football over she returned to Paddy's where she met up with Crystal Chandelier and the Limpet again. Now another hugely ironic thing happened. What is Tricia working on at the moment? Her lips. What is the Limpet's party trick? Snogging you so hard you can't break free. Tricia wasn't sure if this was a good or a bad thing but was clamped to the limpet for a good five minutes. After she had finally managed to break free the Limpet asked whether he could take Tricia home with him. She knew what he wanted.

"Sorry hun, can't do it, working in Sheffield tomorrow". Thank goodness for small mercies.

Tricia also bumped into Tony. She liked him a lot. He was quiet, intelligent, modest and amusing. Tricia thinks he likes her too. The difficulty is that he has not yet accepted that he is attracted to t-girls. He is still clinging on to the hope that he can fancy real girls. Tricia is sure he can't but has to wait for him to give in. Tricia must be patient and not push too hard. She hopes she will see him again in two or three week's time but he said he wouldn't be back for around seven. She hopes he will kiss her and invite her back to his place. She hopes they can start a relationship; she thinks she is now ready. All Tricia's hopes may well get dashed; we shall see in due course.

Tricia was a good girl (isn't she always?). She left reasonably early; but what's reasonable? She had a Chinese meal and walked back to T-Girl Towers. Tina was still in bed in agony. The following morning was very sad. She was going to have to go eleven days without being Tricia. Oh well; she shrugged her shoulders and smiled. At the end of the month she will be Tricia for ten days consecutively. Won't that be fun. And Tricia likes fun. With that thought Tricia's face went into a beaming grin and her eyes lit up. It was good practice.

Chapter 40

Goodbye

Two of my best friends were going away this week. Tina was going hiking in the Himalayas (no, not dressed like that) and Megan was going to India to bowl leg spinners and googlies for the Aussie test team. No, Megan was going to Australia for a school re-union, though the Aussie test team needed her. I went to see West Side Story (the musical) and my outfit got covered in tears because I loved it so much. The outfit wasn't bad either.

So and by the way....

> Goodbye-ee, goodbye-ee,
> Wipe the tear, baby dear, from your eye-ee,
> Tho' it's hard to part I know,
> I'll be tickled to death to go.

Tricia says goodbye to her friends.

Tricia phoned Tina on Thursday. "No chance I'm coming out on Friday" said Tina who needed to be at Heathrow on Saturday. "I need to prepare".

"Shouldn't you have been preparing for the last three months by walking into the village with me rather than taking a cab?" Tricia replied.

"Probably Trish, but its too late for that now. I'll see you when I get back".

Tricia texted Tina on Friday as she was leaving for Manchester. It was just a courtesy text. Tina rang back.

"I'm in Paddy's, what time will you get here?"

So Tricia met Tina, who was with Steve, the one flat mate who knew (and a good mate he was too) in Paddy's in drab.

"Trish, I need you to do me a favour" said Tina. Tricia was going back to the flat to change.

"Can you pick me up the following so I can get changed at Via Fosse?"

"I thought you weren't going out" said Tricia.

"I've changed my mind, and a girl is allowed to do that".

"But you're not a girl yet".

"Only a matter of time Trish, can you do it?"

"Well yes, but I'd recommend you come with me and change at the flat. I may forget something, I won't know where anything is and the light has gone" said Tricia.

Tina wrote out a huge list which would cause Tricia a hernia if she were to carry all of it back. They discussed and paired it down a bit.

"Errrm Tina, there's no make-up on the list".

"That's ok, I'll borrow yours".

Tricia shrugged her shoulders. She knew this wasn't going to work.

"Are you sure you're not coming back with me"

"Certain, I'm fine with Steve here".

So Tricia trudged back to the flat where it was pitch black. Apart from Tina's little light by the mirror (which was hugely useful) she was on a wing and a prayer. She carefully got herself ready and made herself up. Then she started on Tina's list. Nothing, absolutely nothing, was where Tina said it was. After around ten phone calls Tricia had collected together the bizarre mixture of clothes which was to comprise Tina's farewell outfit. But her wig was not on the wig stand. Tricia sighed, her battery was by now nearly spent but she phoned again.

"Oh yes", said Tina, "its in a yellow bag in my rucksack".

Remarkably there was a yellow bag in Tina's rucksack so Tricia crammed it into the plastic bag containing Tina's clothes and left the flat to find a taxi.

Tricia was tired but she should have known from experience. If there was one thing that is certain in life, it was that Tina's wig would not be in a yellow bag in her rucksack. In fact it wouldn't be in her rucksack at all, or in a yellow bag.

Tricia, looking divine as always, returned to Paddy's and gave Tina the plastic bag. Tina took the clothes from the bag one-by-one. "Lovely, perfect, I'm going to look hot tonight" then ...

"Where's my wig?"

"In that yellow bag which was in your rucksack"

Tina peered more closely. "But its not there!"

"Its not where?"

"Its not in the yellow bag. Can't you do anything right?"

"You said it was in a yellow bag in your rucksack. This is the yellow bag, previously in your rucksack."

"I can't go out without my wig".

"Well in that case you'll just have to go back to the flat and find it; like you should have done the first time".

Both girls were getting irritable. Tricia was disappointed though. She wanted to get it right for Tina, and this was Tina's last night.

"Alright, I'll go back" said Tina; who did and promptly fell asleep as soon as she arrived at the flat. She had far too many beers already that evening. So there was to be no farewell performance.

Tina wasn't the only one who had too many beers. Tony was also in the pub (a funny seven weeks Tricia thought). It's amazing how people change when they are drunk. It made Tricia think twice about any liaison with him. Whereas he was quiet and self-effacing last week, this week he was blokeish and boorish. Never mind, thought Tricia, tomorrow is the big day anyway; and she walked back through the City quite happily.

Tina apologised in the morning before setting off for Asia. Tricia quickly got herself ready for a busy day; an important day. Today she was going to the theatre by herself for the first time. So she made sure she had enough time for an early start in Paddy's. The performance was at 14:30 and she had to take the tram (another first) to get there. She met Tom in the pub and had a few, but not too many, beers. After all she wanted to watch West Side Story, not spend all her time in the Ladies. She caught the tram, it was easy, and picked up the tickets from the booking office. She took her seat between two middle class straight couples. Still no problems.

For days afterwards Tricia was singing the songs in her head. The performance was outstanding. The cast was young and vibrant. The singing and dancing were top quality. Of course West Side Story is Tricia's favourite musical because it reminds her of her own predicament. In many, many years time there will be a place for people like her but it's not quite ready yet. The ease of her day so far maybe does suggest that it's closer than she thinks. Tricia cried all the way through the performance; so much so that she had to redo her make-up both in the interval and at the end. Naturally she used the ladies. 'When love comes so strong, there is no right or wrong, your love is your love' and Tricia just loves being Tricia.

Tricia waited an age for the tram to turn up to take her back into Manchester. It was packed solid. It's good that Tricia is so slender as she only just could fit in; but fit in she did. There were no problems going in on the tram either.

She was frustrated however because she wanted to watch the England football match. She ended up missing the first half but that didn't really matter too much as it ended 0-0. She went to the straight pub that is best for football, with the big screen and the atmosphere. She didn't play safe in the village where there isn't much call for football. The girls serving behind the bar like to see Tricia, she shows them freedom. No problems in the pub either; this life is easy she thought. England went on to win 5-1 in the end. It wasn't a brilliant performance but it was more than good enough. Tricia is thinking she is getting more than good enough. Dangerous thoughts girl!

She wandered back to Paddy's for a while. No Napoleons tonight, she was already shattered. She met Wayne whose boss had the operation. She did it in two and a half years he told her. Tricia thought deeply. "I'm just over a year into doing this seriously. I will have the freedom to transition in another eighteen months. Dare I? Can I afford it? Do I want to?" The time will come when she has to make up her mind, but that time isn't now. She is happy where she is for the moment. She is Tricia, she is she, she is who she wants to be!

Chapter 41

You've got to Pick a Pocket or Two

Now this is ridiculous and I've got to sort it out. The Limpet fancies me to death and is desperate to have his evil way with me. He has even phoned Iain at work. He saw me in the pub tonight, made a bee-line for me cos I've got a hive full of honey (warning); attached himself to me and it was like kissing a Dyson. Anyway, he is supposed to be with Crystal Chandelier who is madly jealous. Then there was trouble. I need to kill off this ridiculous quasi- relationship with the Limpet.

Trish be nimble, Trish be quick, Trish jump over the candlestick.

By the way, and this is what the trouble was all about.

> You've got to pick-a-pocket or two, girls,
> You've got to pick-a-pocket or two.

Tricia the tea-leaf

After the theatre and the football and a short time in Paddy's, Tricia went home. She was emotionally and physically exhausted and didn't need Napoleons or even a man to comfort her. She got back to the flat to find no gas or gas cylinders left. She would have to sort that out later; but she was no good at those sorts of things. She was a girly-girl after all.

So the following morning, even though the cock didn't crow at all, Tricia was up bright and early because she had a good night's sleep. She hastily arranged to meet Megan and Becky for lunch; it was Megan's last weekend before going to Australia. The sun was shining and she fancied hitting the shops early; maybe start with a cappuccino. She had to shave in cold water but her hormones are making a huge difference to her beard growth so it wasn't too bad. She felt she looked good as she stepped out; well, as good as she gets.

She got quite a few positive comments and smiles as she walked round Manchester. One guy even complimented her on her figure. "Nice t*ts!". He left it at that but she wondered what she had to be shameful about. Not her legs surely? It was a lovely shop although she didn't buy anything. She is much more confident, much more certain about herself and this is rubbing off on other people she is sure. She would go back shopping later but fancied a couple of beers so guess where, before meeting Megan and Becky who were running late.

Four beers later and Megan and Becky arrived. Lunch was off. They didn't do it at Spirit any more; sad. They had a good chat anyway before Tricia, almost falling over after so many beers, said her goodbyes and staggered off shopping again hoping Megan will have a brilliant time in Oz. At least Tricia would get some air in her nice lungs and sober up a bit.

She returned back to Paddy's and had a huge discussion with Coco concerning how to look after children in difficult circumstances. Then she met the Limpet and Crystal Chandelier. The Limpet immediately positioned his lips over hers and sucked the life out of her. But Tricia is a canny lass. She worked out where he was ticklish. It did at least give her some time for air.

Crystal Chandelier then went to the ladies. Tricia followed slightly later, not surprising after all she was drinking, and noticed that Crystal Chandelier's handbag had been left out by the washing basin. Tricia shouted and warned Crystal then made sure the bag was protected by staying with it until Crystal had finished. She then relieved herself (sitting down naturally) washed her hands and touched up her make-up before going back into the bar.

When she got back to her seat everything was in turmoil. It transpired that Crystal had lost £250 from her bag and she started blaming Tricia. Tricia knows it is a conspiracy. Tricia knows Crystal is jealous because the Limpet fancies her; but she can do nothing about it except protest her innocence. Innocence is not something Tricia does well any more.

The next time Tricia went to the Ladies it was to be just as eventful. A tall, large, arrogant scouse girl grabbed and fondled her while she was re-applying her make-up (yes, again). "I bet you'd like me to shag you, wouldn't you. I'll look out for you honey. I've a very large black strap-on back home which I'm sure would satisfy you". With that she pinched Tricia's backside, laughed and left. Tricia wondered whether the scouse girl had just come into contact with £250; maybe that was why she seemed so happy. Tricia reckoned that was an option. She could prove nothing but one thing was for sure. It wasn't Tricia who stole the money; if indeed any money was stolen at all.

Chapter 42

Raindrops Keep Falling on my Head

Wow, this is it, this is serious. No, I'm not going anywhere hot or sunny but I am going to meet up with Monica Ann, a t-girl from Houston, Texas via Afghanistan. We are meeting in London where I am going to show her the sites then I'm bringing her up to Manchester, hopefully for a bit of fun. What makes it special is that I'm going to do the whole lot dressed.

So, I'm writing this on the train going to Manchester, my home town in drab. It is Saturday 25th October. Sunday and Monday in Manchester bulding up. Tursday down to London to meet up with a work colleague on Tuesday evening. Wednesday meet Monica. Thursday and Friday in London sightseeing. On Saturday back to Manchester and stay there on Sunday and Monday hopefully for some fun. The final Tuesday will be very difficult.

That works out at ten days dressed. Ten days as Tricia! YAY! Mega! It will be interesting to see what I feel like at the end. Whether I still enjoy being Tricia after all that time dressed.

By the way, heavy rain is pouring down outside and is forecasted to do so all weekend, so:

Cryin's not for me
'Cause I'm never gonna stop the rain by complainin'
Because I'm free
Nothin's worryin' me

A Wild Wet and Windy Day in Manchester

It was the start of the most momentous week of young Tricia's life and guess what? It was pouring down with rain in Manchester. Not only that but it was cold and windy too. A good job then that Tricia had come up on the Saturday and not the Friday lugging her winter wardrobe in a suitcase. Tricia had six days off work. Six days (plus weekends = ten days) in which she was just going to enjoy being herself. Tricia was later going to the smoke but was starting in Manchester. To get herself prepared and to get her attitude right.

The trouble with Manchester is the rain. When it rains Trish can't walk the canals because they are too slippery. With the rain and the wind poor Tricia really struggled and must have made an amusing site as she tried to march through Manchester with her girly umbrella and her handbag. She ignored thoughts of a cigarette. She was having enough trouble keeping her girly umbrella up and her handbag over her shoulder. Her girly umbrella was indeed a girly umbrella. At the first sign of any danger i.e. wind; it protected itself by turning half inside out. Tricia then had to feel above her head to straighten it out. In doing so her handbag would fall out of position and all the rain which had collected inside the upside down umbrella was deposited on her head. It was not easy.

It was cold, wet and windy enough for Tricia to wear her winter coat. Tricia's winter coat is very warm and has a fur hood. The trouble is she can't use the hood. She has learnt from experience; after all she is over a year old now. The last time she wore her coat with the hood up she walked into the pub with hair dry, took her hood down and her wig came off with it. Sniggers all round. Not good at all. Tricia thinks she should practice taking her hood down while keeping her wig on. It would be far easier than struggling with this pesky umbrella. Maybe she will have time this weekend before the fun really starts.

Tricia looked at herself in the mirror in the pub. There was nothing wrong. She looked like Tricia. She also looked like the weather though, dull and lifeless. The weather does change things. Why does she insist in living in England? It must be easier where Megan is now, in Australia. Tricia likes wearing sexy short skirts with flimsy tops to show off her body, but hardly ever gets the chance in England. Tricia feels depressed and looks depressed. She hopes things will perk up. Time for another beer which may help.

Actually it didn't really but as you know life is a funny thing. Tricia, looking wan and depressed went into town where everybody else looked wan and depressed. The poor English weather makes everybody miserable. Trish was hardly spotted at all and received no comments whatsoever. She blended in better than she had ever done before. She was just another miserable shopper on a wet and windy Saturday in Manchester, England.

She did some shopping though. She found some size eight calf length boots with a heel which she liked. Size eight was the largest the shop sold but Tricia was size nine or ten depending on the shoes. She tried them on anyway and they seemed to fit. Lucky Cinderella. She saw some size nine shoes which she also liked. She tried them on and they were too small. She tried the boots on again and still they seemed to fit. She shrugged her shoulders and bought the boots. Wait for the screaming in agony, wait for the chilblains; but she was sure they fit. She noticed there were only two pairs of boots of that style left in the shop and they were both size eight. She wondered whether she had found out why. Anyway there is now only one pair of size nine boots left.

She also bought herself two sets of underwear, both very pretty. One white and one black bra and panties set. She had been meaning to buy these for a while and they would be good to wear during the week ahead. She spent three hours shopping and spent one penny in the ladies; of course she sat down.

Tricia spent the evening in the pub before an early night. She knew her attitude was already right and, with the punishing schedule ahead, it was sleep which mattered and not marching the dance floor at Napoleons. She noticed something which, when she thought about it, probably wasn't surprising. Her pout was coming on nicely. She realised why. When she sips a beer she pouts her lips. When she smokes a cigarette she pouts her lips. Most times, whether in straight world or Tricia world, she is either drinking a pint or smoking a cigarette or both. So it should come naturally. Other things are coming together as well. The way she bends down, the way she gets up from a sitting position, the way she delicately treads around the puddles, her hand gestures, the softness of her voice. They are all getting better and that is good. Go Trish go.

Chapter 43

Into Parliament She Shall Go

This was my preparation time for the big excursion to London and back with Monica Ann. There was to be no pounding the dance floor at Napoleons; I had all the attitude I needed. What I actually needed was plenty of rest as the week's schedule was punishing. The song, by the way, comes from Iolanthe. It's about time the English girl used Gilbert and Sullivan again. It represents future pleasures for me.

> In the Parliamentary hive,
> Liberal or Conservative —
> Whig or Tory — I don't know —
> But into Parliament she shall go!

Tricia Prepares.

Tricia was getting ready for the longest week of her short life. She was going to meet Monica Ann (of Afghanistan via Houston, Texas), take her around London then bring her back to Manchester for some fun. Tricia was starting off in Manchester to gear herself up and get some important things sorted out; namely to book an appointment for nail extensions and an eyebrow trim with her beauty consultant; and to arrange a makeover. Her nails and eyebrows were to be done on Sunday, her makeover on Monday. On Tuesday she was going down to London on the train. On Tuesday she was leaving the nest of Manchester. She hoped by then she was perfectly prepared.

The London schedule was massive. Monica Ann wanted to go to Taplow Park in Hertfordshire, the head of the SGI in England as well as do St

Paul's, The Globe, Tate Modern, The Tower of London and the Changing of the Guard. There were also two musicals to fit in. Tricia likes musicals as you might have gathered. The highlight however was to be a tour of the Houses of Parliament. I arranged it for the girls through my MP. A t-Girl in Parliament? Whatever next!

Tricia is as hard as nails on top; she has to be to do what she does. Underneath however, as people quickly find out, she is very soft and cuddly. This came out when she had her ceramic nails attached. She felt particularly feminine with her hands on the pad while Lilli was making her nails glamorous. She now knows how to do a French polish to perfection. You cheat and get someone who knows what they are doing and has the right set of tools to do it for you. Some of the tools seemed more at home in the dentists than the beautician but it didn't hurt at all. It was really very relaxing. It took about half-an-hour. Tricia enjoyed chatting to Lilli during this time. She talked about what she was going to do, what outfits she was going to wear. She imagined that was how any girl having her nails done would chat. She was probably right. She chose a medium length although they were longer than she had ever managed to grow them.

To start off with she had a great deal of trouble finding coins and even writing up her notes. She was dreading fastening buttons. After a couple of days though, they felt totally natural and they were much stronger than she ever believed they could be.

The following morning Tricia went to Debenhams at the appointed time for her makeover. She felt particularly proud as she sat down on the seat with mirrors all around her. Anybody in the large Department Store could see she was having a makeover. She got told off by Debbie (who will now look after Tricia's cleansing routine and her face) for not moisturizing enough. Debbie put on a lighter, fresher foundation and powder than Tricia had been using. The in-look was to be fresh with little make-up. Tricia explained the difficulty she had with eye-liner. "I don't want you using any eye-liner until you have been through the regime I am going to put you on. We concentrate on lips with only minimal eye make-up until we remove the tiredness around your eyes". Trish was delighted. No more panda eyes, well not for a while at least. YAY.

Monday afternoon and evening was a boisterous affair even though Tricia wanted it quiet. She met Mark and Eric, aka Ruby Gaye (the 'e' is important apparently but probably superfluous). Eric was a professional female impersonator who unfortunately lost both his complete wardrobe – at Manchester Piccadilly Station - and the full use of his larynx. The latter was more important as s/he used to sing. He was stamped on by a couple of thugs after a private gig and spent over a month in hospital. Not a happy story. DUM DUM DUM DUM – Trish, remember the danger song and be aware at all times.

Eric had a while back lost his partner of many, many years but he seemed to Trish to be pulling out of the grief. Just how far he was pulling round from the grief she was to find out at the end of her journey. For the afternoon and early evening though, he regaled all who wanted to listen with his stories from the past, of music halls and theatres, of famous people he had worked with. It is all so different now.

On the following morning Tricia added more stuff to her suitcase, carefully; she still wasn't 100% confident with her new nails. She struggled to where she waits for a taxi, but one turned up quickly and dropped her off at Manchester Piccadilly Station. Keep your eye on your suitcase, she thought to herself. The fact of the matter is that the journey to London was totally uneventful. Tricia wore her black jeans with a pretty pink top and her winter coat to save packing it. She didn't try to impress, probably didn't impress, got another taxi to an apartment at London Bridge and arrived in one piece. Signing into the apartment was fun as the girls on reception just loved having Tricia around and finding out what she had planned for the week.

In the evening Trish met Fran, a work colleague who knew all about her and they had a good chat and a lovely time. Trish wasn't sure about Fran calling her "a complete tart" but knew that on occasions that is precisely what she is. That was to be proved later in the week. An early night in the apartment then tomorrow meet Monica, London, sightseeing. What was in store for Tricia?

Chapter 44

Always Look on the Bright Side of Life

This was a very exhausting time for both Monica and I. We walked miles and miles in the afternoon. It was also a pain being on the top floor of a hotel with no lift. At least Monica's trunk arrived and she had a chance to get out dressed eventually. I actually think it helped her that she had a day to see that I was getting no reaction when walking around the City. There were quite a few obstacles in our path which, by the way, the song reflects. It comes from the musical we saw on Thursday night.

> If life seems jolly rotten
> There's something you've forgotten
> And that's to laugh and smile and dance and sing.

In which the girls face challenges, and overcome them.

What was not in store for Tricia, or Monica come to that, was a transformer for Monica's phone. That didn't actually matter because in the end she didn't need one anyway. Tricia couldn't understand it. Nobody seemed to know what Monica actually needed to get her mobile phone charged and working in the UK. We don't have many American tourists in London after all. The girls zigzagged Oxford Street, not looking for skirts and dresses but looking for adapters and transformers. At least Monica could see what London was like, how busy it was, how people would just barge into you without saying sorry, and how it was expected that you did the same back.

Monica's trunk hadn't arrived from the states. This was quite important as it contained her clothes and make-up. Eventually the girls managed to find out that it would be delivered the following day; when exactly had still to be established. So for day one in London Monica had to be in drab so couldn't be Monica. Tricia could be Tricia and looked demure in her skinny white jeans, now with a minor blemish. A tiny stain of nail varnish on her left knee. She did her best to clean it off and felt her best was, just, good enough. The girls had a long discussion about how it was actually easier to 'pass' if you had the odd blemish. Tricia was more than worried about the 'odd' blemish.

The hotel the girls had chosen was also to provide a challenge. Although it was very old; because it was very old, it didn't have a lift and the girls' room was right on the top floor. Poor Tricia was only just strong enough to lug her suitcase containing the kitchen sink up the stairs into her room. It was definitely not a job for girls like her and she had to re-apply her powder when she finally made it.

On Wednesday night they decided to have a quiet meal with a few English pints. The meal itself was superb and very English. Bangers and Mash with onion gravy. Monica was in heaven.

"Its nothing like it is in my pub in Houston, the Richmond Arms, it's just gorgeous". The girls left reasonably early, tomorrow was going to be a long, long day. The pub was showing cricket on television which intrigued Monica and girls discussed the differences between cricket and baseball. The games are remarkably similar.

Monica's trunk duly arrived the following morning, but not early enough for her to go out as Monica. So Mike accompanied Tricia who was looking ravishing in black dress and patterned tights. First stop, Buckingham Palace to see the Changing of the Guard. It was packed solid because the kids were on half-term from school. Tricia managed to get her picture taken with a Japanese family. Who had the slantier eyes? She is starting to quite like the camera now. Funny that, I hate it! The weather was bright, sunny but bitterly cold. Good practice for Monica Ann when in Afghanistan apparently.

The girls (I can't be bothered with girl and boy) walked down the Mall to Charing Cross then took the tube to Tower Bridge. Then they walked and they walked. They saw the Tower then crossed London Bridge getting a good view of Tower Bridge on the way. They saw Southwark cathedral on the right and Tricia knew of a very old English pub called the George where they stopped to have a drink. Monica was impressed when she heard that Dickens had drunk there. Tricia wasn't quite so sure. Then they went through Southwark Market grabbing a Samosa on the way and along the Thames passed the Clink. In days of yore girls like these wouldn't get beyond the Clink. Inside it was arranged into a series of cells and it has such exhibits as a whipping post, torture chair, foot crusher, and other torture implements. Wouldn't mind a few hours in there (the torture chair), or on there (the whipping post) myself, thought Tricia but they had to keep walking. Further on were the Globe and the Tate Modern.

The Modern Tate, I'm afraid, Tricia simply doesn't get; but Monica was in her element. They paid (yes paid!) £10 each to see an exhibition of work by Mark Rothcoe.

"Wow" said Monica, "this is amazing"

"Ow!" said Tricia, "I've paid £10 for this?"

"But can't you see the subtle movement?"

"The pictures just look like bricks; and if there is one thing bricks don't do it is move subtly"

"Look at the borders though, so clever".

"My kids were painting stuff like this at nursery school".

It didn't help Tricia that there was some mad woman following her into every room humming random tunes out loud. This whole thing was too weird, even for Tricia.

"That's it" said Monica, "you can only take in so much Rothcoe in one go; it makes you emotionally unstable"

Tricia mumbled something under her breath which sounded like "about ten seconds".

"I don't think I'll ever understand", sighed Tricia.

"You need to start with something less advanced", said Monica.

"Less advanced???"

One day Tricia may try a bit harder with modern art, but for now she's enough on her modern plate and the Modern Tate will have to wait.

As they were walking out they saw a pretty young girl wearing a gorgeous yellow Elizabethan outfit. It was so cold though she had jeans under her dress.

"Bless her pointy head", said Monica.

"Bless her cotton socks surely", said Tricia.

It was one of a number of very similar but slightly different phrases across the pond.

Back to the walking and the girls go across the Millennium Bridge to St Paul's. They stop for a beer on the way as by now they were parched. Then back to the top floor of the hotel for Monica to become Monica (at last!). The girls were going out that evening. They were going to see Spamalot at the request of Monica Ann. She was a very big Monty Python fan.

Tricia was a little disappointed with the musical. Yes, it was well done but she knew most of the jokes already and it all seemed a bit dated and maybe a little jaded. Tricia thinks Monty Python's time has come and gone. Still, an enjoyable enough evening though.

After the show they needed to eat. They didn't want to encounter too many drunks on the tube so went back to Marble Arch, close to the hotel. What Tricia found surprising was that many of the restaurants were closed or closing. She thought London never slept, but clearly it does. Eventually they found somewhere and the girls had a long philosophical discussion over a pizza. Monica's primary motivation for dressing was to pass because she was a transsexual. She didn't yet realise how well nigh impossible this was. Tricia's primary motive was to be herself. She was a t-girl. Tricia felt it was far easier being in her shoes than Monica's; which were lying unworn under the table. They had caused her agony all evening – and there was more agony to come.

Chapter 45

I am what I am

This was a superb day. A walk down Oxford Street, a tour round the Houses of Parliament topped off with La Cage Aux Folles. By the way this song I have wanted to use for months but I now feel I can, with justification. It has been pinched by the gay community but this one is indeed a transgendered song, even though nobody sings it better than la Bassey.

> There's one life, and there's no return and no deposit;
> One life, so it's time to open up your closet.
> Life's not worth a damn 'til you can say,
> "Hey world, I am what I am!"

A Wonderful Day.

The girls discussed something else over their pizza. They were intending to go to Taplow House, the headquarters of the SGI movement in the UK. The trouble was it was out in Hertfordshire, about an hour and a half away. The girls agreed it was too much and instead they decided to do what any other girl would do if they were in a hotel five minutes walk from Oxford Street. Shop 'til they drop. Well not quite until they drop because they were going to the Houses of Parliament in the afternoon and a musical in the evening, but you know what I mean. First thing on the agenda; shoes for Monica Ann.

Now, those of you who have been paying attention will know what a slow shopper Tina is. Tricia uses her peripheral vision and if she sees something she likes she will make a beeline straight to it. It either works or it doesn't. If it doesn't work Tricia doesn't mind. There are plenty more clothes and plenty more shops selling clothes Tricia will like. Monica however is an advocate of the Tina style of shopping. Inspect every single item of clothing in the shop to great detail. It was for this reason that they only managed to shop in two stores in three hours; Debenhams and Next. Not a particularly successful number even given that Debenhams is a Department Store.

They were always going back to Next because Monica had seen an outfit she liked in the window. They left Debenhams empty handed after two hours shopping. Tricia didn't worry too much. She was well aware that she had so little room in her suitcase she had to sit on it to zip it up; and she had already sorted out her clothes in Manchester at the start of the week.

In Next Tricia had already bought some jewellery, had a couple of cigarettes and a chat with some friendly young girls before Monica finally came out of the changing room wearing the outfit she had seen in the window.

"I'm not sure Trish, do you think its me?" said Monica.

Why do girls keep asking Tricia. You are what you are. She is Tricia she is she. She is not Monica Ann, she is not Tina. All she can say is 'Honey, you look fine to me' and admit that the outfit is not something that Tricia would wear. We are all different. That is what makes life fun and we know Tricia likes fun. Tricia is candid and critical though. She will, for example, tell Tina if the clothes she has chosen are totally outrageous (they usually are). Tina will normally smile, give her the thumbs up and buy them anyway. So what is the point of asking Tricia in the first place? In this instance there was nothing wrong with Monica's outfit at all; it just wasn't Tricia and she said so. The girls had already realised they were different; that is why Tricia dresses like a twenty four year old girl (that old?); that is why Monica dresses to pass. Monica bought the outfit.

"Shoes Monica, shoes, over there" said Tricia and her chain smoking began again. However hard they tried, they couldn't find any shoes to properly fit Monica's feet. The poor saleslady must have gone to the store at the back of the shop a dozen times but no joy. Monica's feet were just too large.

"Its ok Monica, I know a specialist shop in Manchester, I have the same problem" said Tricia. "You'll just have to hobble on until then; its hard being a girl sometimes". And indeed Monica did. She hobbled through the cobbles at Westminster where the marathon runners break down. Monica didn't break down however and they reached the Houses of Parliament in time for their tour, and for a sandwich to keep them going.

The start of the tour was scary for Monica. Everybody had to have their pictures taken for security reasons. Tricia wondered what name would be put on her photo as I had booked the trip for her. Neither Monica nor Tricia needed to worry. They had the pictures, they didn't need the words. The tour was exceptionally good and brilliantly done by an MP who took the girls round in a group of about twenty. There were no troubles at all; the girls even asked some questions. It was apparent that Westminster was well used to t-Girls which is good. It was fascinating going through English history in this, the most English building of them all and then being brought back to the present day. Did you know that the Prime Minister scribbles on the dispatch box, Tricia has seen it! Good girls like Tricia didn't even scribble on their desks at school, never mind the dispatch box (hmm, not sure about that).

After the tour the girls went back to the hotel room to change for the night out. Well, Tricia didn't. It was freezing outside and she was still looking demure in her 'Those shoes look fab, I have to have a pair' pink t-shirt and skinny black jeans. Monica Ann wanted to change and rest her weary and painful feet. Tricia worked out how to get to the theatre from the Internet and went for a beer.

"Back in an hour or so hon" Tricia likes the 'or so'. It gives her some leeway.

"Make sure you're ready because we haven't got much time".

Tricia knew, as sure as eggs is eggs, that Monica Ann would definitely not be ready in an hour So she gave her an hour and a half. They had to be out in two hours and Tricia only had her make-up to top up.

She duly arrived half an hour before they had to leave to find complete carnage in the room. True, there was a half dressed though un-made-up Monica but there were clothes, shoes, bags, pills, make-up and jewellery everywhere.

"I hope you don't thing I'm taking over" said Monica Ann.

"Hon, you do what you must but we only have half an hour to get out and you're not even dressed yet", said Tricia, trying to stay calm.

165

"Do you think this will work with this?"

"Yes, but as I've said before, its not me".

"Thank you, I need a sounding board"

"Aaaaaaaarrrrrrrrggggggggghhhhhhhh!, Ok hon, just get going".

"Don't put me under any pressure, I'm no good under pressure".

"Ssshh, don't tell your employers. You drive trucks in a war zone for goodness sake. You have to be able to take pressure. Now you need move quicker than you've ever moved in your life. It shouldn't be hard".

Tricia, frustrated, was getting bitchy.

"And I thought Tina was slow!"

But she relented, she realised that being bitchy was no good and that she needed a plan. She started tidying up, lent Monica her foundation and things started to move again. She was also well aware that Monica had no chance of dressing up in Afghanistan so it was difficult for her. Tricia, using all her woman management skills, cajoled and encouraged Monica to such an extent that they managed to get out in forty five minutes. There was still enough time.

Tricia had established where the theatre was. It was easy. Take the tube to the Strand, left and then across the road and right towards Charing Cross. The trouble was that there were approximately twelve exits out of the Strand so the odds of her getting the right one were, well twelve to one. Not surprisingly she didn't win the bet so she needed time to find her bearings.

"Are you sure I look ok in this Trish?"

"Do the shoes go with the outfit?"

"Do you think it suits me?"

"Do you ...."

"Monica, will you just shut up for a moment. It's a bit late to worry about your outfit and you've just travelled on the tube for goodness sake. I need some space to find out where we are going".

Tricia was exasperated again but spotted a signpost to Charing Cross. She knew where she was going and who was coming with her. She relented.

"You're looking fine, you're outfit is fine, the theatre is two minutes away, all is good".

Tricia smiled, Monica smiled, and all was indeed good.

In fact things were better than good. The show was absolutely fantastic! Tricia thinks it was the best she has ever seen. I think it was the best I have ever seen. It helped that it was all about girls like Tricia. It helped that the girls went dressed. At the end of the first act, when the signature song of the musical was sung, it was given out with such feeling, such guts, that tears started welling in Tricia's eyes again. She must stop crying in the theatre. No, she mustn't stop crying in the theatre, it's good for her. Crying with emotion is fun.

Absolutely knocked out by the show, the girls had to go back to the hotel to pack for the next leg of their journey, Manchester. They had done London, the history, the heritage, the theatres. Now for some good old fashioned English theatre. The farce that was to ensue over the next couple of days made La Cage Aux Folles believable. But you are promised one thing. It will definitely be fun!

Oh, and by the way, I am what I am too.

Chapter 46

Let's Face the Music and Dance

This was tricky for me. I had messed up the booking arrangements and it was important to me that Monica was happy. So I had to give up the room for a night. I did strike it lucky though. I think it was because I had other people on my mind and not myself for once. So, by the way, it was time for me to face the music.

> there may be trouble ahead,
> but while there's moonlight and music and love and romance,
> let's face the music and dance.

How Does Tricia get out of this one?

It was cold, very cold again as the girls woke up on the Saturday morning. It was the day of the transfer to Manchester. It was the day when the history lesson ended and the fun should begin. Did it? You bet!

"Its cold enough to freeze the balls of a brass monkey", said Tricia, not immediately realising that she was talking to a girl from Houston, Texas.

"What does that mean Trish? But I'm interested". Monica took notice; certain things interested her a lot.

Tricia patiently explained as she always does.

For the last couple of days the girls had been puzzling over a thorny conundrum. What could they do with Monica's trunk? Actually, we know precisely what Monica wishes to do with her trunk, it is Tricia who is struggling to decide what to do with hers. But it was neither of those trunks that concerned the girls. It was the trunk in the corner of the room, open and winking at them, full of Monica's clothes. This was a trunk they could not get to Manchester. The girls decided to find out what the hotel could do for them. And the hotel came up trumps. Monica could leave the trunk there and booked back in for the Tuesday night when she could sort out shipping it back. It would be an important time for Monica, Trish knew. Monica would be trying to get back to straight mode on Tuesday night. Tricia didn't want to think about it. Too painful.

A taxi to Euston then the train up to Manchester. Monica, laden with bags and rucksacks, bringing only one drab outfit but a lot of drag; Tricia, suitcase overflowing, dressed conservatively in jeans and yellow top. She doesn't dress over the top when travelling, we know that. Her winter coat covered everything up anyway. There was no way it would fit into her suitcase and anyway, it was cold enough to freeze ......

On the train a young boy (around 14) couldn't take his eyes off our intrepid travellers. He had never seen anything like them in his young life. Hopefully as he grows up more of them will be around. Tricia is working on it but it's hard on your own. No problems or incidents on the train, but there was to be a problem, but not an incident, checking into the hotel room.

Manchester was supposed to be all about fun and be more chilled than London. With this in mind Tricia booked two rooms; one (smoking) for her and one (non-smoking) for Monica. When they checked in the hotel could only find the smoking room despite looking wide and far. Tricia, who had bought every bit of documentary evidence she thought she needed had not brought her confirmation email. She had cocked up (a position she was quite used to). She was frustrated and there were no more rooms available on the Saturday night, so the girls again had to share. There may be trouble ahead, thought Tricia who, using her by now well developed feminine intuition could see into the future. Tricia phoned Tina who came down to drop some clothes off for Saturday night. So many clothes, so little room, but all went well thus far.

Monica wanted some sleep and a little space so Tina and Tricia went together to meet Megan and Becky at Paddys. The girls had a fun afternoon talking. There was much talk about. Megan wanted a bed containing chains and handcuffs. Tina volunteered to help; after all she is a steel worker during the week. Tricia volunteered to trial it. The afternoon turned to early evening. The early evening turned to late evening. Where was Monica Ann? Tricia had given her directions from the hotel to the pub (three minutes at most) and was starting to get worried. Just as she was starting to get worried Monica turned up. It transpired she had been hobbling about in ever decreasing circles for the past twenty minutes. Monica is never short of words except when they are important. A simple question to anyone of 'Do you know where Paddys Goose is?' would probably have got her there quicker. Never mind, she was with us.

The next problem for Tricia was the changing bit.

"Tina, we need to make sure Monica is welcome so we need to change in shifts. You or me first?"

"I'm having fun Trish, so can you go first?"

"So am I Tina, but we have to sort this out so I think that would be good. Look after her though".

Tricia went back to change. She changed from fairly provocative bitch into fairy princess in her sparkly gold dress.

Later, Tina went back to change. She changed from fairly provocative bitch into very provocative bitch, wearing her white outfit which leaves nothing, whatsoever to the imagination.

"I'm going to pull tonight Trish, I can feel in my water" she said on her return.

"Remember its Saturday night and the competition is stiff, all the girls are out. And I suspect your water is mainly alcohol now, anyway", said Tricia.

"That's all right Trish, I'm good at stiff." Tina always took the part of the conversation which most interested her.

And with the girls jabbering away inanely, they arrive at Napoleons and Tricia's potential nightmare begins.

A pause now to set the scene. We have three horny girls and one hotel room packed with sexy clothes. If Monica pulls tonight, she has to have the room, thinks Tricia. If Tina pulls tonight, how am I going to keep her away from the room? If I pull tonight? Don't even go there. Thoughts of threesomes, foursomes, fives, sixes went through her mind. I must play it by ear, she thought. That will be a novelty.

Now, one of the reasons for bringing Monica up to Manchester was to give her a chance to talk to the transsexuals who had been through what Monica intended to go through. The TS's meet downstairs in Naps on a Saturday night and talk amongst themselves, although Tina and Trish are quite welcome to join if they want and are sober enough. So they took Monica downstairs and introduced her. Monica was immediately at home and was having no trouble integrating, so Tricia went upstairs for a dance and Tina went for a prowl. There were plenty of men about.

Time passes. It is now 2:00 in the morning and Tricia returns to the downstairs bar where she meets Monica with a blonde girl around her neck.

"Amy and I are going back to the hotel, is that ok?" says Monica.

"You got your key hon?" says Tricia, a little surprised that Monica is taking a girl back, but each to their own.

"Yes Trish, see you later" and Monica and Amy were off.

DUM DUM DUM DUM, now what about Tina, thinks Trish, this is the scenario which worries me. Tina turns up downstairs with a guy in a Stetson hat (don't believe absolutely everything written here but what happens does).

"Hi Trish, just pulled with a Canadian"

"Can see that hon; oh shit you can't have the room because Monica has gone back with Amy"

"No worries, he's taking me to his"

"What, Montreal?"

"No idiot, he's got a house in North Manchester, we're getting a taxi now".

"Yay", says Tricia, the main problem resolved. "Have fun".

A relieved Tricia goes back to the dance floor, she is sure she can sort it all out from here. She has been so busy worrying about other people she needs to think about herself. What is she going to do? The option that pans out before her is to go back to T-Girl Towers. It will be cold and unwelcoming but it will solve the problem. She walks downstairs to the main bar and somebody talks to her.

"Hi sexy, can I buy you a drink, you look dead hot".

"No", said Tricia, "I have to go home now".

What?

"Yes", said Tricia, "I'll have a pint of bitter".

Half an hour later Jed and Tricia were in a taxi together.

Forty five minutes later Jed and Tricia were in bed together.

Half an hour after that Manchester suffered a mild earthquake and all three girls had smiles on their faces.

Isn't life fun?

And the fun was to continue the following day. And the farce was to continue the following day. This now though was to become a farce of English proportions.

Chapter 47

I'm Just a Girl who can't say No

If last night was farcical today was even worse. By the way, this one's fairly obvious as well! I suspect it's more for Tina than it is for me. I can say no, but — it would appear, only after I say yes!

> i never make a complaint
> till its to late for restraint
> then when i wanno i caint
> i caint say no

The Sexual Proclivities of not so young Ladies

Tricia leant over to give Jed a final peck before getting up. "Told you. It's always better in the morning", she said.

"Morning, afternoon, evening", any time suits me" said Jed.

Tricia was about to find out how true to his words Jed was.

"What about the American girl, will she be up for it do you think?"

"She's been with another t-girl all night, she might fancy a guy for a change"

Tricia replied thinking that she quite likes the expression 'easy come, easy go'.

"Can we go to the hotel and see?" Jed was clearly still keen and eager.

Tricia had a dilemma. She could hardly wear her sparkly gold dress on a Sunday lunchtime, and most of her other clothes were back at the hotel. She started reciting a little ditty she learnt when I was growing up.

"What can I wear today, today, what can I wear today".

Jump suit or denims, skirt or wool dress, what can I wear to play"

"Let me dress you", said Jed.

"Bet it will take longer than it did to undress me last night" said Tricia, tongue in cheek for once.

"That wool dress hanging in the coffin would look great on you"

Tricia put on her red wool dress for the first time. It had been a speculative buy and she wasn't anticipating much. She went into Tina's room and looked at herself in the full length mirror.

"Wow Jed, this is sooooo sexy"

"Told you, got any fishnets"

"Think so"

"That black belt will go well"

"I'll change my shoes when we get back to the hotel. The gold flats will have to do for now. Coat is a problem though".

"Wear the sheepskin jacket hanging there. You'll need to be warm".

"I thought that was your job?"

In half an hour flat Tricia was ready, which was just as well because her phone beeped. It was a text from Tina.

"Morning Trish, great night, Paddy's at 1?"

"Am at the flat, great night here too, going back to hotel, see you at 1"

They noticed something strange when leaving the flat. On the door, in an arranged manner, were cloves, bulbs of garlic and silver balls. Spooky stuff. Tricia and Jed went to the flats downstairs. No silver balls, no garlic. Very spooky. Maybe someone in the flats doesn't like t-Girls. An investigation will have to take place.

So it came to pass that Tricia and Jed took a taxi to the hotel where Monica was just waking after her own eventful night with Amy.

"Ask her if she's up for it Trish"

"Up for what?"

"You know, a threesome".

"Count me out hon, I've people to meet".

"Ok then, just me and her"

Tricia asked. Monica's face lit up.

"Yes, but can she have some time to get ready. About three days will do! Only joking hon. What about if you come to the pub with me for an hour or so which will give Monica time to get ready".

"That sounds good". Jed's face lit up.

Tricia changed her shoes and found an even better belt to go with her sexy red wool dress and left with Jed.

Pause for some slushy music. Think hundreds of violins. Think Tchaikovsky. Think Romeo and Juliet.

Unlike in London, the girls' room was on the first floor of the hotel. There were two ways down; either the lift or the huge carpeted red staircase with the enormous chandelier hanging above it. No not Crystal Chandelier but it was crystal and it was a chandelier. Jed took Tricia's arm as they descended gracefully down the staircase to the foyer. Tricia felt like a screen goddess; but which one. She thought deeply. Liz Taylor in Cleopatra, that's who she felt like. As we know she has a very vivid imagination. Julia Roberts in Pretty Woman, maybe not quite so pretty, was probably more to the mark. Tricia smiled at Jed.

"Thought you'd like that" he said.

Now, some things in life are hard and some things easy. Though equally some things are hard and some soft. Some things Tricia used to find hard, she now finds easy: like putting on a necklace for instance. It used to take her fifteen minutes and a lot of bad language; she now does it almost instantaneously. Tricia was about to introduce Jed to Tina. Jed was a man who liked t-Girls. Tricia suspected that the easiest thing in the whole world was for a man like Jed to catch the eye of a transvestite like Tina. As sure as eggs is eggs the plotting began.

"We could do a threesome" said Jed.

"But your going back to Monica" said Tricia.

"We could do a foursome" said Tina.

"That would not be fair on Monica" said Tricia, "anyway you have only just returned from a previous romantic liaison".

"So have you, and anyway you know me Trish".

"I certainly do Tina".

"How about we let Jed have his time with Monica, alone though, then we can think of options for later". Tricia was finding it hard to maintain any semblance of control, but that got the nod in the end.

An hour passed. "Time to go" said Jed.

"Get another beer in" said Tricia, who knew "she won't be nearly ready".

Jed left a further hour later and returned with a flushed Monica a couple of hours after that.

In the meantime Paddy's was very full for a Sunday afternoon and plenty of people who knew Tina and Tricia, and plenty who didn't, crossed their paths. The girls were quite happy.

Jed didn't waste words on his return to the pub.

"What about our threesome?" He was clearly on a roll.

"I can't leave Monica here on her own" said Tricia. "I have to look after her. You take Tina back".

"That sounds good". Jed's face lit up.

"That sounds good". Tina's face lit up.

"Can we borrow your key? It's a shame to waste that lovely hotel room". Tina had her foot in the door already.

"Having fun?" said Tricia.

"You bet" said Monica, "but what do we do now. I don't want to drink too much".

"Neither do I" slurred Tricia, "but what we do is go for a leisurely curry. I bet you haven't eaten today."

"Well, not that sort of eating".

So while Jed and Tina were getting to know each other, Monica and Tricia enjoyed a genuine English meal. Not like the Richmond Arms in Houston, Texas at all. The Ashoka in Manchester serves up wonderful food.

The girls went back to Paddy's for a couple more beers and a chat before returning back to the hotel where Tina and Jed were still at it.

"Don't turn the light on" said Tina.

"I can see why not" said Tricia, "but I'm going to have to blow the whistle for half time. This is our room and we need some sleep".

"Do we have to, can't you join us" said Jed.

"No" said Monica and Tricia in unison.

"I know", said Tina, we'll go back to my place".

"You already know where it is" said Tricia.

"Are you coming?" said Jed

"No, I need to be here with Monica. And it doesn't look like you are either".

"I will" said Jed, confidently.

"He will" said Tina, even more confidently.

Jed and Tina left. The room was a complete mess and didn't smell particularly healthy. Monica and Tricia didn't worry too much. They were sated with beer and food and ... they would have a good night's sleep.

Only one more day left and it was time to unwind, relax, and start the horrible process of reverting back to their straight lives. Tricia went to sleep counting; not sheep but days, days and nights she had been herself. It was now eight. Only two more to go and she still loved being Tricia. That was important to her.

> *Now Trish, Mon and Tina were three fine whores*
> *Who gave Jed a time he had never known before*

Chapter 48

Hive Full of Honey

And the farce continues. Hard times for Monica and I as we had to start transitioning back after such a long time enjoying ourselves. We were both by now though absolutely shattered! The song, by the way, could be about me but is more about Eric (roll back a few chapters, before London). It is from Calamity Jane and you will have to watch the film to establish its relevance.

> I've got two wonderful arms,
> I've got two wonderful lips,
> I'm over twenty one, and I'm free!
> Oh, I've got a hive full of honey
> for the right kind of honey bee.

Eric's Finger

The girls woke up late on the Monday. They were very, very tired; it had been a gruelling week. The original plan was to search for Monica's roots. The trouble was that Monica didn't really know where her roots were. They could have been in Herefordshire, they could have been in Wales depending on which side of her family she believed. It is ironic therefore that Amy and Jed knew more about Monica's roots than Monica herself.

"Honey, we can go to Herefordshire, we can go to Wales but we can't do both. Either will be about four hours travelling, two there two back. I don't know which to do?" Tricia was far from enthusiastic.

"Neither do I" said Monica " and I'm tired and I need some new shoes. Let's go shopping instead".

"And I know where to get you some shoes that fit". Tricia was very relieved. "Take your time getting ready, there is absolutely no rush".

Tricia got ready quickly and went for a beer. She knew she was better leaving Monica to do her own thing at her own leisurely pace. But what's leisurely? Tricia returned to Paddy's.

"Still here love?" said Steve behind the bar, pouring Tricia the umpteenth pint of Unicorn this weekend.

"I'm not sure where I am" said an exhausted Tricia.

"Lovely to see you again darling" said Eric.

"Do you know what I want?"

It then dawned on Tricia precisely what Eric wanted and it wasn't just another pint of beer. He apparently had a lovely bijou pad. Tricia lives and survives in a hovel though, she doesn't need etchings. The farce continued. Eric wanted to put his finger where no finger should ever go. Tricia didn't want anything bad to happen in the pub. As soon as Tricia got up however, to go to the ladies, for a smoke, or to the bar; Eric chased her, finger poised. Fortunately Tricia was too quick for him (except once in the smoking shelter). Eric was once again though entertaining and fun.

"I'll have to introduce you to my American friend" said Tricia.

"I'd like that" said Eric.

So, having given Monica plenty of time, Tricia returned to the hotel.

"I've got someone I'd like you to meet and he would like to meet you".

"I've had a nightmare" said Monica who had had a nightmare. "I can't decide what to wear, my make-up's wrong, can I borrow some foundation, I'll try again, and don't rush me?"

Tricia is used to Tina. Tricia doesn't rush anyone except herself,

"There you are, my foundation, meet me in the pub when you are ready".

"My darling, where is she?" Eric's finger continued on its quest as Tricia tried to wriggle and squirm out of its way.

"Just wait you greedy so and so, and she'll be here later"

Eric's finger hit a nerve. Tricia wished she had changed from her denim mini to her jeans.

"Can we take it slowly?"

"I don't want slowly Trish".

"I know, but remember where we are".

Tricia smiled, Eric smiled.

"Life is mostly about anticipation anyway" Tricia suddenly became serious.

"Life is about enjoying yourself. And I am you sexy beast".

Tricia gave Eric a kiss. "Time hon, in time, time matters – and keep that finger away from me for now".

"Alright" said Eric, "but remember I'm at the end of my career".

"And I'm at the beginning of mine, so let's wait and see how things develop".

"My things already developed".

"I don't wish to know. Can you un-develop it?"

"Not easily"

"But you are happy with me?"

"Yes, very happy"

"Alright. Look after me and lets take our time".

Eric smiled.

Monica walked in.

"Its been a complete disaster, nothing goes with anything else, my make-up's still all wrong and I feel wrong!"

"You look lovely darling" said Eric

"Sssshh, don't encourage her" said Tricia, the voice of experience.

"You're my girl" Eric patted Tricia approximately where his finger had been earlier". "But let's talk about America"

And talk they did, on and on. Eric had performed many times in America, including Houston, Texas.

"Monica hon, we're supposed to be going shopping". Tricia was drinking far too much again and felt she had to intervene.

"You go girls, I'm fine" said Eric, hand moving up Tricia's leg.

So finally, on the last day of the holiday, Tricia steered Monica around the centre of Manchester to Long Tall Sally. Monica bought a pair of shoes and a pair of boots. Both fitted well. Tricia bought some dead sexy black patent stilettos and Monica gave Tricia her old pair of shoes which fit Tricia because her feet weren't so wide. Tricia's footwear was developing. She now had:

1 pair of ankle boots, black, half inch heel

1 pair thigh length boots, black, three inch heel

1 pair sexy black patent stilettos, black, four inch heel

1 pair mules, black, two inch heel

1 pair flats, black

1 pair flats, gold

1 pair flat strappy sandals, white

1 pair stilettos, black, six inch heel, for burlesque (there's a thought)

The girls were not quite dogs but were dog tired so did only a little more shopping, had a Chinese and went back to Paddy's for a few pints, but only a few pints and then an early night. Monica had to go back to London the next day, Tricia to homes various. It was a difficult time.

In the morning Monica, in the only drab she had with her, made friends with the porter which was handy for Tricia, who looked dead sexy in her purple outfit, and arranged to leave her suitcase while she thought about the nutty problem of how to get her ceramic fingernails removed. She had become quite attached to them, and them very attached to her. The only option, as she saw it, was to go back to the beautician. She kissed Monica goodbye then booked an appointment. There was time for a quick drink in Paddys while she waited.

"Still here love?" said Steve.

"Sadly not for long" said a sober Tricia.

It was a good decision to return to the beautician. It took about twenty minutes and all sort of horrible implements before Tricia's nails were back to their normal size.

"What do you want to do with them now?" said Lilli.

Tricia shrugged. "What do you think?"

"How about a manicure"

So for another thirty minutes Tricia had her first proper manicure from Karen.

"It must be different making nails unglamorous", said Tricia.

"Its fine" said Karen, "what colour nail polish do you want?"

"Sadly, it will have to be clear".

Tricia still quite enjoyed the manicure though.

She trudged back to the hotel to pick up her suitcase, then got a cab back to the flat. Tricia would not be out tonight. Tricia was absolutely shattered. She unpacked her suitcase and hung up her clothes. She separated the dirty clothes for washing during the week. They just about fitted in her holdall. She was feeling very low, but then she thought for a moment. Hang on Trish, its Tuesday already. Only three days at work and I will be back. She smiled. She could manage that. What was important was that after all the time spent dressed, she still desperately wanted to do it again. She so loved being Tricia.

Chapter 49

The Way you Look Tonight

"So here it is Merry Christmas Everybody's having fun". Hmmm, not so sure I am. This was a very dangerous weekend and I was a v.v. naughty girl after being a v.v. good one. I think consistency is my major problem, well that and probably alcohol. It was the Northern Angels Christmas lunch (me an angel?) so at least I got some good food down me this weekend. I wore my sexy (Father Christmas) red wool dress. It's about as close I'll go to celebrating the festive season which, for me, is the worst excess of modern man — or even woman come to that. By the way:

> Some day, when I'm awfully low,
> When the world is cold,
> I will feel a glow just thinking of you...
> And the way you look tonight.

Wild and Dangerous times.

Friday was a bit wild and Tina got particularly drunk, she did pretty well at that on Saturday night as well. On Friday this manifested itself in a huge row with Marie behind the bar about whether George Best was a good husband or not. Apparently he put his son through a plate glass window. Whether he did or not is just hearsay, but the argument raged on for over an hour. Tricia shook her head. How can you possibly argue when you don't know the facts? George Best was of course Tina's hero as he played for Manchester United. He is also the best footballer I have seen in the flesh, but I'm not at all sure of him as a family man. Tricia kept out of it, sensible girl that she is.

At Naps later Tina joined Tricia on the dance floor; well for two minutes anyway. The first minute she tried to gain her balance, the second minute she lost it again. Tricia, being the considerate girl, held her upright and they decided to leave and get a cab back to the flat. They were safe and sound and that was important.

Important because the following day all sorts of strange things happened. At lunchtime the girls went to get some cigarettes from the shop in the village which should be safe. Tina's handbag wasn't quite shut as they left up the stairs. The guy following her had his hand in her bag which fortunately was noticed by the girl who had served them. She shouted and chased the guy out of the shop. It only shows how careful you need to be, but no sob stories this time at least.

In Paddy's they met a somewhat subdued Paula. She was drinking black coffee not beer or wine. "I'm getting too old for this", she said. "I need breaks from alcohol, and anyway tonight I'm going to wear my fairy costume and I don't want to be too drunk. No, a drunken fairy is not a good idea at all, agreed Tricia.

Later that afternoon the girls hit their favourite store; the wig shop. Tricia still thinks she wants a short wig but can't pluck up the courage yet. Tina was determined to spend again and she got two more wigs. Tricia thought they were very similar to her old ones, but what does she know. Tina did manage to haggle with the prices so she ended up getting two wigs for the price of one. It was either that or the girls would hang around in the shop frightening off the other customers (only kidding).

So to the meal in the evening and the girls got themselves glammed up. Tina wore a long purple dress (surprisingly extremely sophisticated for Tina) and Tricia wore her red Santa dress. Girls came from all around; it was like Bethlehem. Tina and Tricia were on a table with Natasha and Deirdre from Dublin. On the next table was a girl from Aberdeen. No wise men but plenty of not so wise Queens. The food and conversation were excellent as was the organization by Lisa.

After the meal everyone went their separate ways before meeting up in Naps at the end of the evening. For Tina and Tricia that meant a return to Paddy's and a hook up with Paula in her tutu, still sober. After a great time they were approached by Colin and Robert at the end of the night. If anything didn't seem right to Tricia then this didn't. They wanted a foursome of course. Initially Tina was up for it but Tricia managed to talk her round. There may not have been a problem at all but the way Colin was talking to them seemed all wrong. They managed to make their excuses, got out of Naps – looking behind at all times, and lived to fight another day. For Tricia it may only have been for another day as we shall see.

So Tricia, the very good girl on Saturday night, was wholly content to have a quiet Sunday. She was not to get one, or a quiet Monday come to that. Tina went back to her parents as she now tends to do on a Sunday. Tricia met Tony from the Isle of Man in Paddy's after shopping. She also met the girl from Scotland again and they discussed travelling on public transport. Tricia could share her experiences and confirm that there were no problems. Then she met Patrick.

Patrick was charming, Patrick was funny, Patrick hit a nerve. Patrick wanted Tricia, Tricia wanted Patrick. He had been eying her up in the pub for about an hour, but when they started talking everything seemed fine and, well, nice. Tricia had no idea about Patrick's circumstances. Tricia and Patrick walked back to the flat and climbed into bed, where they were to remain until mid-morning on Monday, by which time Tricia had missed her train back to work. Tricia made her excuse, at work (fortunately she had a day's leave left) and then got up to get them some cigarettes. She left Patrick gently snoring. Boilers are so unreliable!

Now, what you don't know about all this is that while they were kissing and cuddling on Sunday night, Patrick dropped a bombshell. It wasn't just Tricia who failed to get back. Patrick lived in a secure unit and needed to be back there by seven o'clock on Sunday night. Tricia wasn't exactly sure how safe she was but Patrick had been the perfect gentleman. "Just a little theft", he said.

Where is my purse? Thought Tricia, the slightest bit of knowledge makes all the difference. But throughout Sunday and Monday, Patrick was the perfect gentlemen. Where he is now, goodness only knows, likely in prison. Tricia gave him her number but does not anticipate a reply. Never mind. She had a lot of fun and ended up safe and still had her purse. That is what it's all about isn't it?

Chapter 50

Hair

This is the worst part of being a t-Girl. I really hate Thursdays though once I've got through my routine the weekend looms large which is brill. The song is the only one I could think of, its from a good hippy musical though so will suit Tina for once. The quote is the only hair I like. And its not even mine!

> Gimme head with hair
> Long beautiful hair
> Shining, gleaming,
> Streaming, flaxen, waxen

Hair (today gone tomorrow)

What's interesting is that Tricia doesn't need any hair at all since she wears a wig. That is any hair anywhere. It is a source of constant frustration for her that she constantly has to remove the damn stuff. Not only that, but having removed it she then has to tidy everything up. As all girls know, removed hair gets everywhere.

Tricia always likes the bad news first, the bad news before the good news. So we'll start with the worst news and go (so to speak) bottom up. Well it makes a change from bottoms-up which quite frequently happens in Tricia's life. Yes, we could be talking about drinking.

Every two weeks she has to do the job she hates most in the world. Every second Thursday, before going to Manchester the following day, Tricia has to remove her body hair. She calls it Nair day but could be called Veet day because she uses that as well. She runs the bath first (she seems to get better results in the bath than in the shower although it is a bit harder to clean up afterwards). Then the worst thing of all. Back to her (my) bedroom, undress, and open the horrible squirty tube. It is actually better than it was a few years ago because it doesn't smell quite so much. It still smells though.

There are certain things which always happen with Nair or Veet. She can predict them:

A big blob of it will go on the floor which she has to clean up afterwards.

Loads of it will disappear into her finger nails, never to be seen again but it makes her feel uncomfortable for the rest of the night.

It will very nearly work well.

She will end up with a little bit left in the tube.

Tricia starts with her chest and works down. Since she's been on Estroven it has gradually become easier as her hair grows back much less coarsely. Yes, she does put it on those, but very carefully, then she does her thighs and calves and then her feet. So far she has only used her right hand but she has to Nair her right hand. The sticky, squidgy, smelly, stuff is now coated to her right fingers, nails and palms. As her left hand joins in the fun, she screams to herself inside. This is ridiculous, there has to be an easier way. Having done the back of her right hand and arm, she poses like a baboon to remove the hair under both arms. She is not an Italian girl after all, she is an English rose. She finishes with her neck and the dimple on her chin (did you know she had a dimple on her chin?) Her body is now covered in the slime and needs to remain so. She has spent around three minutes putting the stuff on and it should only be on for three minutes. She knows from experience that it works best if she gives it another three minutes. She goes a little red and blotchy for a while but by the morning she is fine.

Now, what does Tricia do for the three minutes, and how does she measure it? Her hands are now coated with sticky goo so she washes them, dries them, then lights up a cigarette. A cigarette takes Tricia precisely three minutes to smoke if she is indoors and concentrating. The cigarette gives her some solace. While she is smoking she thinks how ridiculous the whole process is.

Cigarette finished, time for the spatula thingy or whatever it is called.

Tricia tests her left breast first; if hair comes off she will be ok. It normally does and she has to admit she gets a little secret pleasure watching the hair being removed onto the spatula thingy.

Tricia then goes into the bath. The slimy stuff is too slimy for the water to remove it so she works with the spatula thingy to remove every bit of hair she can. The bath starts filling with pieces of hair and white blobs of nair. The bath in fact gets so greasy she will have to have another bath afterwards. Having done her arms, body and feet she gets out to do her neck and dimple because she needs the mirror to see them. Having finished that task she works on collecting all the hair from the bath and putting it in the bin in the bathroom. She does the best job she can then empties the bath and ooshes all the remaining hair down the plughole. Using a flannel she tidies the bath completely. She then has a proper bath to remove all the slime.

Tricia hates every second Thursday.

Tricia also hates her facial hair although that again is growing far less following the girly tablets. If there is a God (and Tricia is far too immature to enter that argument) why would he wish to take hair from her head, replacing it with more hair in her nostrils and on her ears? It makes no sense at all.

Iain shaves every day in the morning. Tricia shaves whenever she gets back to the flat, except when becoming Iain when she doesn't shave at all. Tina and Tricia have an ongoing joke together when they switch back to drab. Will they pass? It's getting harder.

When Tricia shaves she has to use that horrible camper gas lighter to boil up her water because there is no electricity in the flat. It normally explodes twice in her pretty face before the water is ready. Tina told Tricia to listen for hissing when changing the gas. If it hisses it hasn't been done correctly. Tricia doesn't really understand what hissing means, except that she sometimes gets it on the streets of Manchester. Surely it has to hiss a bit or no gas would be coming through. Sometimes it does work perfectly though until the cylinder runs out.

Water boiled, Tricia puts it in her pot noodle container and goes to her bedroom. Now it gets dark early she shaves by candlelight. Surrounded by six candles she lathers her brush and then her face. She waits a moment for the very hot water to soften her skin then takes her Bic razor to the stubble. She is very careful. She doesn't want to cut her face; even the best concealer can't cover that. Sometimes she does as conditions are far from perfect but she knows she has to live with it. She waits a while after shaving before moisturizing and doing her make-up. Her skin needs time to settle down, or so she thinks.

The only good thing about hair is her wig. She's just got a new one which is causing her problems because it hasn't yet settled down. Isn't it ironic that she loves everything about hair that isn't hers and nothing that is. She shakes it out before brushing it for a while then leaves it to settle. Then she will style it using Tina's full length mirror and her fingers. When she takes it off she uses her reserve make-up bag number three (she has to be desperate to go into there) to hang it on. It makes life easier when she returns. She can take as long with her wig as the rest of the make-up put together. The wig is the most important thing. The wig makes Tricia herself – and Tricia likes being herself.

Chapter 51

Christmas Day in the Cookhouse

The dark nights and the cold are coming home to roost now. When I get back to Manchester I have to do my make-up by candlelight. Christmas is upon us in earnest. I hate it, Iain hates it. It gets in the way of everything. The false hopes. The artificial excitement (even Tina was at it). The let downs. So, by the way,

It was Christmas eve in the nightclub,
The admirers were standing round,
And hundreds of beautiful trannies
Were stretched out on the ground,
When in strode the Bad Dominatrix,
And onto her throne she sits,
Saying, 'What do you want for Christmas, girls?'
And the trannies answered...
Tidings of comfort and joy, comfort and joy,
Oh, tidings of comfort and joy!

In which making up is hard to do, Tina gets very excited. Dawn rises, as does Josh and there are danger signs for the two girls.

Tina has a theory. Like many of Tina's theories it would likely not stand up in a Court of Law. Tina likely would stand up in a Court of Law provided there was a burly policeman in the dock with her. Tricia thinks she would be particularly attracted to the right arm of the law if the finger of suspicion was pointing her way too. Tina's theory is that pulling is far easier on a Friday night. This, she claims is due to the fact that by the Saturday night she is totally shattered and too drunk. She does not, she always adds, put it down to the increased competition on a Saturday night. Tricia doesn't particularly subscribe to that theory. After all, only a couple of weeks ago, three girls all pulled on a Saturday night. As we know, Tricia is pragmatic. Last week she pulled on a Sunday evening and she wasn't even in Naps. Sometimes you do and sometimes you don't; it just depends. Tina's theory was however proved this weekend.

Tricia arrived in Manchester at the normal time on Friday evening. You've probably guessed by now that the rain was really lashing down so she had a couple of drab pints before making her way to flat. Her feminine intuition again was proved correct. The rain had pretty much stopped after her second pint. The door was opened by Josh. Tricia knew Josh was there and had told Tina to leave the door unbolted. Tina forgot. One day Tina will forget her trousers; but that probably won't matter as she hardly ever wears trousers these days. On the front of the door were some strange hieroglyphics. This was obviously a continuation of the silver balls and garlic which Tina had cleared up the week before. The girls were clearly being put under a curse, but what did the hieroglyphics mean?

Tricia had a predicament. Josh was in Tina's room getting up to no good and Tricia didn't want to disturb. She's good like that. She needed to get her make-up on however and get dressed. The only port in the storm she could see was lying on her table; a bag containing fifty candles. Tricia carefully made a circle of candles around her make-up mirror and got moving. It wasn't perfect but Tricia didn't mind. She would be herself, after all, warts and all, in an hour or so. She was happy. She put her radio on to drown out the noise coming from the other room. She was not nosy and, in any case, knew exactly what was going on in there. She hummed along to the music while she was getting ready.

Tricia had almost finished when Tina knocked on the door.

"Are you ready Trish? I'm feeling lucky tonight and it's a Friday. I always pull on a Friday".

"But you've only just finished with Josh. Where is Josh?" Tricia smiled, she knew Tina's appetite was insatiable.

"I'm in the mood now Trish. Josh has left to meet Marie. I just need to top up my make-up".

"Can you put any more make-up on your make-up? I'll be ten minutes".

So the girls hailed a cab and went back to the village. It was clear from Tina's demeanour that she wanted more of what she had just had. Tricia just wanted a few more beers (well, a lot more beers), a dance and to see if anything developed. Well it did; for both girls. You see, Tina is right sometimes.

Knowing precisely what they are, we will leave Tina to her own devices for now. What was his name? Where was he from? These facts are not remembered so cannot be documented. He did however leave his key at the flat so goodness knows how he got in to his house. By all accounts he was disappointing.

Tricia bumped into Dawn (not literally, she had remained sober) on the dance floor. Dawn was supposed to be dressed in all her finery, but it all went wrong for her in the hotel. It was her first time and she had no-one to help. She wanted Tricia to stay in her hotel room in the village with her and help her dress. Hot water, electricity, warmth, how could Tricia refuse. She did a few twirls and transformed herself into the good fairy she occasionally was. They left Napoleons as it was closing and went back to Dawn's hotel room where, with Tricia's encouragement and help Dawn changed, well into Dawn.

An hour later a little head poked around the hotel entrance in wig and make-up.

"Trish, there's someone there".

"So, follow me. I'll give you strength inside you, courage to win your battles" Tricia wishes she wouldn't keep quoting Genesis at every available opportunity, particularly post Peter Gabriel. Out of the door went Tricia followed by a very brave Dawn who was struggling with her heels.

"Relax Dawn, I'm here, I've done it a thousand times before and I won't take you anywhere you don't want to go.

The girls walked around the village for a couple of laps. There was still a crowd outside New York, New York. Tricia wanted to take Dawn through the crowd but Dawn wasn't comfortable so she steered her away. They walked for about half an hour before returning to the sanctuary of the hotel.

"Enjoy it hon?" said Tricia.

"I think so, but its all so much, so hard and so different".

Tricia knows it will take Dawn some time for everything to be absorbed but she is there for her. What was left of the rest of the night went pretty well as well.

So Tricia could have a wash with water but not a shave, as her razor was at the flat and had to walk back through Manchester at nine o'clock with a nine o'clock shadow on Saturday morning. It wasn't raining so she took the canal route with a smile on her face. Then she went straight to bed.

"Trish, are you ever going to wake up!" Tina was getting impatient. Tina getting impatient!

"It's Christmas and there will be a brilliant atmosphere in town". Tina was keen and eager, but at least she wanted to go into town. That was a turn up for the books.

"Its Christmas, It's a Saturday, it will be manic, I don't want anything to do with it." Tricia, as ever, was cynical.

The volume on yet another Hawkwind record (apparently they have written more than any other band in the world which may explain, thinks Tricia, why none of them are any good) increased. Tricia turned on her radio to drown out the noise. Tina came in and snatched the transistor.

"Will you get up, and how can you listen to this rubbish when the greatest music of all time is playing in my room".

"Hon, give me time. I am moving albeit slowly. The music I am listening to is from the 16th Century. I doubt Hawkwind will last four hundred years". Tricia tried to keep her calm.

"You don't know what you are talking about!"

"Possibly not, but give me an hour". Tricia does not wish to offend followers of Hawkwind, but was a girl of her word and after a massive effort was ready in an hour. By now it was starting to get dark again.

"Let's go and enjoy the Christmas atmosphere in town". Tina was enthused, or infused depending on your point of view.

"Anyway, I need some new knickers and I haven't been to the thrift shop in ages".

Tricia sighed, deeply. "Come on then, but let's go for a couple of pints first. I need waking up properly. Tricia drank quickly. If the thrift shop was an option she needed plenty of resolve.

Chapter 52

When Tricia Comes Marching Home

What I have noticed is that the more often I do this, the better and more confident I become. This makes it far easier for me to communicate with the straight world and helps them communicate with me. Things aren't as bad as people think, so, by the way,

> The old church bell will peal with joy,
> Hurrah Hurrah
> To welcome home our darling girl
> Hurrah Hurrah
> The village lads an lassies say, with
> roses they will strew the way,
> And we'll all feel gay
> When Tricia comes marching home

In which Tina spends the gas bill again and shows her attitude, the girls get good greetings from straight people but there is writing on the wall and Tina transforms into Bet Lynch.

The girls were lucky; a cab turned up straight away and whisked them to Paddys Goose. There Tina donned (if that is the right word) her Santa hat.

"I love Christmas Trish".

"Take that ridiculous thing off Tina".

"Bah humbug" said Steve from behind the bar, and he meant it.

They were sitting at the bar on stools, provocatively crossing and uncrossing their legs. Tina went out for a smoke. Tricia looked up and noticed, by the fruit machine, a shifty looking man staring at her, his hands in his pockets. That's odd thought Tricia, its warm in here. A minute later the shifty man disappeared to the Gents. Ten minutes later he re-appeared. A minute after that he drunk up and left. Aren't men strange, thought Tricia.

Tricia was drinking for England. The thought of visiting the thrift shop had suddenly made her throat very dry. Four pints and about ten minutes after the four pints, the girls arrive at Primark.

Now, some things in life defy all logic. Tina is in Primark, the cheapest shop in all of England. She needs some knickers, fair enough, ten pairs at most? Knickers are on sale at £1 a pair. So how, on earth, can Tina end up spending £65 in Primark on knickers?

"That'll keep me going next year Trish".

"That'll keep you going for life hon". Tricia smiled. That was Tina for you.

While Tina was paying there was a slight altercation. Tricia, who had bought nothing, was having a video taken of her by some pretty Asian girls when all hell broke loose at Tina's check-out.

"Mind out of my way!". A young lad was intent on causing trouble as he passed through.

"Who are you talking to you ******* little ****". Tina later said she could have handled him if it came to it. Tricia just put her finger to her lips. The Asian girls' cameras quickly switched to another angle. They didn't realise there were two t-Girls in the store, one with a major attitude problem. Still, there was no further trouble and Tina left the lingerie section with a big smile on her face and around fifty pairs of knickers.

Tina was determined to spend today. "Forgot Trish, I need a warm winter coat as well, is it ok we look for one?"

"Ok hon, but ten minutes max". Tricia's bladder after the earlier four pints was beginning to fill. If Tina was looking for coats she didn't hold out much hope of being out of the shop in ten minutes. She was wrong again though; but that's Tina; unpredictable.

Now, there is a long running English soap opera called Coronation Street, which you may, or may not have heard of. Although still on air today, its prime time was probably in the seventies and eighties. Then, (and remember that is the era Tina likes to dress) there was a character who stood behind the bar in the pub called the Rovers Return.

"Trish, this coat screams Tina". Screamed Tina, excitedly.

"Tina, that coat screams Bet Lynch". Tricia hesitated. "and Tina".

"Look, its warm too".

"I'm not sure that entered into the equation". Tricia knew Tina well.

In a matter of seconds the cheap leopard skin faux fur coat was whisked to the check-out by a smiling Tina. Tricia was relieved it all had happened so quickly but even so urgently need relief herself. Tricia deflected the need by wondering how long it would take before Tina bought some cheap faux fur skin-tight leopard skin trousers.

Tina was still determined to spend. "Now let's go to the thrift shop Trish, I'm enjoying my shopping". After the four earlier pints, the thought of standing outside the thrift shop for an hour smoking cigarettes was superseded by another thought. Tricia smiled; she had found a way out.

"Tina, you go to the thrift shop. I will go to the pub we haven't been in for a while. There is something on my mind. Well, my bladder actually".

"Ok Trish, get me a lager, I'll see you in fifteen minutes"

"Hon, if you are going to the thrift shop you likely won't see me for at least an hour, maybe a day. I'll buy you one when you appear".

"Ok Trish, see you later". The girls went their separate ways. Yet again though, Tricia's thoughts were to be proved wrong.

Tricia walked into the straight pub and immediately got a wonderful reaction from behind the bar where three girls were serving.

"Great to see you again"

"Thought you'd forgotten about us"

"Where is your friend?"

198

The cynic in Tricia thought she may be good for business. She was certainly attracting attention in the pub as any budding supermodel would, but, after a relief as long as that of Mafeking, she realised that the girls were genuine and enjoyed serving and chatting to her. The charity shop was closed so Tina was at the bar when Tricia returned from the ladies. Tina got the same reception. The back door was unlocked for them and the girls went out for a smoke. Tricia and Tina felt very welcome and natural in the straight pub. They enjoyed themselves, and if it happens to help business so what?

Laden with over fifty pairs of panties and a Bet Lynch coat, the girls walked back to their normal drinking haunt and a full pub at Paddy's. They met Mark and Jade. They met a straight couple; the female of the two (what's that?) took a particular and a peculiar interest to the girls. The male of the two (what's that?) had a go at Tricia's wig.

"You should spend more time on it like your friend here!"

Tricia had just checked her wig and was happy with it. The difference between her wig and Tina's was that Tina's was a mass of curls whereas Tricia's was wavy. The guy thought Tina had spent an age putting the curls into her wig. Ha-ha, as if! Men, what do they know, that would have taken Tina a day or more!

While they were chatting, they were joined by the man with a goatee beard. The man with the goatee beard normally comes to chat with them but he very rarely has much to say, hence the reason he has not been mentioned before. Tina, who hadn't learned her lesson from the week before, was now in full "wine and lemonade" mode. Tricia disappeared to powder her nose. When she returned there was a full blown argument going on concerning Greenpeace, the roll of America in modern society, the British Government and the amount of money Manchester City had available in the transfer window. Tricia did her best to calm things down. Tricia always does her best. The man with the goatee beard apologised but it was not his fault. By the end of the evening things were ship shape and certainly Bristol fashion but why on earth argue about things you have absolutely no control over. Tricia shook her head and smiled. That's Tina for you!

Another Saturday night in Naps and again the girls didn't pull. Maybe Tina had it right after all. Tricia didn't mind though. She had had fun the night before and enjoyed her dancing. She was, in any case, shattered after Friday.

On Sunday Tina disappeared back to her parents leaving Tricia with a quiet day to wander around town. A lovely wander it was too. The shops were far less manic than the day before and there was a chilled atmosphere in Manchester. Tricia bought the Christmas presents she needed, for the first time as Tricia, so she was happy. Later she went into the second straight pub where she hadn't been for a while to watch the football. Again she got a lovely welcome and had a long chat with the barmaid. Tricia is beginning to realise that most people like and respect her, because of what she is doing. And so they should, after all she is a very brave girl who is getting more and more confident all the time.

Chapter 53

Polly Garter's Song

Let's look in for a change so this is a joint effort by Iain and myself (Tricia). I've just dug up my pass to Westminster which I suppose proves that girls like me may have a place in society after all. But then what is society? By the way yet another role reversal song but this time slightly different. From Under Milk Wood by Dylan Thomas. A play for voices now, whatever next! Don't you just love Richard Burton's voice!

> Now Mon, Trish and Tina were three fine whores
> Who gave Jed a time he had never known before

A view from the other side.

Narrator:

It was eleven o'clock in the morning when the dark side of the City aroused from the jumpy, humpy, rumpy-pumpy shenanigans of the night before. The less enlightened City dwellers were already awake; cutting their lawns, washing their cars, cooking Sunday lunch. Over the garden walls the gossiping began.

1st Straight:

Were you woken up again at the crack of dawn this morning?

2nd Straight:
Yes, those gays again. It is immoral

3rd and 4th Straight:
(Nodding in agreement)
Immoral

2nd Straight:
The Government shouldn't allow it, or them; they should be sent to prison.

1st Straight:
And some of them weren't even men!

3rd Straight:
And some of them weren't even women!

4th Straight:
Having fun like that is a disease.

5th Straight:
And I bet nobody has measured the effect it is having on global warming.

4th Straight:
Or on their families, or the lives of law abiding citizens like us. (4th straight was a banker).

1st Straight:

And it sets no example for our children. What must they think?

All Straights:

It's disgusting, it's filthy, it's immoral, it shouldn't be allowed.

Narrator:

And the gibbering, jabbering, garbling, gossip goes on as the other side of the City get ready; honest, happy and open. Eyes open, minds open, legs open, they go about their abnormal day with a smile in their lips and a song in their hearts.

Tricia Dale was smiling as she was making herself up. She was wearing her favourite black dress with some sexy patterned tights. She loved wearing patterned tights. She was meeting her friends for plenty of drinks at lunchtime and was looking forward to it.

Not quite dead yet, Captain Iain was slowly waking too after a heavy session in the pub the previous night. He used to skipper a cricket team and the reminiscences from afar echoed around his alcohol soaked brain.

Most famous living English all-rounder:

Remember me, remember me. I hit you out of the ground from the third ball of the match. You were very young then.

Aussie Fast Bowler with Walrus moustache:

Remember me, remember me. I was too fast for you. I beat you four balls in a row. I said I was going to nail your f****** head to the f****** sightscreen.

Indian Indoor Team:

Remember us, remember us. Remember when you opened the bowling with your devious leg spin. At the end of the first over, the score was 18 for 3.

Anonymous Bowler from Epping:

Remember me, remember me. I hit your box twice in two balls. I was only medium pace but you were in agony.

Narrator:

Captain Iain never recovered in a cricketing sense from that. He didn't have the balls (metaphorically). He anticipated every delivery sent his way for the rest of his career would do the same thing. But what if he didn't have the balls physically?

He didn't want to think about that though. Those were bright, light days when the sun shone on the sightscreens of his life. Days of fun, sticky buns and tons and tons of runs. Captain Iain dozed gently off again with a faint smile on his face. *"And the run stealers flicker to and fro, to and fro"*

Tricia Dale, after umpteen pints with her friends in the pub that never closes snapped out of her daydream too. She was dreaming of her first lover. She left him fourteen months ago and hasn't been able to get in touch since. He had very bad flu at the time.

"And I always think as I tumble into bed"

"Of Man City Tony who may be dead, dead, dead".

She walked out from the pub into the rain-sodden, gloom-ridden Manchester Street next to the bus station, called Bloom Street ironically. She was happy though, happier than she has ever been. She lit up a cigarette, had a drag and smiled to herself. *"And the rent boys flicker to and fro, to and fro"*.

By now though the straights were in their element. It was Sunday lunchtime! Mother and daughter were having a chat.

1st Straight:

Lovely to see you again Mum, was it really that long ago?

2nd Straight:

Yes, you really must do better keeping in touch with me.

1st Straight:

But I have a busy life; there's far too much to do.

2nd Straight:

Your Mother and your family are important too: Anyway, we've cooked a lovely meal for you. Sunday roast, all the trimmings.

1st Straight:

I'm looking forward to it. To change the subject, I'm a bit worried about your grandson. He's a bit, how shall I put it, effeminate. He likes to play with his sister's dolls.

2nd Straight:

He's only young yet though.

3rd Straight joining in:

If he doesn't get over it soon I'll clout him to Kingdom come. That'll teach him.

Narrator:

The misinterpreted, misunderstood, mish-mash of common sense continued, to the detriment of the poor boy who just wanted to be himself.

1st Straight:

After all, what would the neighbours say!

Narrator:

Tricia Dale and Tina Trevain had the afternoon planned. They were both going to improve their appearance. Goodness knows they needed that. So a trip to the wig shop was the next event on the horizon; horizontal being something the girls' understood.

Ali Barber:

Now girls, you know the rules, buy a cap and you can try on three wigs.

Girls:

What's a cap?

Narrator:

Girls like these in a wig shop? Only three wigs? As we know, Tricia Dale only knows about laws, not rules. Cricket only has laws, not rules. So the girls put on wig after wig after wig.

Ali Barber:

Girls, can you please make sure you put the wigs back where you found them.

Tina Trevain:

But that's the problem. I never know where I got them from in the first place.

Tricia Dale:

Maybe if you just took one wig at a time that would help?

Tina Trevain:

Yes Trish it would, but they are all slightly different colours and I need to be able to see the difference immediately. What do you think of this?

Narrator:

Tina Trevain put on a wig so resplendent that there was nothing left of Tina Trevain. The loudest, gaudiest syrup in the whole shop.

Tricia Dale:

You're a drag queen now are you?

Tina Trevain:

No, but I like the volume.

Tricia Dale:

You like the volume on Hawkwind, it doesn't mean I do.

Tina Trevain:

It's a no then?

Tricia Dale:

It's a no. But you don't do no's do you?

Tina Trevain:

Thanks Trish, I was thinking the same thing.

Narrator:

Fittingly fitted with wigs that fitted, Tricia Dale and Tina Tresvain returned to the house that fuels their hopes and fills them with hops. There they meet, amongst others their best friends: wife one and wife two.

In the other world, the world away from the village, the straight world, it was all systems go for Monday morning. The sullen, spoilt, selfish children were called away from their playstation; not in from their play. The next round of the x-rated x-factor would have to wait. They knew they were going to win anyway. They had won every day of their boring life for the past two years. They always win. They always lose.

The teenagers, sighed and weighed down with the unfairness of it all, have to turn their face on Facebook and start the essay they meant to start the previous Monday morning.

The parents, in different houses in different towns with different partners and different children have their baths, watch a house being redecorated and the play that follows about celebrity. No Church for this generation, few morals either. But before retiring they carefully re-cycle their cans and bottles. They are good people after all. They go to their beds and dream; of fast cars and kitchens and extensions and money.

No school or work for the grandparents though, isolated and lonely, far away from their children, their grandchildren and their great grandchildren. Everybody is living longer now but there are fewer and fewer reasons for growing older.

In the alcoholic, light, white, bright, smoke-free pub on the other side of the city, the party was in full flow.

1st Wife

So you can make me a bed which I can lock second wife in and give her access to music and light if I want?

Schoolgirl

Why would she want access to music and light?

2nd Wife

Because it gets scary when all is turned off.

Transvestite

Its fun being scared. It increases the pleasure.

T-girl

The trouble is, how far do you go before you go over the edge?

1st Wife:

That is why I, first wife, am so important.

Dominant Gay:

We do look after you subs you know.

Submissive Gay:

Sometimes, though I prefer it when you don't

Narrator:

The party was to continue until the early hours before the gays went to bed and dreamed; not of fast cars and money but of how to further their lives, how to engage more, how to realise their own dreams. Dreams which were not artificial but very real.

The light slowly died on the City. Outside all was far quieter than the night before. The residents were safer on a Sunday night. Tricia Dale, secure and snug in her soft, single, shag-me bed slowly dropped off. In her dreams?

Captain Iain:

Remember me, remember me?

Chapter 54

Send in the Clowns

For the first time I didn't really enjoy myself. It was so cold and I had a row with Tina which put a dampener on the whole week. I worry though that it's me though, that I am not as happy as I was. I suppose time will tell. By the way I love this song to death and it reflects my mood during the week.

One thing though, it is next year; a new year a new challenge? Where am I going to end up.

> Isn't it bliss?
> Don't you approve?
> One who keeps tearing around,
> One who can't move.

A time for freezing, worrying and changing. Tina and Tricia have a fall out. Tina gets another fur coat and Tricia gives up for the first time.

Tricia was spending her first New Year's Eve as Tricia. She was going up to Manchester on the Wednesday night and staying until work on the Monday morning. She didn't make it to the Monday though. She went back on Sunday. It was just too cold.

No heating at the flat; minus eight on New Year's Day, Tricia never really warmed up all week after that. It is not good waking up in the morning with condensation coming from your still painted lips. Tricia desperately wanted a hot bath and to just get the cold out of her bones. She wanted to shop, she wanted to hit the sales, she wanted her eyebrows shaped but because of the cold, the drive had gone from her. Was it because of the cold though? Her journey thus far had been great fun and she had immensely enjoyed every bit of it. Maybe though the journey was over and you know what they say. "It's better to travel hopefully than to arrive". Maybe Tricia had arrived, she had certainly come often enough. Maybe the novelty had worn off. She can do anything now as Tricia but is that really what she wants. Worrying times but this week could be put down to the cold. Couldn't it? For once it wasn't her bladder that was on her mind.

Delayed on Wednesday afternoon due to work, and the fact that the direct train between Sheffield and Manchester had been stopped for engineering work (Tricia did wonder how much work was actually achieved on New Year's Eve afternoon), she eventually arrived via Leeds. She had plenty of time on the trains to decide that it was a night for her Chinese yellow dress. She had only worn it twice before and likes to get her moneys worth if she can. After all, if you can't wear what you want on New Years Eve, when can you? Maybe she should have waited until Chinese New Year's Eve though.

Tricia felt she looked pretty good after getting herself ready in the freezing cold, and this was despite the fact that Tina put the generator on for twenty minutes. The girls were due to meet up with Georgina at eight. They didn't arrive until half past but Georgina was impressed. Tina was normally at least an hour late. Georgina's job in Milan had fallen through; something to do with the global economy, and she was looking for jobs in the UK and making her flat in Manchester more habitable. So Georgina should be about more often.

Double taxi fares? Tickets to get into your own pub? Tricia did prefer the New Year to Christmas, but only marginally. At least for the £2 Paddy's ticket, everybody got a hotpot. A traditional Lancashire hotpot at that! Perfect for the cold weather. The pub was healthily crowded, the atmosphere was good as was the conversation.

So, onto Naps and Tina and Tricia have their first major fall-out. To be perfectly honest Tina fell out with Tricia. Tricia doesn't really understand why, particularly since Tina used a scattergun approach to attack her but Tricia shrugged her shoulders, left early and got on with her life. The gist of the argument appeared to be that Tricia never listened to Tina. She should have worn a yellow belt with her Chinese dress. Apparently Tricia looked pregnant?? The fact that the line of the dress was vertical and in any case, Tricia didn't have a yellow belt, seemed to pass Tina by. As for Tricia not listening to Tina, Tina doesn't get it. Tricia listens to no-one. Tricia ignores indoctrination of all types. She learns by her mistakes. That is her experiment, that is what makes her free, that is what makes her the person she is. She still has more conditioning to remove, but it's about removing conditioning, not gaining additional Tricia layers.

Tricia trudged home in the early hours of 2009. She wasn't pleased about the row and realised that things would now be different and that she'd likely be more on her own in the future. That didn't worry her too much and she felt that it may in fact be a good thing. She just hoped she could patch things up in the short term.

When she got to the flat she had another predicament. Bolt on or bolt off. Was Tina returning or not? Either way she would undoubtedly be told off. She sighed. Bolt on, Tina always says bolt on. She was in a deep sleep when she heard furious banging on the door (makes a change from banging in the flat). Tina had apparently been trying to get in for the previous hour and blamed Tricia for being petty following their bust up. Tricia wasn't being petty; she was just in a very deep sleep. Things were to get better over the week but the girls ensured they kept their space. Tina went to stay at Georgina's; hot water, electricity and food, while Tricia remained in the freezer. That was probably best all round.

The trouble with sleeping in a freezer is that you don't want to get out of bed. Tricia woke relatively early for the rest of the week; saw the condensation on her breath, felt the cold so she just turned over and went back to sleep. It was absolutely freezing getting up and getting dressed and required a major effort. She did some shopping, but nothing like what she was anticipating.

On New Years Day, Paddy's wasn't open until late so Tricia had to go into straight pub for an hour or so. She was a very brave girl and chose the Wetherspoons on Oxford Road. She needn't have worried though. There were no problems there at all and she quite enjoyed her quiet pint(s) while reading the paper. She later went back and found Paddy's open. Tina and Georgina were there as was Suzy. The previous week Tina had asked Suzy about her fur coat and Suzy replied that she had a spare one she would give Tina. Rumour has it that Suzy is on the game but what are rumours?

213

Tina therefore now had two fur coats. One very long and glamorous, the other which made her look like Bet Lynch.

Now, before you say "all fur coat and no knickers" remember that this line was used many, many times throughout the evening. The fact of the matter was that Tina had prostitution very much on her mind. As a result of the credit crunch her business wasn't attracting too many customers so she had to explore other avenues for money.

"What am I good at and what do I enjoy doing?" she asked Tricia.

Tricia didn't need to reply. Suzy told the girls that the bill of fayre on the streets, so to speak was £30 a blow, £50 full and where to stand, as it were, so maybe the rumours are correct.

Tricia and Georgina had a chat following the argument with Tina the day before. Tricia assured Georgina that that there were no ill feelings from her end. Georgina made the point that there are enough enemies outside so why make more inside which Tina and Tricia agreed. Things were getting slowly patched up. Tina went back to Georgina's. Tricia went to Naps for a dance. She needed to re-build her confidence and attitude.

On the Friday Tricia hit the sales. She was extremely frustrated because the only things she liked, she couldn't find in her size. She was getting used to that though. Sales are not all they are cracked up to be, a little like Christmas and the New Year. Empty-handed, she came back to the pub. Georgina had bought this super duper web cam which could follow you wherever you are in the room. What precisely Georgina wished to do with the web cam I will leave you to contemplate. Tricia has some ideas but she may be wrong. Georgina was now on the hunt for an internet connection and phone line.

On the Saturday Tricia again couldn't get out of bed. It was about three o'clock in the afternoon, about time to get dark, when she entered Paddys. Becky and Megan were already there and were to be joined by Georgina and Tina for a drunken few hours. Megan had quit her job but a couple of opportunities had come her way. She was currently throwing herself into designing a new menu for a café in Gorton. It is a great challenge for her but Tricia is sure she will make it work and it may just be the beginning of something big. Tricia's only concern is that Megan may overdo things and get ill. She will watch out for her though, as will Becky. Becky, a bit like

Tricia, is having a few problems of her own at work. So in a few months goodness knows what they'll all be doing. Georgina's job didn't materialise, Tina is considering prostitution, Becky and Tricia are thinking of new starts and Megan already has one. Times, they are a changing. Needless to say Tricia got very drunk, had a Chinese buffet and wandered back through the freezing streets of Manchester into the freezing flat with funny writing on the door where she curled up like a ball under her blankets. This is no good she thought; this is no fun at all.

The following morning was just as cold. Tricia couldn't take any more of it. Tina came back to pick up her drab.

"I'm going back home" said Tricia. "I can't take any more of this weather. In any case the village is going to be dead quiet tonight". At least she had some warm tights to put on under her trousers. Sometimes being a girl helped. Tricia wanted warmth, she wanted a bath, she wanted to see her daughters again. She wasn't worried at all about being Tricia for the first time. Should she worry? What does she really want? She doesn't know but she will be up next weekend when it is Tina's birthday.

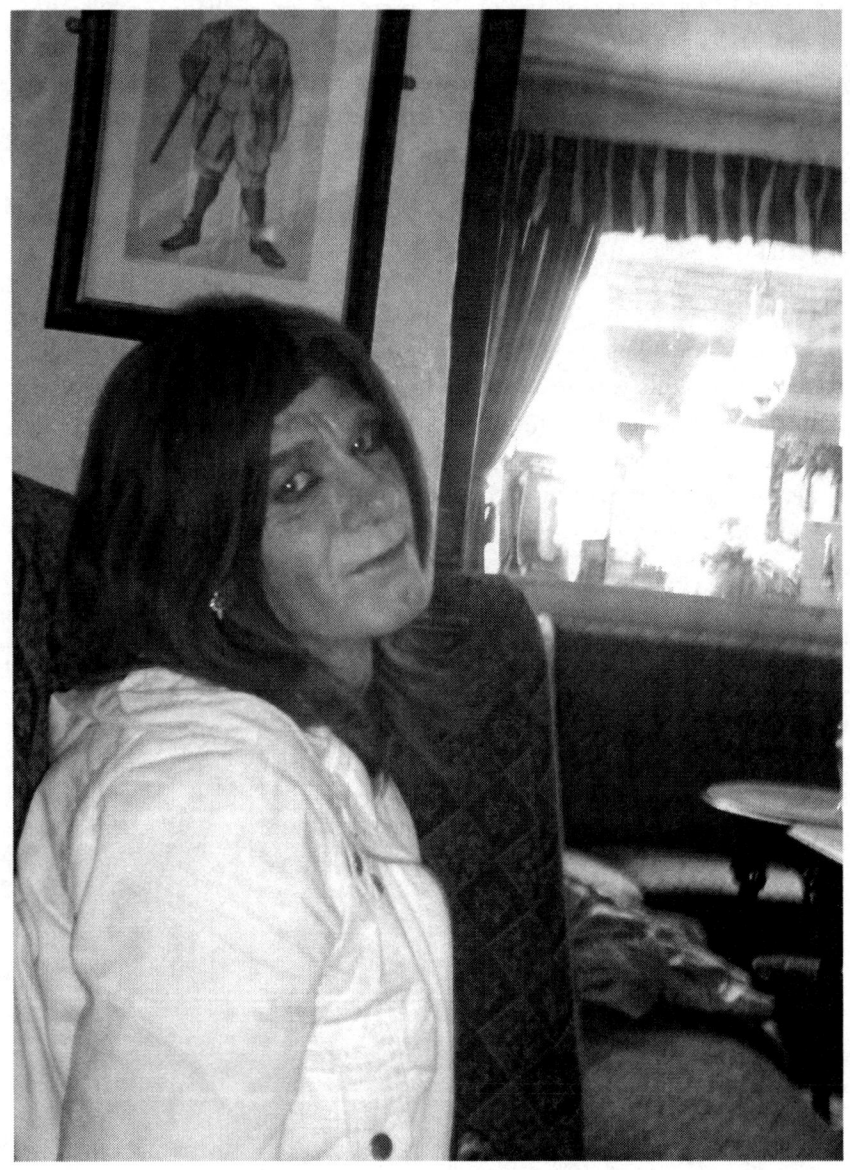

Somewhere Over the Rainbow

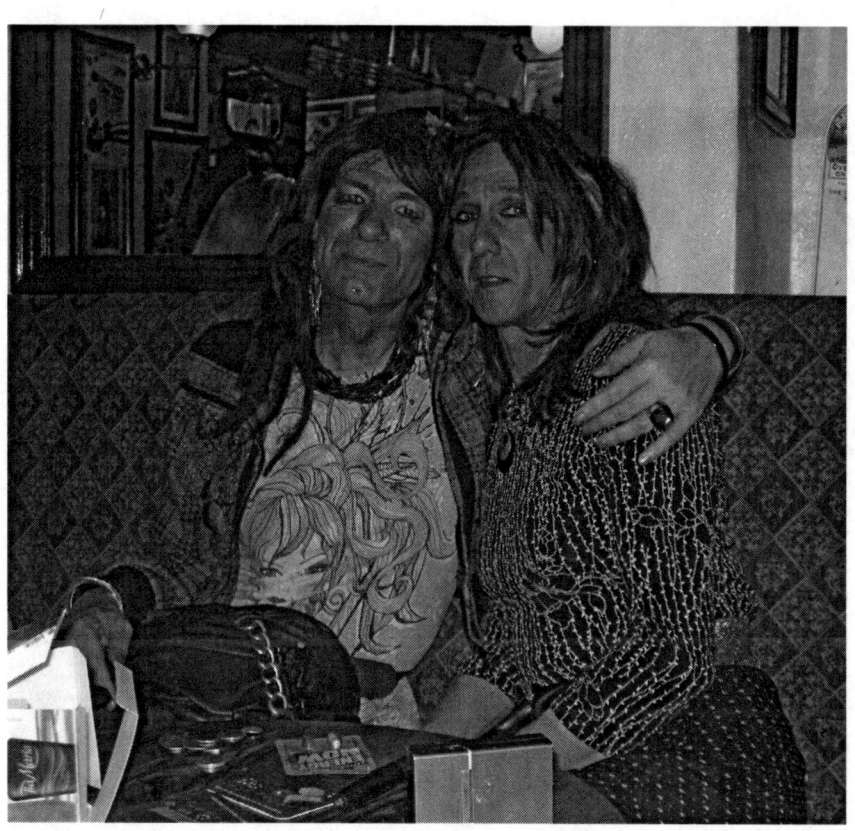

Two Ladies

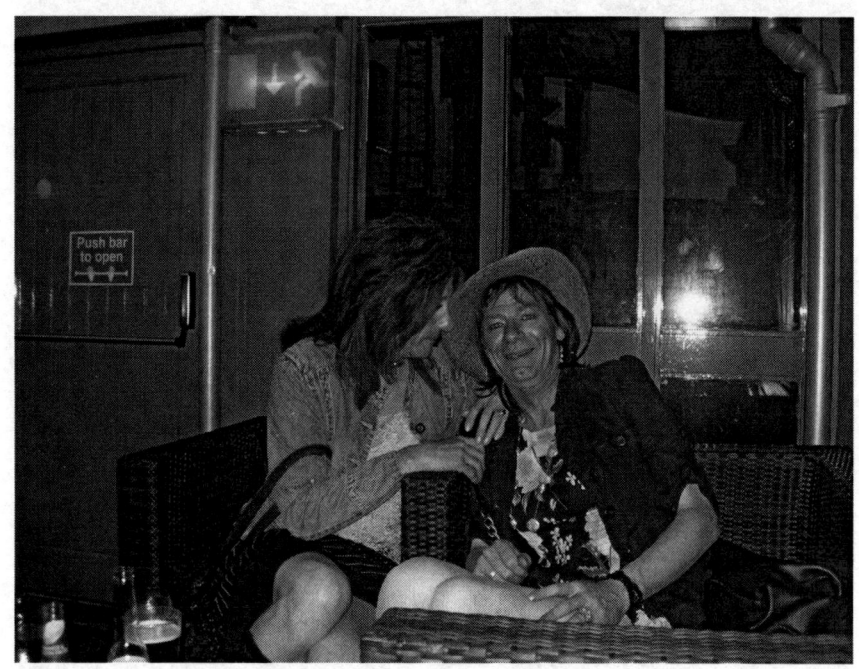

The Sun has got Her hat on

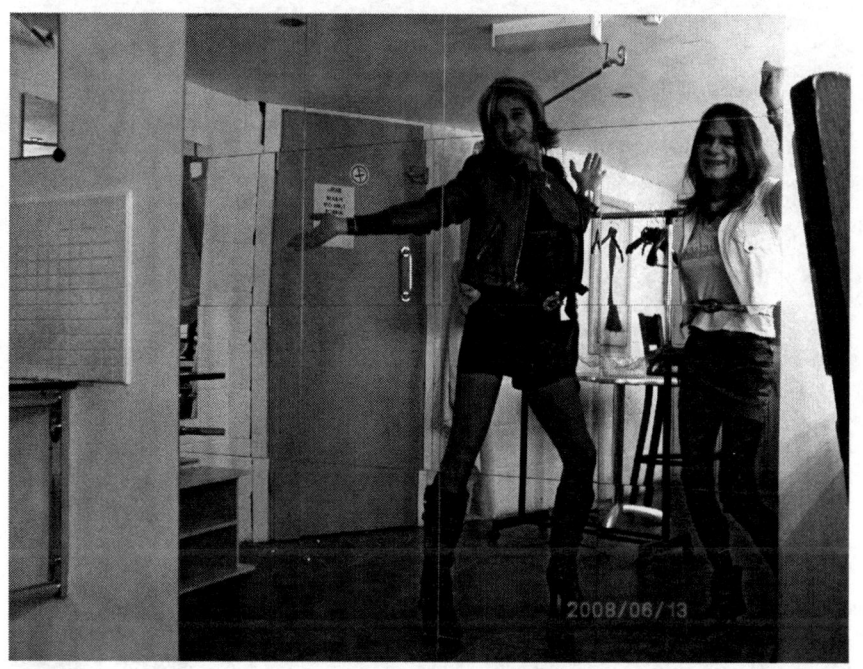

Your tiny hand is Frozen

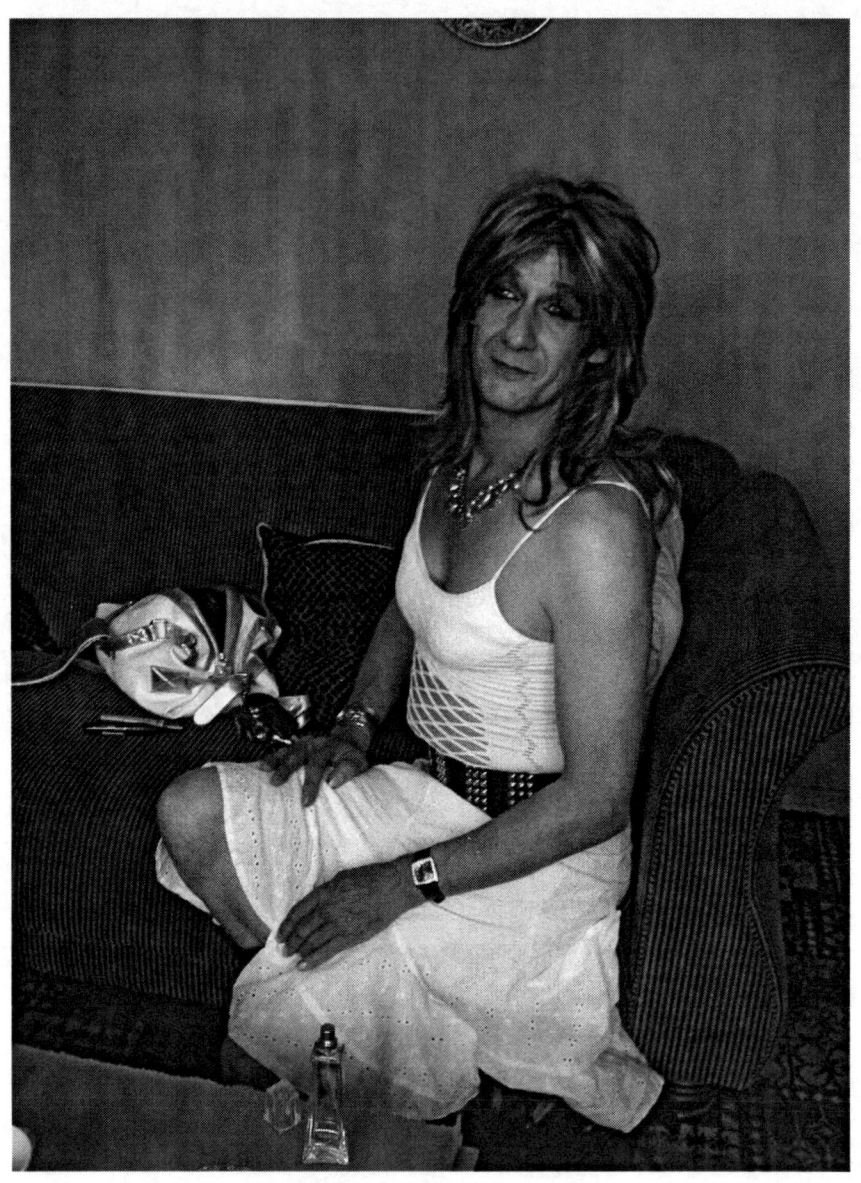

Oh What a beautiful morning

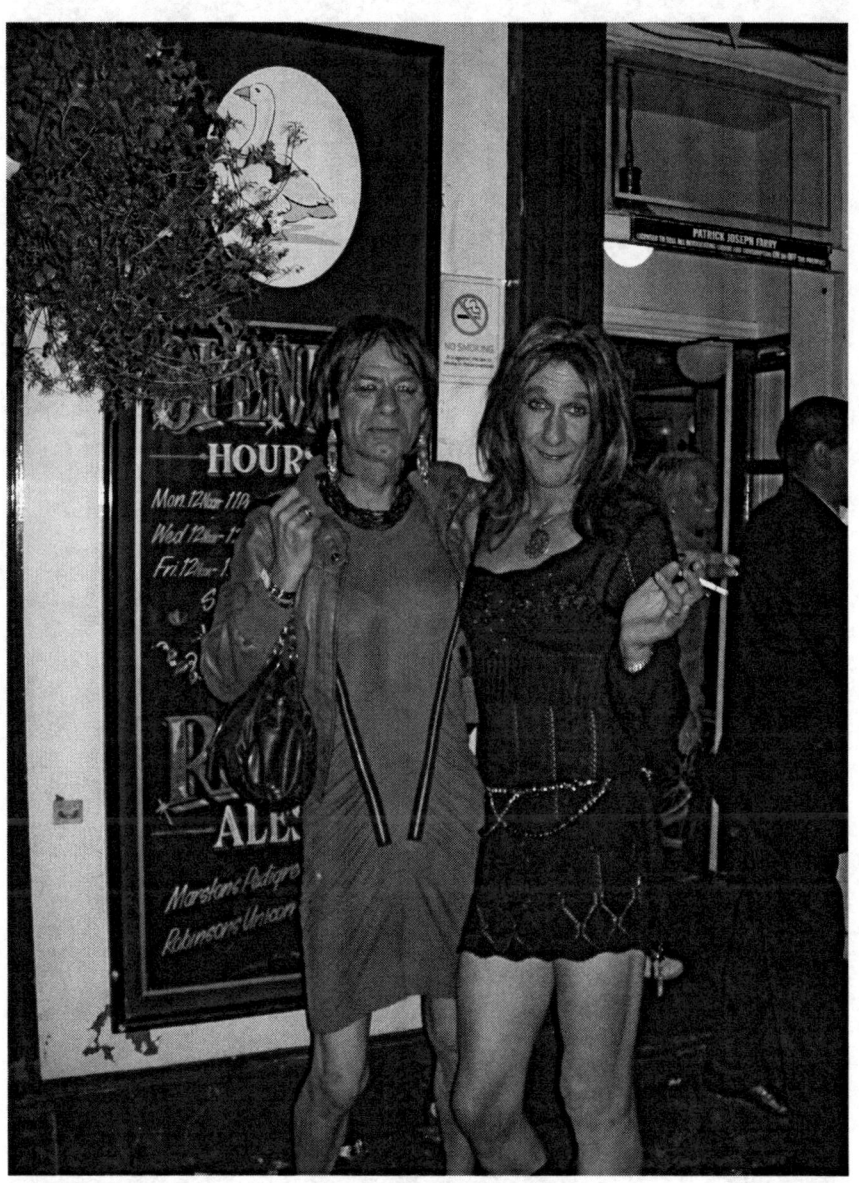

What a wonderful world

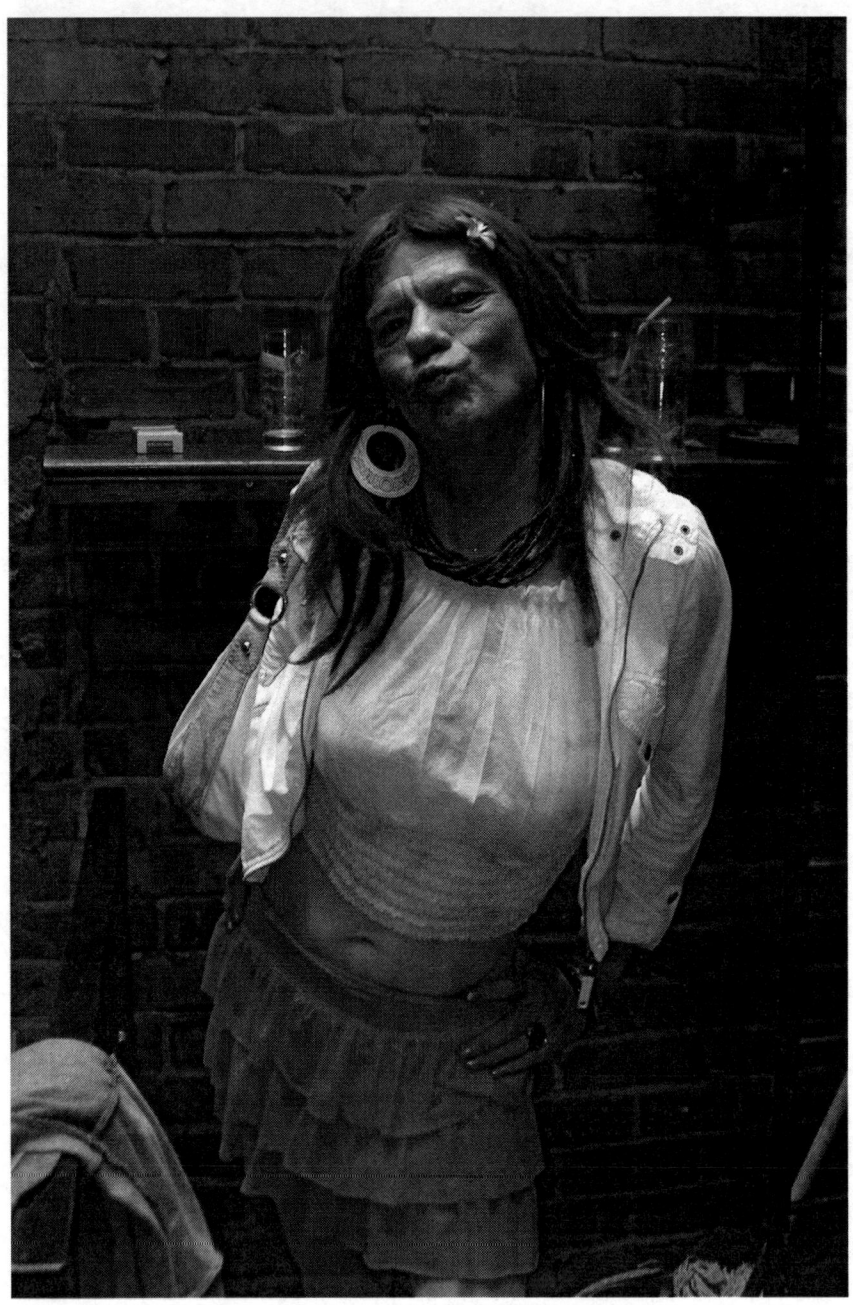

There's no business like show business

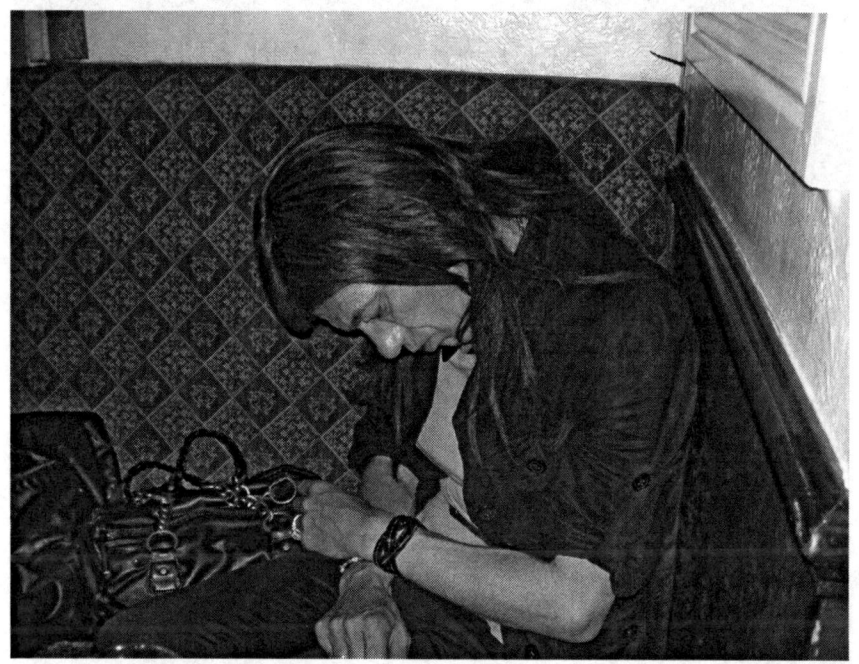

Summertime

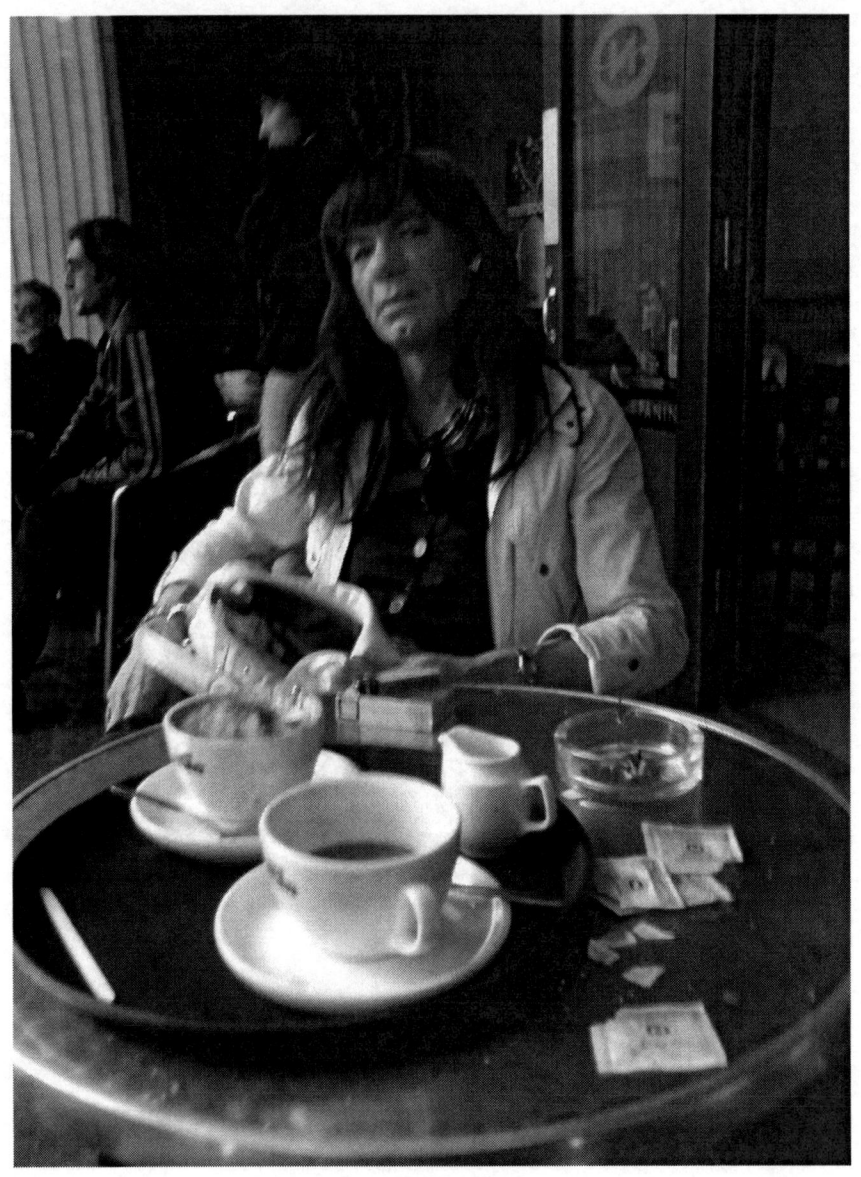

Ladies who Lunch

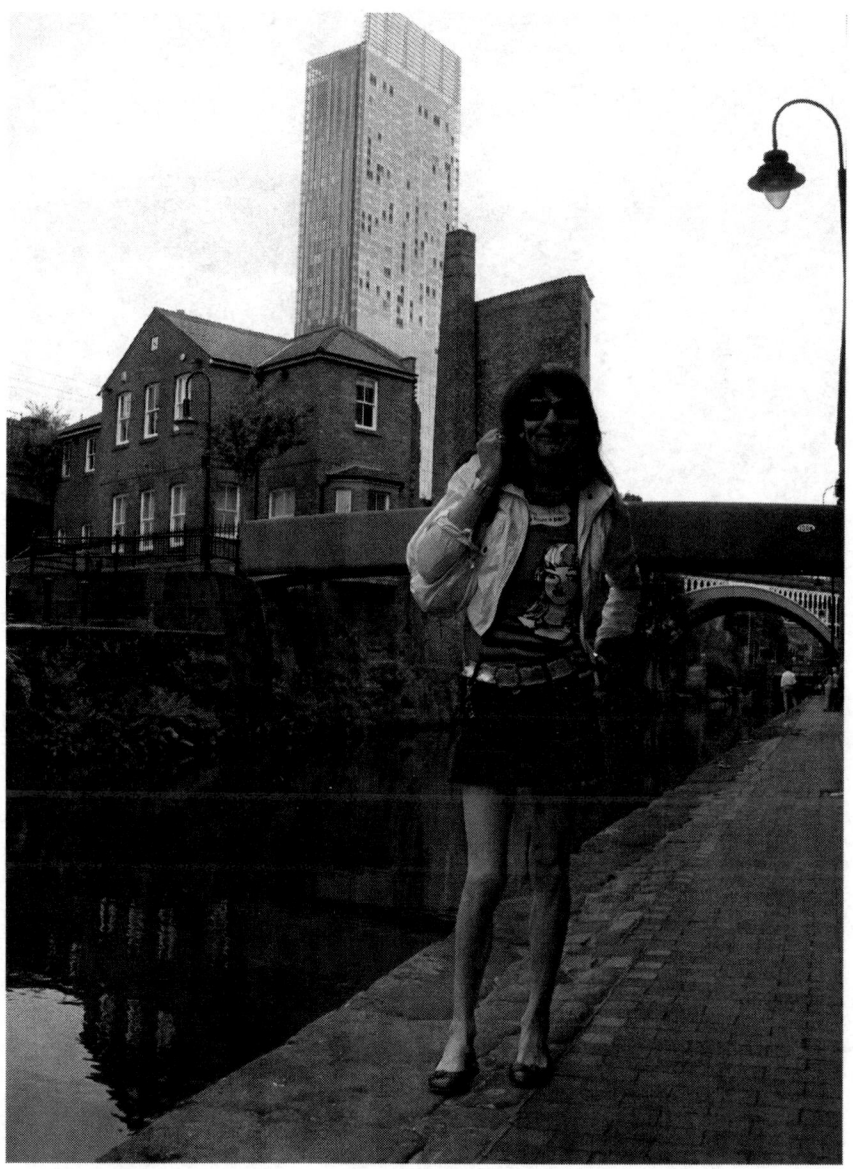

Secret Love

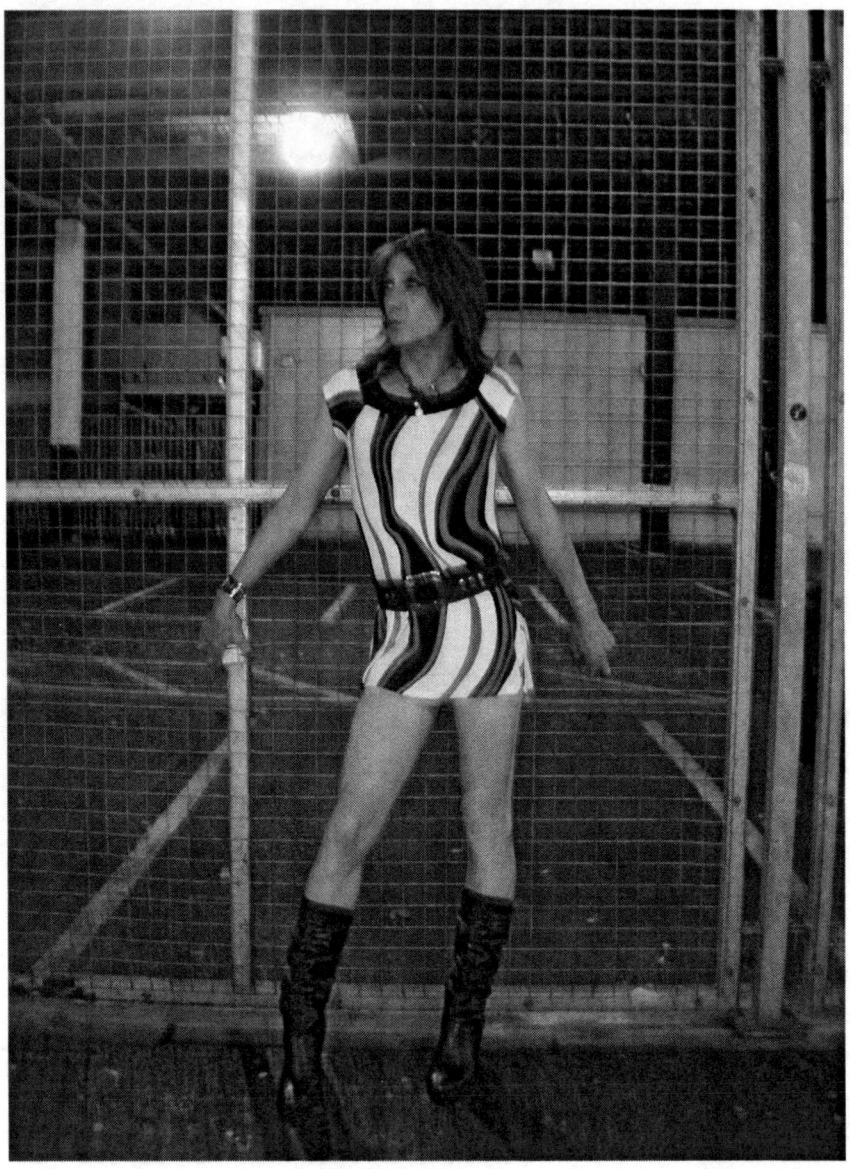

Lily Marlene

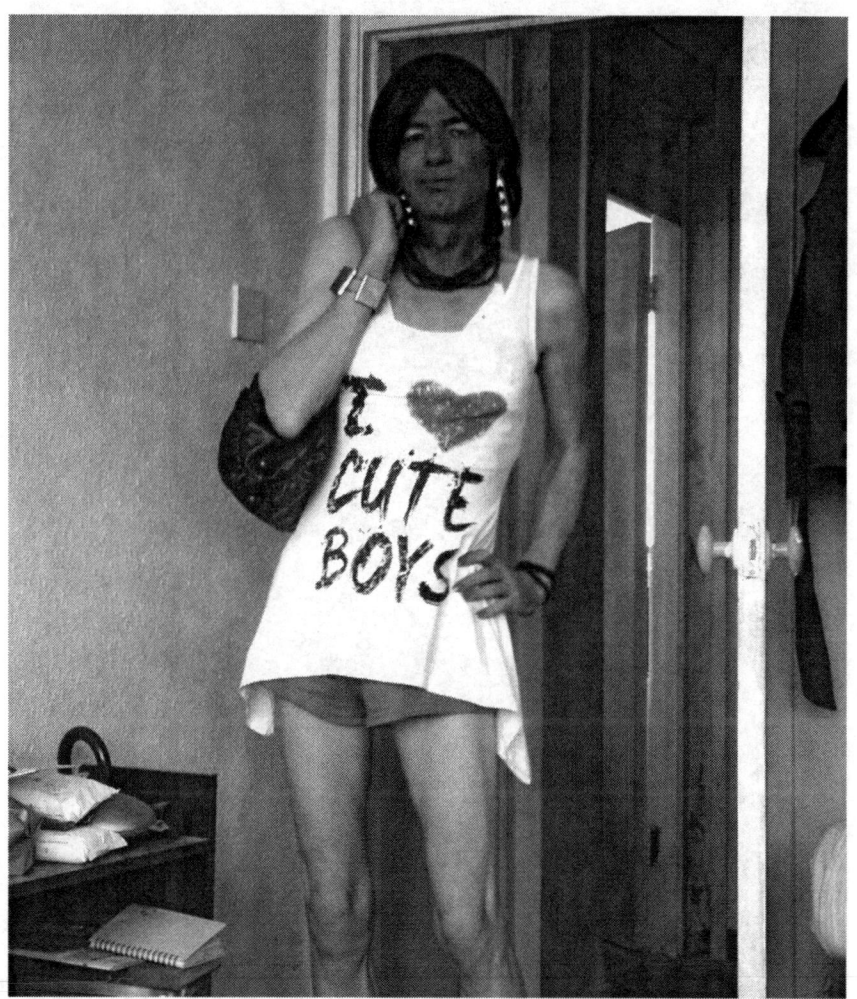

Officer Krupke

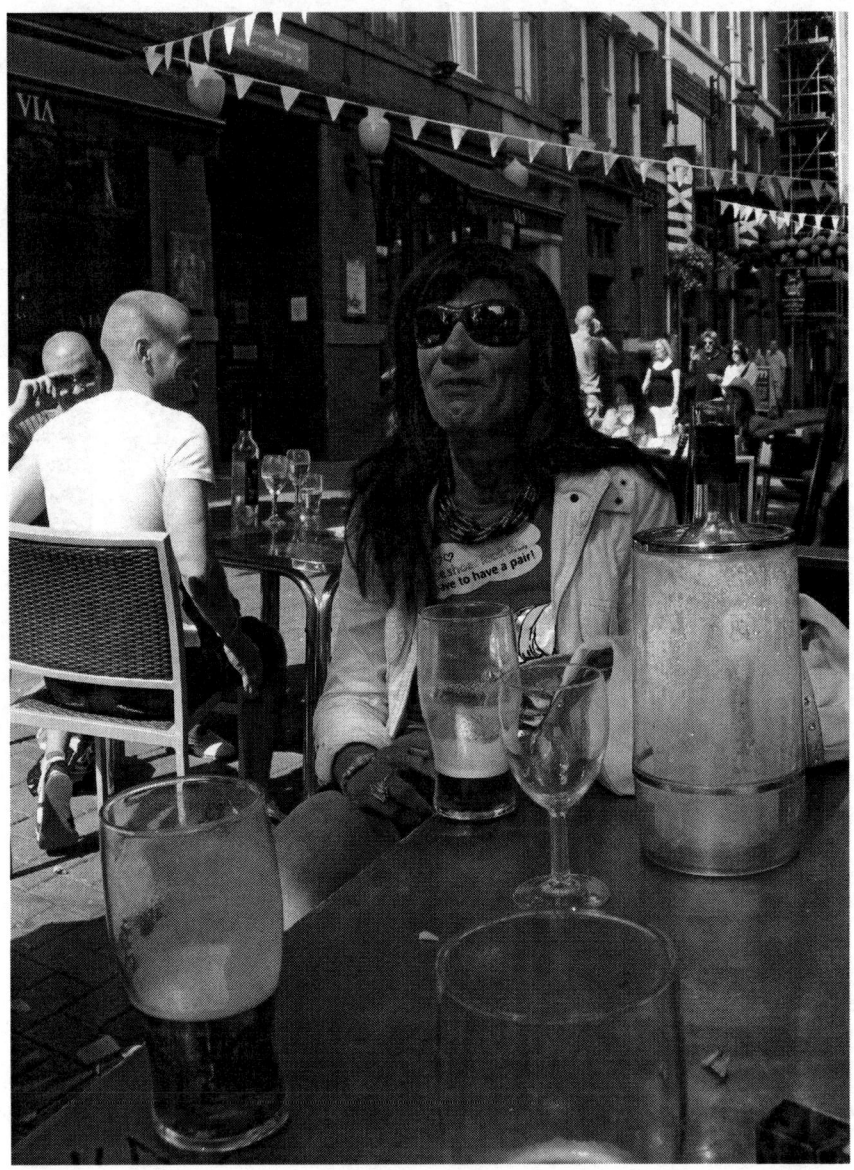

I enjoy being a girl

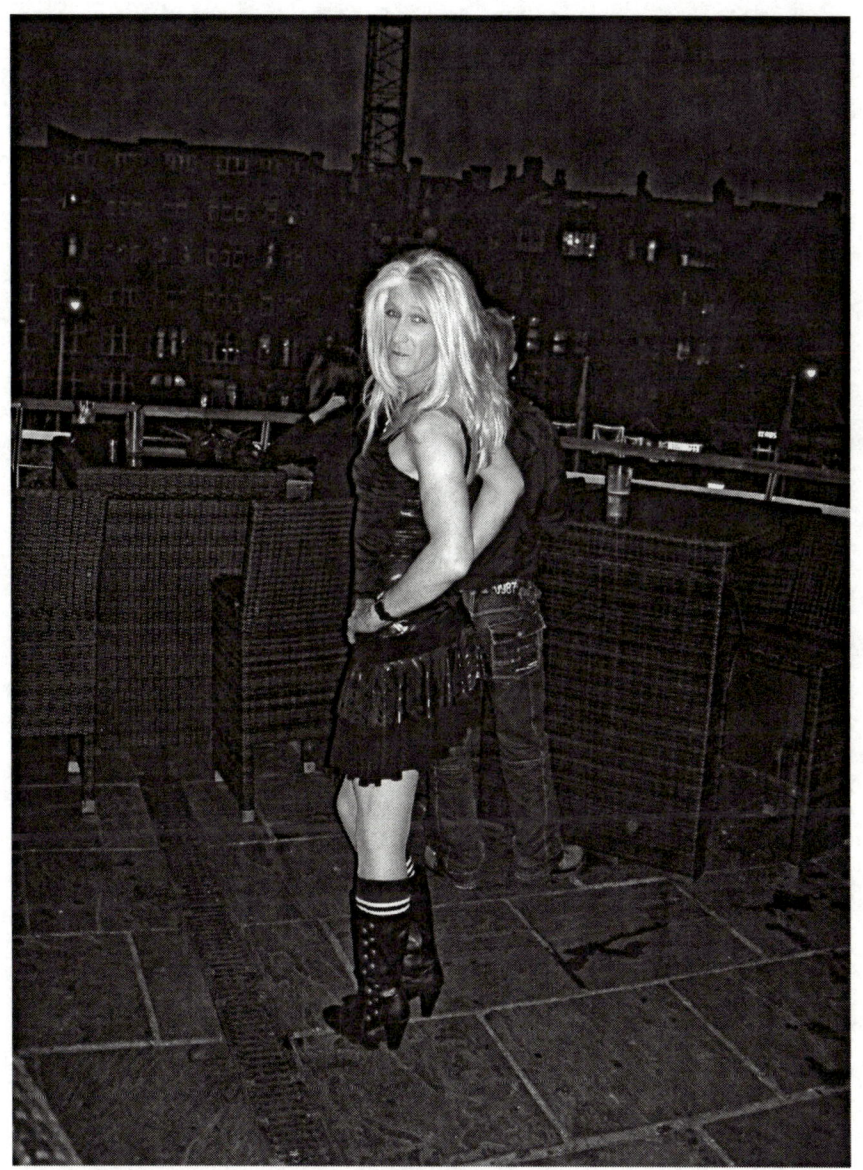

There is nothing like a dame

Tricia Dale

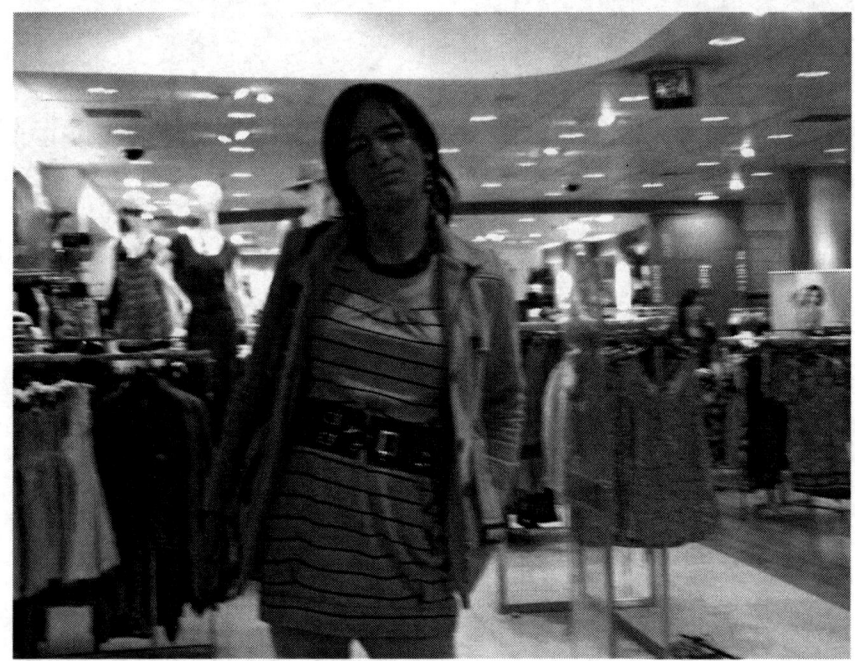

I had a dream

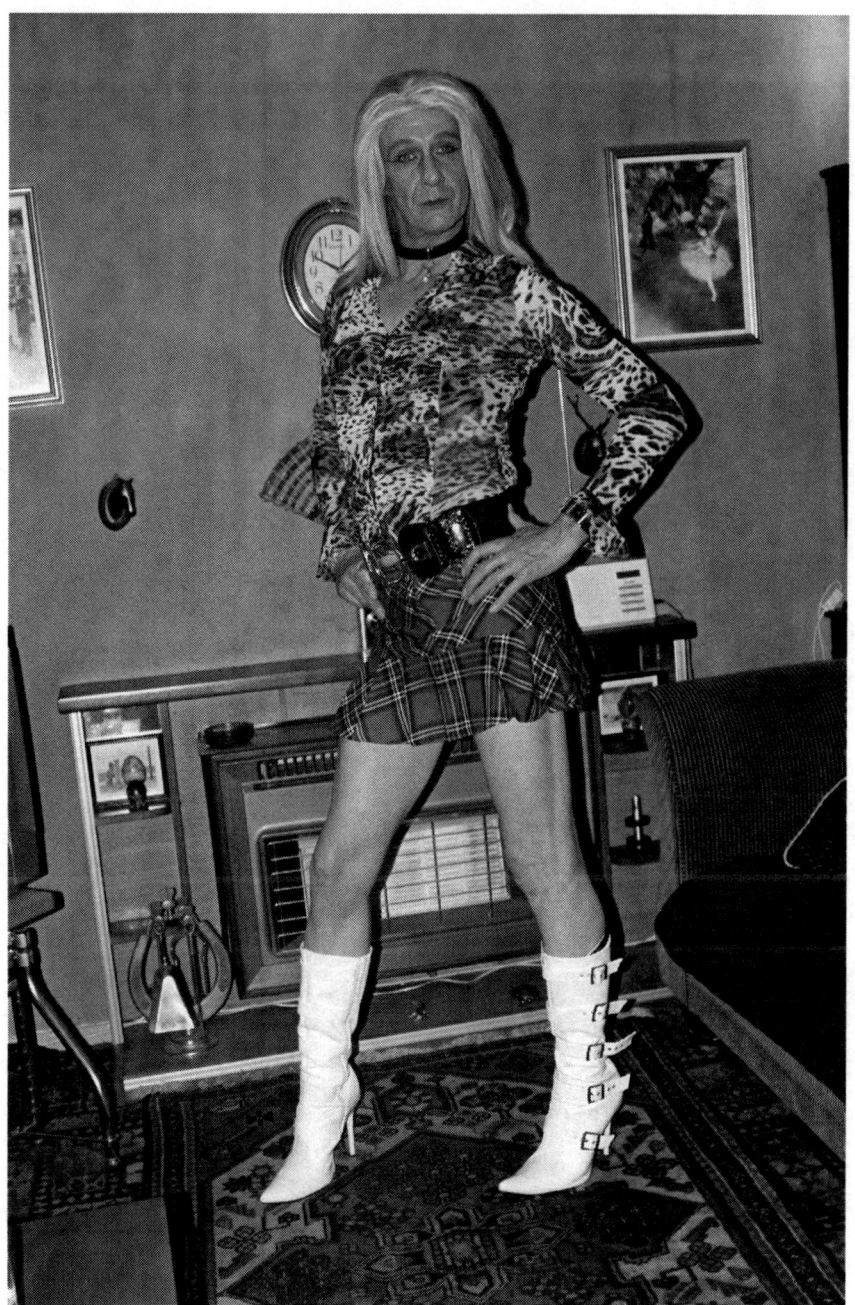

I do like to be beside the seaside

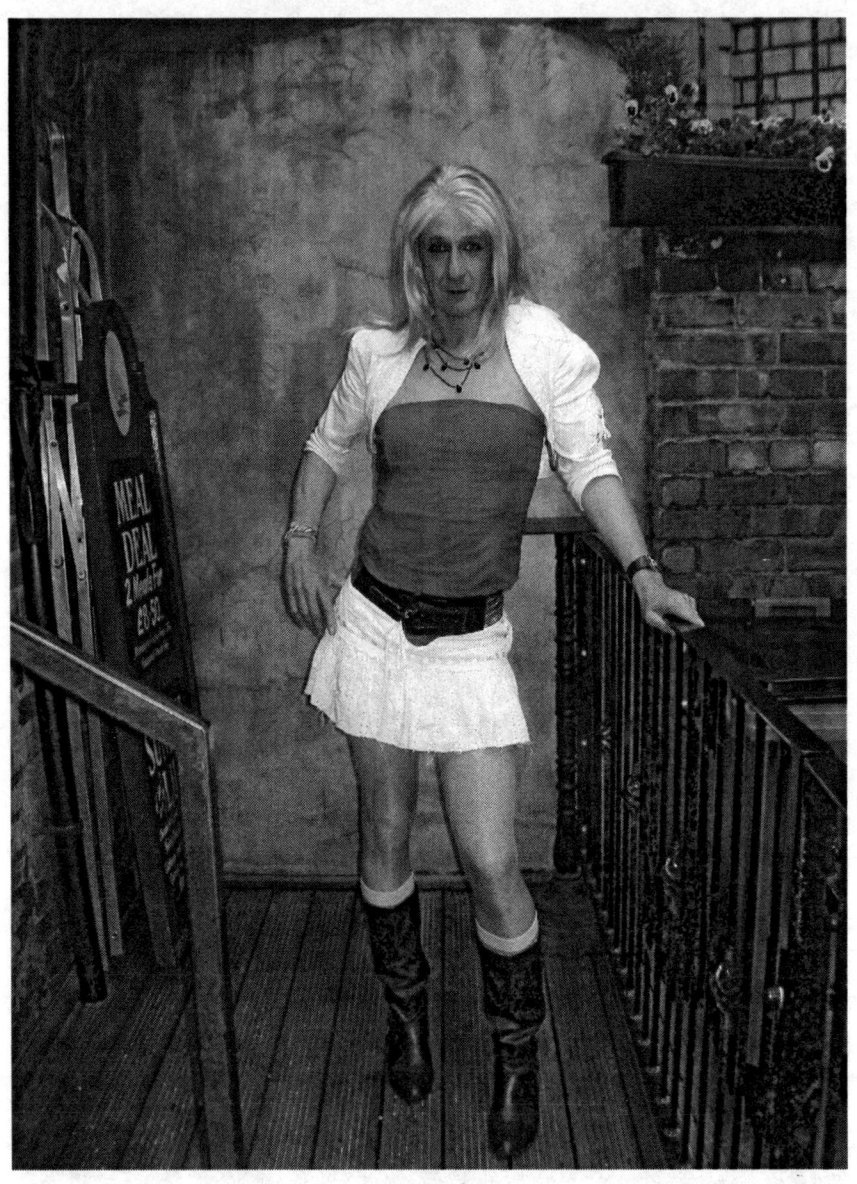

Friends

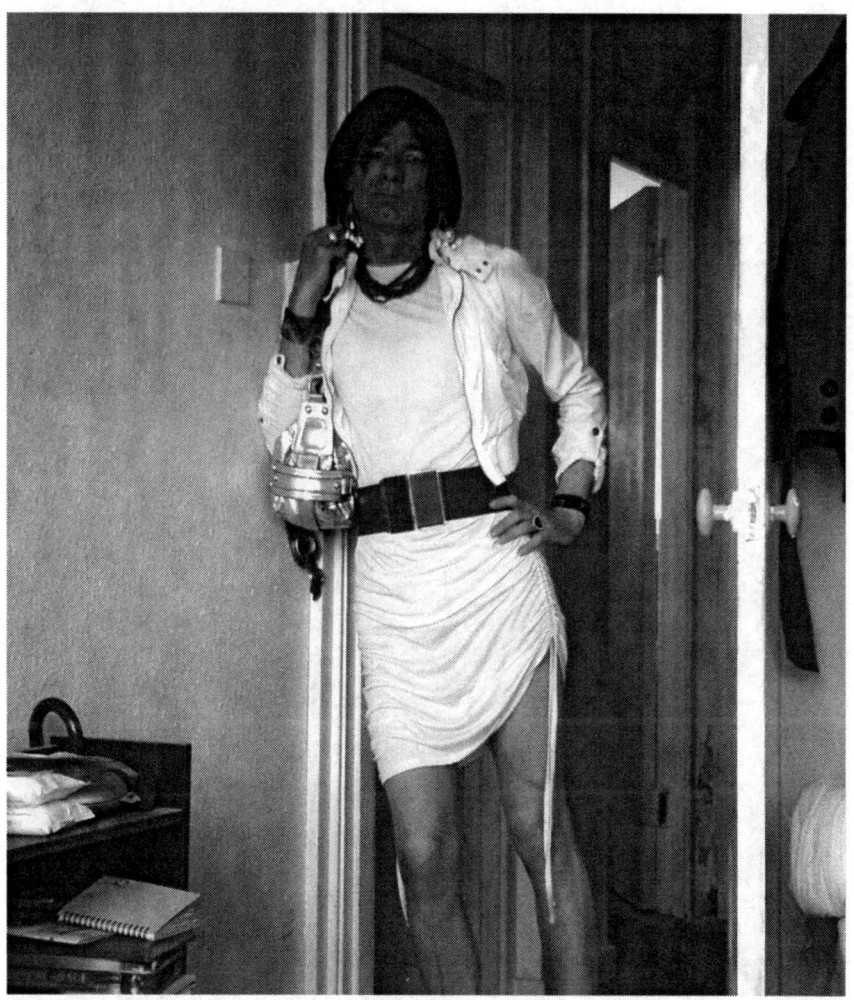

Pretty Woman

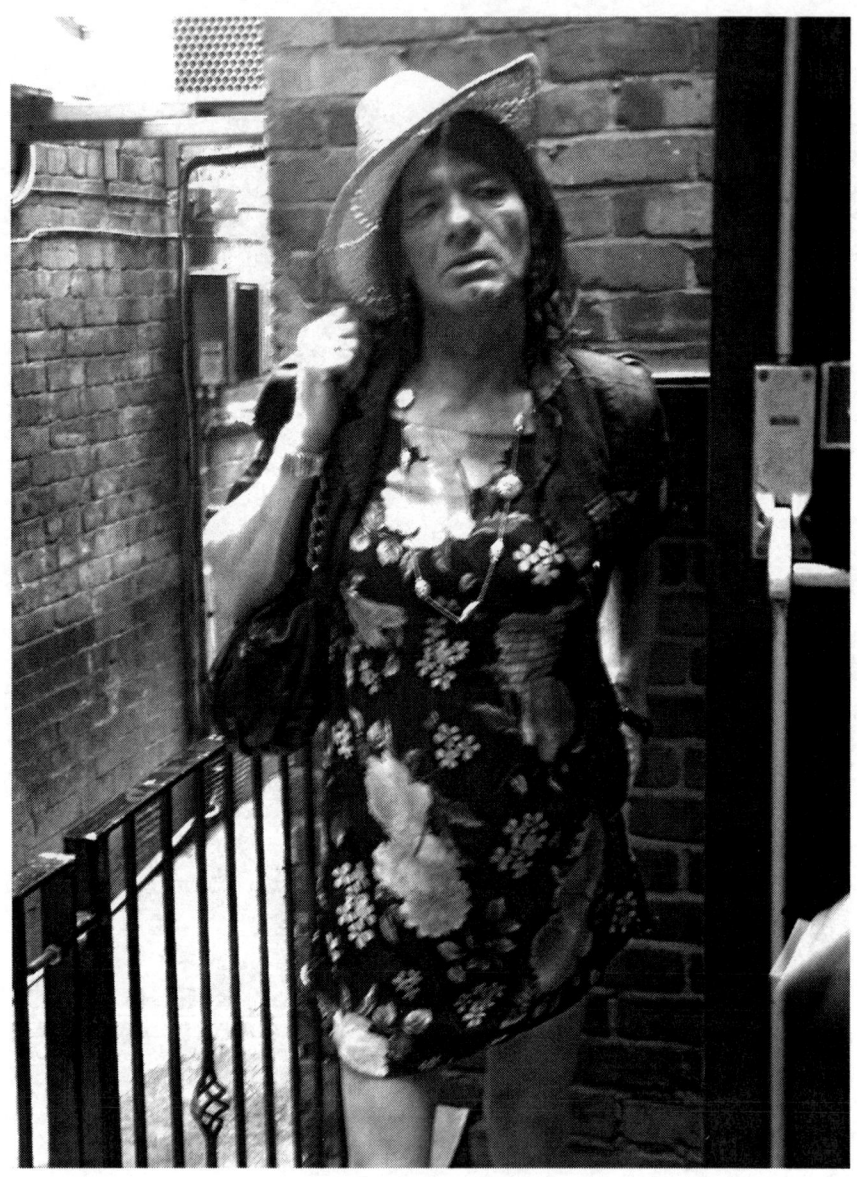

Easter Parade

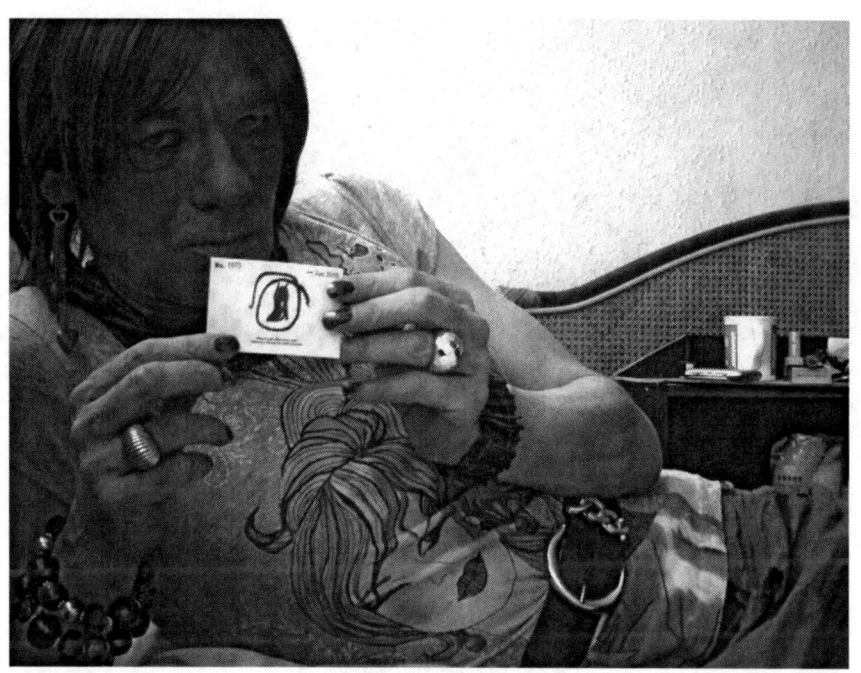

Suicide is painless

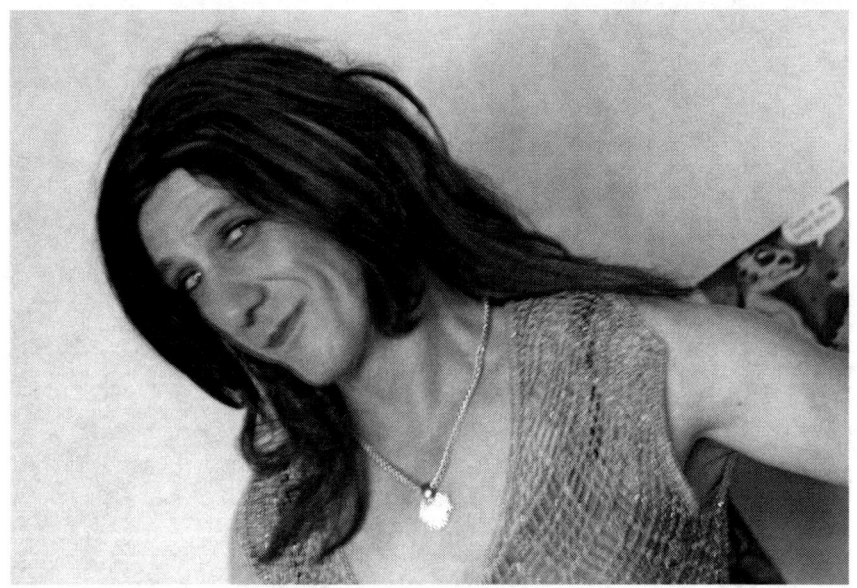

Mad Dogs and Englishmen

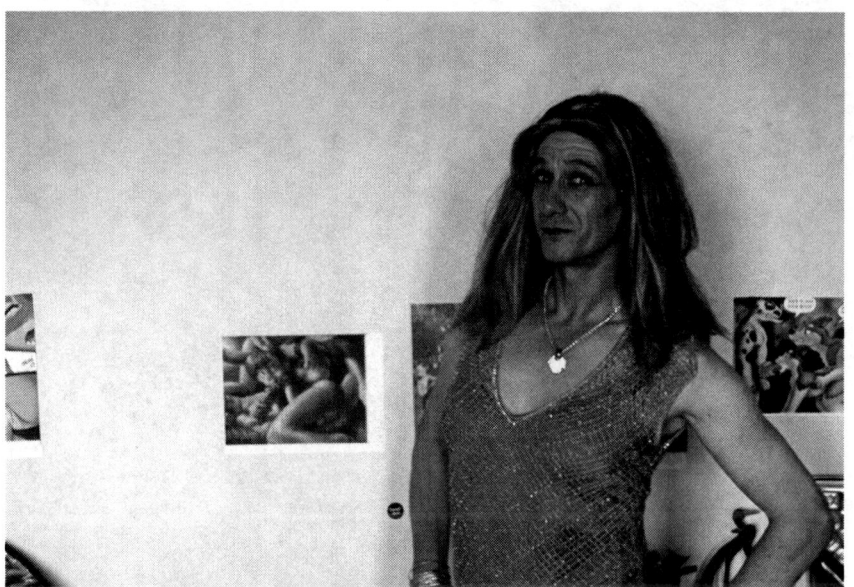

Ding Dong the witch is dead

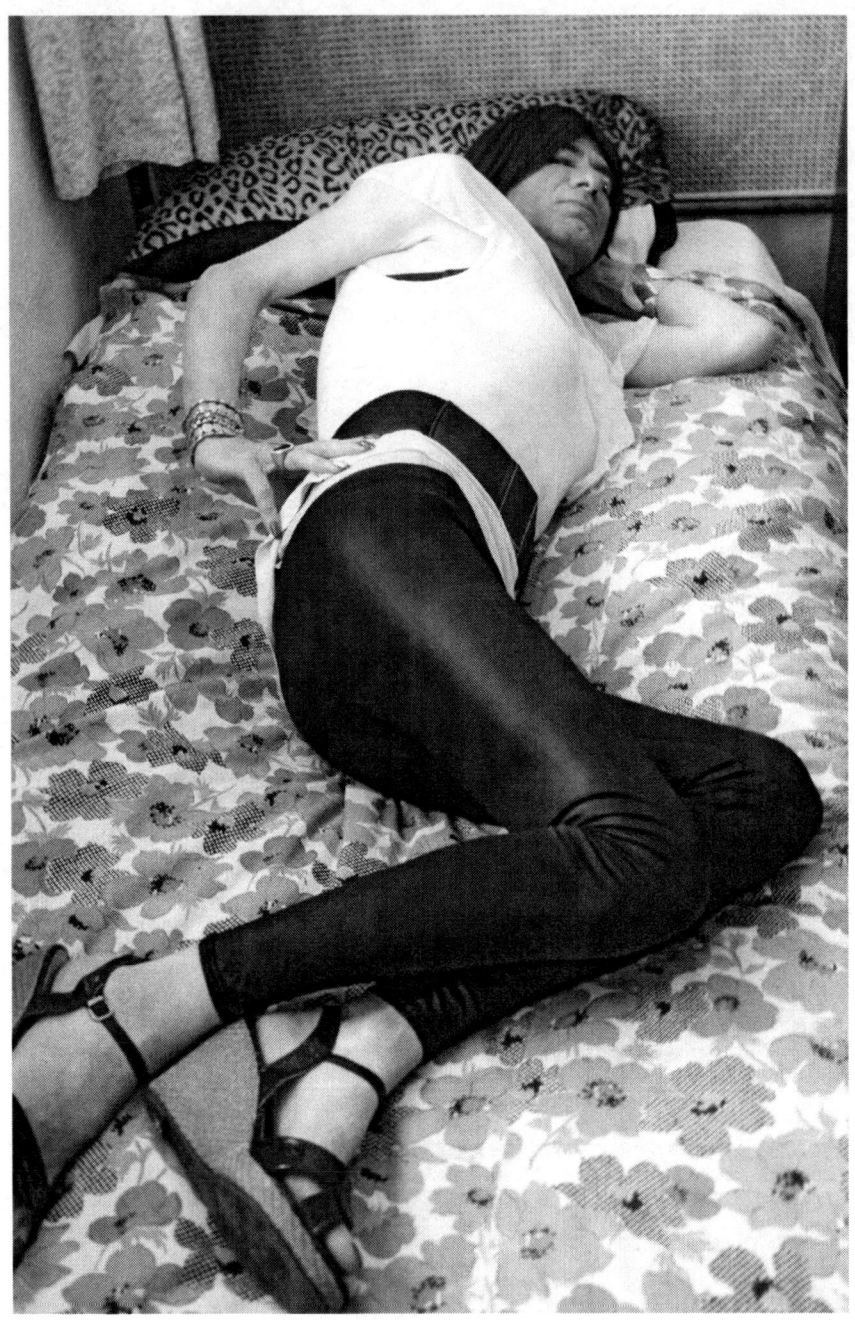

Cheek to cheek

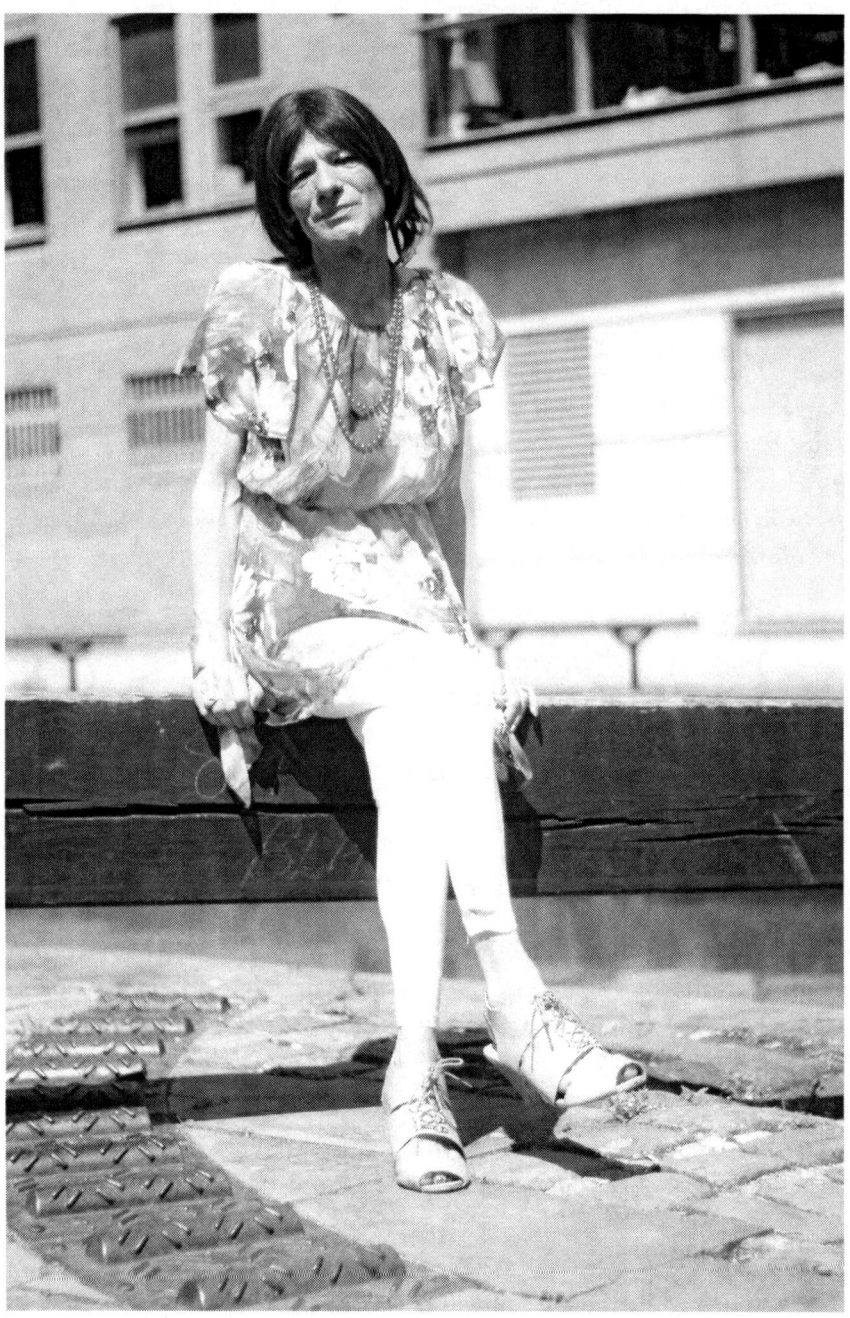

Always a Woman to me

Chapter 55

Bridge Over Troubled Water

Both Tina and I struggle to kill off relationships. I'm not sure why that is. Maybe its because we're that desperate, or maybe its just our girly side. I will leave things hanging, Tina will ignore them completely hoping they will go away. They don't of course, they just get worse. This weekend Tina as the birthday girl. By the way, and I'm sure there's more of this to come! Most of my life is spent in the village after all.

When youre weary, feeling small,
When tears are in your eyes, I will dry them all;
Im on your side. when times get rough
And friends just cant be found

Tricia the Peace-Maker, Tina the Inebriated Woman.

Despite worrying all week neither Tricia, nor myself, should have worried at all. Yes times are a changing, but just not as dramatically as we thought. Come Friday afternoon and Tricia was ready to travel. Megan sent her a text just after lunch.

"I am @ Paddy's already r u coming tonight"

"Am on my way. Are you still in Paddy's? Due at Piccadilly 17:05"

"I am here"

"See you in a while then. Trish will have 2 be patient"

"Aint she a saint?"

"Ha-ha, for now, tonight she hopes to be a sinner"

"From Saint to sinner in 3 easy steps, maybe 2"

"From Saint to sinner in 4 pints of Bombardier?"

"Hell I'm on Bombardier 4! Never fear"

"Then you must be a sinner too. Good, much more fun than being a Saint".

Tricia was to meet Megan and Becky, but not as Tricia. The easiest way was to go straight from the station rather than walking back to the flat, changing, and going in the reverse direction back to the pub. Tricia interrupted, you might say. She phoned Tina who was just starting to get ready after being at the flat since 15:00. What does she do? She could be forgiven however because today was her birthday.

The downside of drinking in the pub not as Tricia is that you do occasionally get propositioned by the rent boys as sadly happened to me that evening. Megan has been drinking all afternoon and slowly disintegrated leaving wife one to take wife two back safely. Tricia could become Tricia earlier than she thought. When Tina arrived at the pub all girls had gone which meant she was the only t-girl (or straight girl) around. Very rare for a Friday night.

Tricia literally flew back. Got changed in Tina's room where there was slightly better light, slapped on her make-up and flew back out again. She's becoming quite a decent bird. She hadn't noticed that Tina had set out a new make-up area for her.

Although she dressed, made-up and walked back in record time, she was too late for Paddy's so went straight to Naps. She got let in with no problems so the break must have done her good. She looked everywhere but no Tina. Very strange. Finally she returned to the middle bar to hand in her coat and get a drink. Sitting next to the bar was Tom. Tricia quickly put two and two together and, for once, got four.

"Hello Trish, have you seen Tricky?" Tricky was Tom's nickname for Tina.

"Hi hun, she may be locked in at Paddy's. I've noticed the doors are shut".

"She ain't, I've just been there".

Now Tom and Tina had fallen out. Well that's not totally accurate. Tina had fallen out with Tom but Tom was still carrying a torch for Tina. Tina considered Tom to be too possessive. Tricia tried to smooth things out. She sent Tina a text while she was talking to Tom. Not that talking was doing much good. Tom was going to flatten anybody who was with Tina. 'That's all I need' thought Tricia. She was still talking to Tom when when a half cut Tina arrived on the arm of someone who looked a bit like Bernie Ecclestone. Tom looked daggers. Tricia tried to smooth the troubled waters.

"Tom, he's older than you, he's smaller than you by over a foot, he's even got less hair than you. I can't imagine there's anything in it".

Tricia wasn't being entirely honest there. With Tina there is always something in it. There is always some ulterior motive. Tricia's phone beeped.

"See you in the downstairs ladies in two minutes".

Tricia duly excused herself to excuse herself and a frantic conversation ensued in the privacy of trap two, Napoleons, Manchester 1.

"Tina, you've got to sort this out. And who, on earth was that dwarf on your arm?"

"Its all right Trish, I reckon he's only got an hour to live, but he might already be dead from what I've seen. He's just camouflage for Tom".

"Camouflage for Tom? He's only five foot two for goodness sake! And he's not having my wardrobe."

"I need someone on my arm. I don't want to talk to Tom".

"I'm well aware of that but you've got to talk to him. You've got to tell him its over. He wants to knock the dwarfs block off".

"You not sorting out the limpet very well, are you. Anyway, how can you knock a corpse's block off".

"Fair point, bit of a waste of energy I suppose. You get hiding downstairs with the dwarf and I will try to sort Tom out. Then we will have some time to hatch a plan".

Tricia returned to Tom. Tina re-united with her friend.

"Tom, just leave it. I don't think Tina's interested at the moment. Necrophilia seems more on her mind". The comment was lost on Tom.

"Its getting late hun, get back home and have a good night. I don't think there'll be much action with Tina tonight".

"I think your right Trish, I'll just have one more beer".

Damn!

"I'll go and have a dance".

When Tricia returned forty minutes later, both Tom and Bernie Ecclestone had gone. She hoped there was no blood on the streets.

Still, it was Tina's birthday, Yay!

Tina's birthday, it appeared, consisted of drinking as much white wine and lemonade as she could and meeting as many blokes as she possibly could.

"Trish, I could have pulled anyone, but its my birthday and I want a drink".

"I can see that hon. But you will end up pulling no-one. Anyway you will be incapable so there will be no point".

"That's ok Trish, I've got some Viagra".

"Enjoy your birthday". Tricia smiled.

Tricia went up to dance again and danced as well as she ever had before. She was getting a lot of nice comments and plenty of dancing partners. Tina joined her.

"Trish, will you dance with me?" Tina slurred.

"Of course hon"

This was to prove difficult however.

Now Tina has a unique dancing style based on the hippy movement (her favourite era of course). She plants her two feet firmly on the floor and does weird things with her hands and body around them. This time she had a problem. She tried to plant her feet but she kept falling over backwards. It was the alcohol.

"I've found the solution Trish, look".

She had indeed. She had positioned herself about one foot from the wall and leaned backwards into it. She juggled her hands and shoulders a bit but the position was far from ideal for dancing. She had a big smile on her face so Tricia went downstairs for a smoke.

Half an hour later Tricia returned, she had got talking. Tina was in exactly the same position as when Tricia left her. Still with a smile on her face.

"Couldn't manage wall creep I see" said Tricia.

"No, but I feel great Trish".

"Want to go home yet?"

"Can you get me downstairs for a cigarette, then we can go home".

With extreme difficulty Tricia peeled Tina away from the wall and guided her carefully down the narrow stairs. They had their cigarette and went to get a taxi home.

The taxi dropped them just outside the flats but they had to walk across the lawn. It was about a seventy yard walk. Tricia let Tina go first just in case she fell over. Tina started off going in the wrong direction. Tricia called her back, she was enjoying this.

"Right hon, I will go first. Listen to my voice so you know which way to go".

With Tricia walking diagonally to the flat occasionally shouting 'Tina, this way', Tina zig-zagged across the grass covering about half a mile. It was definitely time for bed. No boing for either girl tonight. Tricia removed Tina's clothes, got her into bed and kissed her goodnight. Tomorrow was to be another day, but then isn't it always?

Chapter 56

There is Nothing Like a Dame

The easiest thing for me to do is to go into the pub, start talking to people and not leaving. Then going to Naps drunk. This weekend was like that and I must stop it. I want to be out in Manchester. That is one of the reasons I do what I do. There is a time for friends but also there needs to be a time for me to be myself. By the way, the song reflects the different types of ladies I meet, be they straight, t-girls or gay; of course I also love being a dame too. I love them all and I'm happy to be with them all. I think they are happy to be with me too, and that is brill.

> There is nothin' like a dame,
> Nothin' in the world,
> There is nothin' you can name
> That is anythin' like a dame!

Inebriated Tina again, and Inebriated Tricia too. Tricia discovers Tina has a lot of heart and she also overcomes one of her greatest fears.

Another Saturday and the girls get up at the crack of dawn. Another Saturday and the girls actually get up after Dawn has eaten her breakfast, lazed on the sunbed for an hour, got rid of her breakfast, and started on lunch. It was freezing cold but the girls did get up. Tricia needs some more winter clothes; she had to wear her red wool dress again with leggings and tights. Her utility outfit. If there's one thing Tricia is its utilitarian.

As she slowly awoke from her long deep sleep; Tricia noticed, in the corner of her Japanese eye, in the corner of the room, that Tina had set out what looked like a commode with a new make up mirror.

"Hey Tina, that's brill, thanks"

The commode seat was however against the wall and Tricia struggled to sit on it.

"But how do I sit on it? It's against the wall and I can't get my leg over the other side"

"For goodness sake Trish, you stupid bitch, you're a girl aren't you? Girls don't sit with their legs astride. Do it side-saddle".

Tricia, blushing furiously, did as she was told.

Tricia was struggling this morning; well this afternoon actually. Her boobs were causing her trouble again. Her right one had started to leak sticky silicone goo. It could have been her left one come to think of it; they were interchangeable. She decided it was her right and actually had some logic behind her decision for once. Logic which is about to be explained.

As we all know, Tricia is a resourceful girl, so she bought some sellotape and some sandwich bags (actually she had been tipped off about this, its helpful knowing other t-girls). She carefully sellotaped up the splitting boob, taking much more care than she ever did over Christmas presents, and wrapped it in the sandwich bag. Perfect! The one trouble was that when she fondled it , it made a sound rather like a soft sweet in a wrapper; though a soft sweet in a wrapper was pretty much what it was (as was she). It certainly wouldn't convince the guys very much. It was then she had the novel idea of always making it always her right boob. That way, when the guys wanted a quick fumble, she could turn herself to the right, offering up her left boob, which was fine. She didn't really want the bloke to feel a right tit, after all.

Tricia's breast region sorted the girls headed for town, which turned out to be more fun than usual. They were waiting for a cab at the usual place, near the lights, when they were spotted by a driver going far too fast. Tricia had seen the expression on his face many times before. Were they prostitutes? Where they transvestites? Just then the lights changed to red and the poor guy had to slam on his brakes, swerved all other the road, and there was a strong smell of burning rubber. The girls recognised it immediately.

"That's burning rubber", they said in unison and blushed. But not as much as the guy driving.

Having duly got their cab and been deposited outside Paddy's they were lighting up when some tramps over the road noticed them.

"You're not good girls are you?"

"What do you mean, were as good as gold!" Tricia was telling a half-truth again.

"We don't believe you".

"Remember to invest in gold in the current economic climate". Tina was pushing her luck.

"We'll invest in cider love, cheers!"

Inside the pub and who should be there. Why Megan and Becky of course. They all spent an age discussing the length of Megan's hair. Should she have it cut off?

"I'll cut mine off if you cut yours off" Ha-ha, only joking", the cheeky Aussie re-emerged.

"I think you would be happier if you did have it cut off", Tricia became serious.

"I am seriously thinking about it Tricia".

Tricia wonders what all the fuss is about. Megan normally has it tied back and anyway it will be hidden under one of those funny chef hat things. The thought of hers being cut off did make her shudder though, maybe Megan had a point after all. Some cuts go deeper than others.

Megan had picked up another new job which is located just over the road from t-Girl Towers. The girls have agreed to have a meal there soon and offer their professional judgement. I'm not sure Megan need worry too much. Tina has all her meals out of a can and Tricia doesn't eat at all, so I'm sure she'll be fine. Keep your hair on Megan.

Manchester United were playing on Setanta (also hopefully on grass, or not on grass – well you know what I mean) which Tina and Tricia wanted to watch. Tricia (and Tina) knew where you could get Setanta in Manchester pubs.

"Its ok Tina, we can go to the straight pub, its got a great atmosphere".

"I don't want to go to the straight pub Trish, I don't feel comfortable".

"Have you tried Coyotes"?, Becky came up with a solution. Sometimes it helps being a lesbian.

"Will we be safe?" Tricia would sooner be in a straight bar than a lesbian bar where some of the girls scared her to death. They had muscles she could only dream of (actually she doesn't) and sometimes look down on t-girls like her.

"You will be fine", Becky laughed.

Tricia needn't have worried. She very much liked Coyotes. Even though there was no bitter on draught for her, she wasn't bitter. There was however a very chilled atmosphere, cushions spread all around the bar, two big screens to watch the football and a pool table in the middle of the room. The lesbians she talked to were friendly and fun (though she certainly wouldn't want to get in a fight with some of them) and seemed quite happy to have Tina and Tricia amongst them. It was probably good that we both supported Man U though, and even better than Man U won comfortably. Tricia wonders whether she should be supporting Woman U but quickly realised that she actually does, in her own way.

Back to Paddys, back to Naps and Tricia thinks she has wasted the weekend. Both girls get drunk again. Tina again chats up man after man without actually pulling.

"Tina, its the same as last night, I think we need a new plan".

"Trish, I'm not worried about tonight, lets relax and have fun. I'm happy, you seem to be too".

So they did and Tricia got intrigued by Armanda, a genuine girl, who seemed to be intrigued by Tricia. Tricia had to go home the following day to get in to work early on the Monday. She did, but she is thinking hard.

Chapter 57

Uninvited

By the way, this is my danger song. Dum Dum Dum Dum. It is from the film City of Angels but I have spent hours dancing to the disco version of it. It has helped give me my strength and my confidence. It comes into my head when I think, see or hear anything that may harm me. It is also relevant now because I have become much more choosy with who I go with. I think I'll leave the story to explain how things are changing for me in other areas too. Maybe I'm growing up at last?

One thing I have noticed which pleases me, is that I've seen a number of girls wearing outfits and carrying handbags exactly like mine. These girls are young, sexy, chic and trendy; just like me :)

> But you you're not allowed
> You're uninvited
> An unfortunate slight

Dum Dum Dum Dum

Tricia was right to be worried a couple of weeks ago; but not over-worried. What was happening was always going to happen. She can see it now, it was natural. Tricia now understands the law of diminishing returns; it's easy. The first time you buy a dress dressed you are both very nervous and very high. When you have accomplished it you are positively euphoric. The second time you buy a dress dressed you still feel brilliant but not quite as high as the first time. The fiftieth time you buy a dress you're still happy but the thrill, the excitement is diminished. The same is true of walking around town, of going to straight bars, of anything you do.

Tricia was discussing it with Tina at the weekend.

"The trouble is Tina, I don't get the same buzz of excitement any more; I don't greatly anticipate doing things as a girl that I did. I have done them all before, I can do them all again. Also, the more I do it, the better I become, the better I pass and therefore the less fun it is."

"Well Trish you did go a bit mad last year. I'm finding things difficult too. The weather is so cold and it gets dark so early".

"Although those things are true, I can't use them as an excuse. The fact of the matter, I think, is that I am going through a different phase of my life where I suspect I need to consolidate being myself. It won't be as much fun but I still love wearing dresses and make-up so it shouldn't be a problem".

"Maybe you should not do it for a while. Maybe stay at home a few weeks. Then you can see if the fun will come back".

"I could try Tina, but I don't think it will make any difference. I will still know that I can and have pretty much done everything I want to".

"What, gone into the Stretford end dressed?"

"Dum dum dum dum there are limits to everything Tina. Safety is the most important thing for both of us. I just have to get used to this new stage of my life. Maybe I will take a couple of weeks off, I need to get a grip of things at home in any case. Two things I am definitely looking forward to though. Some warmth, and not having to do my make-up by candlelight".

"It will be a while before that will happen Trish".

When the weather gets warmer Tricia will return to Liverpool again. She will try to get to the Halls of Residence I used to stay in. That will be a big challenge for her. She also needs to go back to the theatre. The theatre is good for her. She will find out what's on when and where. She suspects though she is a little blasé with it all and that is showing in her manner. This weekend, like last, she went back home on the Sunday. She did not dress even though the weather was good for the time of year; quite mild and no rain. The problem she has though is that it is extremely difficult to go back to work in drab when you have to take your nail varnish and make-up off by candlelight. Its actually easier putting them on in the dark than it is taking them off.

Tina nudged Tricia. "What about sex Trish, surely that is still exciting".

"I'm much more choosy now Tina, I turned down a guy last night for example".

"Why?"

"Well for one thing he was only five foot four, and for another he smelled".

"That's not his fault"

"The smelling probably is although I do understand it can be hereditary. Anyway, I didn't want to bring back a half cut dwarf who smelt of stale socks for him to fumble and grope me".

"I would have"

"You were too drunk yourself. Ha ha, it would have been the blind drunk leading the blind drunk. I had to help you out of the taxi last night".

"Did you? Damn".

Tricia now understands that the law of diminishing returns doesn't work with drugs. That is why she and Tina find it so hard to stop drinking and smoking. She has heard that the first 'e' you take is the best ever, and she has only taken one, but hard drugs frighten her, they make her sing dum dum dum dum. Tricia also understands that Tina is a transvestite and that for people like her, sex is also a drug.

Tricia returned to the conversation.

"I'd probably have to help him .... No, I won't go there, suffice it to say that it was probably best all round that you two didn't meet".

"But I didn't pull again!"

"Never mind hon, there is always tonight".

"I never pull on a Saturday night".

"You never know what will happen tonight. That bit of it is still fun".

Actually Tina may well have pulled on the Saturday night. We just don't know yet. The trouble was that it was with a straight girl. The other trouble was that it was with the only person in the nightclub more drunk than Tina. Who knows what, if anything will develop?

Tricia will definitely be around to find out though. She also needs to find out who dezauk is. Tricia can't remember but she found the email address in her notebook. On the drinking front she is far from whiter than white herself.

Dum dum dum dum.

Tricia growing up?

Chapter 58

When You're Smiling

I think I get it it! This bit of my life is all about learning to be who I am, not getting to where I want be.. I experimented on Sunday. I got out over the weekend as I said I would. I got some dead sexy sparkly gold leggings for the dancing queen, Tricia. Walking back from my shopping I imagined I was a supermodel (well, I've got the figure) and not a t-girl. Loads of people smiled at me and I smiled back. It was great. So, and by the way, its back to a smiling song. Its all about attitude and all about smiling. When Iain was young he used to love the program this song introduced, so I'm sure he'll support me.

> When youre smilin....keep on smilin
> The whole world smiles with you
> And when youre laughin....keep on laughin
> The sun comes shinin through

Tricia goes back to basics.

Saturday was Valentines Day. That was not lost on Tricia as she headed back to Manchester on the Friday evening. She was going to buy a Valentines Card and give it to some lucky man on Saturday night. I will leave the 'it' to your own imagination. Things didn't go entirely to plan however and Tricia still has the card. It reads:

It is a matter of fact that a young lady with a vigorous sexual appetite will burn through an enormous quantity of calories over the course of a 'romantic' evening ......

.... it is therefore essential that the consumption of large quantities of expensive chocolates should be considered as foreplay.

Inside was '*Happy Valentines Day*'. I will leave the 'it' to your own imagination.

Looking sexy as ever in her blue dress, Tricia went out to have a cigarette at the back of Paddies, and who should she bump into. It was Eric. Eric had just come back from Gran Canaria.

"My darling, how lovely to see you". Eric was as ever polite, but also as ever, drunk.

"Eric hun, I thought you were brown bread". Tricia was as ever subtle.

They talked and they kissed. Eric's hand again disappearing where no hand should ever go, but at least Tricia's backside warmed up.

"Darling Trish, I want to say those three little words, but I daren't. I have been thinking about you all the time while I've been abroad".

Tricia knew precisely what the three little words were, but was totally unprepared.

"I am going back to Gran Canaria, I know your circumstances, and I will wait for you, however long it takes."

Tricia was now totally taken aback (a position she was used to).

"Hon, you have to give me some time to think it through. Life isn't easy at the moment".

Eric did tell Tricia those three little words. He did tell Tricia he loved her. Tricia went back into the pub and Eric couldn't find her. Tricia was in a bit of a whirl. Tina reported that he had walked out looking totally devastated. Tricia went out to find him but he was gone. She doesn't wish to hurt people but she does need time to think. She felt sad. She did buy the valentines card for Eric but was not to see him again during the weekend. She hopes he is ok, she's sure he is and she thinks there's more to come. We'll see.

She rejoined Tina (well Tina is a joiner after all), who tried to take her mind off it, and certainly succeeded.

"You'll never guess what I did on Thursday Trish".

Tricia knew that whatever Tina did on Thursday would have a sexual connotation.

"I'm all ears hon".

"That makes a change. Well, you know outside Georgina's is a red light district".

"Yeeeesssss"

"Well, I walked it. And guess what, I pulled!"

"Did he know what you were?"

"Yes, but it didn't worry him".

"And ....."

"I got into his car".

"I thought you weren't supposed to do that!"

"Its ok, he was a gentleman".

"Tina, you don't meet gentlemen!"

"He drove away to a safe place, he had obviously done this before. I felt safe, and fine".

"And ....."

"It was great, I started off by ...."

"I don't wish to know the gory details. I probably already know the gory details. How much did you charge him?"

"That's it, I didn't, because I'm new. But it proves I can pull a guy".

"You were probably right not to charge Tina"

"I was desperate for it Trish. When he dropped me back there were loads of others, I could have done it again".

"Oh Tina!"

"I may need another outlet. I'm getting no work".

"Not that surely Tina, its fraught with danger. Did you use a condom?"

"We did to start off with".

"Oh Tina. Tina, Tina, Tina!"

Then who should appear. It was the limpet and Tricia got very cross with him.

"Never, never, bombard me with phone calls and text messages when I am at work. If you don't know my position you do now". This certainly wasn't Tricia's normal position.

"Sorry Trish but I needed you."

"No! You wanted me there and then. But I was not there and I need some time for then. You're going to have to be very patient now".

"I know, I'm sorry".

Tricia knows he is going to have to be a lot more patient than he thinks. No valentines card for the limpet.

Onto Naps and Tricia bumps into the three dead sexy Puerto Rican TS's.

"Its Mama! Hi Mama"

Tricia is not so sure about being called Mama. But then with three such attractive daughters? They danced and chatted together. They had a great time.

Georgina was off to Berlin, the sex capital of Europe, on Sunday so the girls met her for an early drink. I'll rephrase that, Tricia met her for an early drink; Tina, as ever, wasn't ready in time. Nobody needed to worry though because the girls from Birchplace were in town. Early drinks however play on Tricia's mind now so she only had a couple, well three, well four... and then had the common sense to go into town. YAY Tricia, at last you know what's good for you. She wanted to get her eyebrows waxed but was too late. Too long in the pub again but at least she was out there where she should be. She had a great shop, earmarked some stuff she wanted to buy, had a coffee (she loves doing that) and went back to Paddys. Tina had moved on to play pool and when she returned she was far more drunk than

Tricia. Eventually Tricia had to get her in a cab but she got home safely. They knew the driver.

Tricia, after even more beers again, went into Naps. She should not have been let in. She was too drunk. She met Mark, Glenda and Jade; spilled a drink over Jade and decided to go back to T-Girl Towers. Walking back past the cinema she fell over. Her right tit remained in tact but there were titters all round. Tricia, behave yourself. But at least she showed a little common sense, going home when she did.

Tricia decided to stay on the Sunday, the first time for a while. Tina was struggling for money so went back to her parents. Sunday was not baking hot, but warm enough, so Tricia could dress at least a little bit sexy. She was determined to do some shopping around town so she paced herself. Only three pints in Paddys then fly girl. Guess what. Half way through her third pint , having got rid of Tom (nicely), Ray and Phil walk in.

"Darling Trish, that's the best I've seen you" said Ray.

"You can't be drunk already Ray. I'm not really sure about this outfit". Tricia was wearing her denim dress.

"Denim suits you Trish". Even Paul, who was normally as cynical as anything agreed.

Tricia cut her losses, had one more beer, agreed to meet up later in Coyotes, where she knew she was safe and went off shopping.

"Remember", said Phil "When your smiling .... the whole world smiles with you".

"Trish knows" said Ray "she's sound".

"I know" said Trish, smiling.

Tricia really enjoyed her shop. On the way there she met three young, pretty girls in their early twenties.

"Your beautiful"

"Your gorgeous", Tricia was worried, they were taking the piss,

"You show us freedom and what people can do", Tricia need not have worried, they were not.

They all kissed and Tricia marched on. She eventually found a great shop. Everything upstairs under a tenner and she saw some dead sexy gold leggings. She had to have them. She asked the assistant if she could try them on. No worries. Plenty of worries getting them on though, they were completely lycra, but she did. Dead sexy they were too. She found a blue woollen dress to go with them, white handbag, gold flats, she had another sexy Saturday night outfit and a blue dress she could use in other ways. Go Trish go! Very Abba, she needs a little hat to go with it she thinks, but next time. Tricia will truly be the dancing queen!

Walking back from the shops Tricia changed the way she thought about herself. She imagined herself as a super model. Not too to far a flight of fancy since she has the stature and the figure for it. She stood up as straight as she could. Following all the dancing she was doing, her hips were moving right and the rest of her body was following. She walked past three black guys at the corner of Picadilly Gardens.

"Hi beautiful", one said.

Tricia turned, winked and smiled.

The guys winked back, and smiled.

Tricia understood. This part of her life was about getting used to her own skin. It will be different, it may not be as much fun, but there is definitely fun there to be had. Enjoy being yourself Tricia.

Chapter 59

I Have a Dream

Having missed last weekend I was literally itching to be myself again. I wanted to be out and about, to go into town, to try on clothes: to be myself, Tricia. Men and sex aren't as important to me now, although that Limpet still won't leave me alone. Tina was skint and had arranged to meet a bloke anyway so I was on my own and that suited me. By the way, I had Abba on my mind for various reasons and have already used dancing Queen, so .... and you know this already

> I believe in angels, something good in everything I see
> I believe in angels when I know the time is right for me

In which Tricia flies solo again, evades the Limpet, buys some more sexy clothes and survives agonising pain.

Tricia was awoken at half past five in the morning by a very drunk limpet. No, it was a text message. Needless to say she didn't answer it. Five voice mail messages later she understood that he loved his sweetie-pie. How will his sweetie-pie respond? We shall see later. She has another fling going on with what seems like a nice guy from Burton-on-Trent (where they brew beer Tricia likes). Internet only for now but she can see some mileage. He likes Gilbert & Sullivan so Tricia is on common ground; but she will see. She knows not to get over-excited where the internet is concerned.

She had missed not being Tricia the previous weekend and wanted to make for it. The kids had gone to London so I took the Friday off work. A leisurely journey up, change in the light for once and a few beers sounded good. But then Tricia's phone lit up and her ring tone, Dancing Queen by Abba of course, started to play. It was Tina and because it was Tina there was bound to be a problem of one sort or the other.

"Trish, what time will you be up?"

"Just after lunch, about two, why?"

"I have a problem".

"You have more than one problem hon".

"No Trish, the gas man's coming".

"I bet he's enjoying himself. Have you given him some of that Viagra stuff?"

"No stupid, he is coming to check for gas".

"Well he is a gas man I suppose". Tricia thought for once.

"But hang on, we haven't got any gas; apart from the camper gas which always blows up in my face".

"I know that you daft cow. But they have to check for leaks anyway. He will be here between twelve and four. I will be at the flat at twelve but I need to get out, I'm meeting Graham".

"So do I need to get out. That's why I've taken the day off".

"Can you man the fort if he doesn't turn up until after two".

"Man the fort? You're talking to Tricia not Rambo!".

"You know what I mean. More like Bimbo not Rambo!".

"Well, I can tiptoe around the flat looking dead girly in my skimpies if that counts as manning the fort".

"That's all you have to do, and you'll need some time to get ready anyway".

"Leave it with me, I wonder if he likes oral?"

"So Bimbo will man the fort?".

"Bimbo will be up for two, yes hon".

Tricia got to the flat at 14:15. Sadly the gas man had already been but, according to Tina who wasn't yet dressed as Tina, hadn't come.

"Pity he hadn't waited for Bimbo" said Tricia who was a little disappointed. The thought of Tricia opening the door in her undies to a startled gas man amused her. Never mind, there will be other times.

Tina had an appointment with a man she met on the internet from Sale. The irony of this fact being that she wasn't selling. So Tricia was free to be herself. Both girls free? That can't surely last.

Tricia carefully got ready. She put on her turquoise wool dress for the first time. She looked at herself in the mirror. As ever she looked divine, but what were those things above her eyes? Were they caterpillars? Did they move? She knew what she had to do but was not going to get them waxed this time. She was going to try something else. She popped into Debenhams but there was nobody at the counter. "Back in twenty minutes" the sign said, so Tricia checked that the shop shut late and went looking for a sexy green top to go with her skin-tight gold leggings. She wanted to be like the tone on her mobile on Saturday night. She wanted to be, as well as dance the part of the dancing Queen on Saturday night. As if to remind her of that fact her phone woke up.

"You can dance, you can dance having the time of your life".

It was the limpet. Tricia left it ringing, the limpet left a message.

"Can I see you at yours, or you can come here. You have my address".

Tricia, having bought a dead sexy green dress which zipped up the front for easy entry and presumably unzipped at the front for easy exit, kept her calm and replied thus.

"Martin, if you want to meet me then I suggest you arrange something neutral. My flat is shared with Tina and has no heat so its not a good idea. I'm not averse to going back to yours but lets meet up first. Be sober! I am in Manchester now looking gorgeous. Text me only, my phone battery won't last".

After that message, Tricia's thumbs were sore (a novel experience for her) and she was struggling to eat her cheese and ham toasty in the Arndale when ...

"You are the Dancing Queen, Young and sweet, only seventeen".

Well, sometimes you really do need to use your imagination.

It was another plea from the Limpet. Tricia texted back thus:

"Hon, I've given you some rules so follow them. You need to meet me first. I'm getting my eyebrows done shortly then will go to Paddy's. Maybe see you later, hugs Trish xx".

Tricia is not such an easy lay; not as far as the limpet is concerned in any case. For the record, Tricia was not to meet up with the limpet all weekend.

Tricia returned to Debenhams and was positioned in a comfortable reclining leather chair. Now threading is where the girl takes two strands of cotton and literally pulls the hair out of the roots using them. The right eye was no problem, Tricia was being very brave, as we know she always is.

"I'm just dropping you down now dear". The seat reclined as it was told to do.

The left eye was agonising. Tricia could hear the hair being ripped away by the roots. She gritted her teeth and survived. Its was worth it. She had arched, feminine eyebrows again. She could just about get away with them at work, she knew that, but that was good enough.

Back in Paddy's sipping a well deserved pint she received a text from Becky. They arranged to meet for Saturday lunchtime and have a meal at Megan's bistro. Tricia would have to be careful tonight so she would be up for it. She did go to Naps, but only for an hour. She was a good girl! But then we know that too; don't we?

Chapter 60

Food Glorious Food

Yay, Iain's letting me write this one. Tricia the food critic? Whatever next! So, by the way, this one is too easy.

> Food, glorious food!
> We're anxious to try it.
> Three banquets a day --
> Our favourite diet!

Tricia Eats for Once

The binary chop sits underneath a large residential block of apartments, generally populated by the young, aspiring middle classes. It is not a place where I would expect particularly good food or service but I was pleasantly surprised with the quality of the food. It is slightly out of Manchester, to the South, but is well worth a visit while the presiding chef is in occupation.

My charming companion Ms Rebecca and I managed to find some seats and looked around the Bistro to take in the atmosphere. We could smell food cooking in the kitchen which heightened our appetites. Behind us, the big screen showing Sky Sports 1 was turned off, to be replaced by some very loud, heavy music on the loudspeakers. Behind the bar Will and Grace, yes they were actually called Will and Grace, were working with a purpose. The purpose being to finish their shift and get off home as quickly as they could.

The seating area was bright and clean. Although the Bistro was far from full at this time, late Saturday afternoon, the busy tapping of people on their laptops could be heard between the songs. Rebecca and I decided to forego a starter, and we both opted for the cheeseburger. We were quite full up from hops consumed earlier on.

The aperitifs to get us started were excellent. The small glasses used to serve Rebecca's gin and tonic and my pernod ensured we had the precisely the correct amount of alcohol prior to the meal. The ice used was in excellent condition. It had been expertly frozen and tasted cold, though pleasantly slippery on the tongue.

The cheeseburgers arrived in good time. Presented on two plates, the burgers were of generous proportions, underpinned on a bed of salad and topped with a healthy portion of English cheddar cheese. The food did indeed look good enough to eat. The taste was exquisite. The crunch of the onions perfectly complemented the smoothness of the mince, giving a rounded, grounded flavour which was a delight to savour. There was a pleasant after-taste which worked perfectly with the accompanying French fries; small, slender and cooked to perfection. Very different from the salty, creamy diet I am used to in other areas of this cosmopolitan city. The burgers really tasted exactly like my Mother used to make them in the sixties and seventies. When burgers were burgers not McDonald's.

I found out that my charming companion, Rebecca, had a great love of modern art; something unfortunately lacking in myself as you will know if you have read my earlier columns. Rebecca put the two burger buns together having topped the burger with a large dollop of the delicious tomato chutney served as an accompaniment. She bit into the heavenly concoction. I immediately noticed a change in the ambience of the place. On the wall beside us appeared a beautiful bright red hue, like the sun going down. It reminded me a lot of Rothcoe. It was perfect for the atmosphere of the bistro. It fitted the surroundings ideally. My companion had left her mark, and the place was the better for it.

We were lucky enough to be joined at the table by chef, Megan Van Dyke and we complemented her on her culinary skills. I was a little alarmed about the length of her hair, surely too long for a top chef, but she assured me it is always tied back. I think this is a young chef who can go far, but whether this particular bistro is the right place for her to showcase her abilities is debatable. While she is in residence though, I have no hesitation in recommending a visit. It is, after all, the food that matters.

Service 3 (Will wasn't willing and Grace didn't appear to know her name, so didn't say it)

Atmosphere 2/3 (White, bright and modern. I missed the string quartet)

Food 9 (I enjoyed the meal immensely)

P.S. The binary chop is a technique Iain used at work earlier in the week to ensure 19,772 not 3,577 out of 19,773 students got paid. I bet the odd one out was a transgendered :)

Chapter 61

I Got Plenty of Nothing

I must stop thinking so much, I must stop drinking so much.

I was thinking, I know Iain says its dangerous, but in Manchester I've not really got anything. A flat with no gas or electricity (which is Tina's), no car and no mod cons at all. I have got lots of friends though and some lovely clothes and make-up. I am very happy, so what's life all about?

> I got plenty of nothing
> And nothing is plenty for me.

Musings and Meanderings

For once Tricia worked up bright and early; well early anyway and carefully got herself ready. She decided to wear her newly bought green dress which zipped up the front with leggings and tights. She was meeting Becky for lunch at Megan's bistro and wanted to go around the shops first. She had seen something else she wanted and decided to buy it. Tina texted.

"Trish, he was all over me last night, it was great".

"Tina, I suspect you were all over him last night, but I'm glad you enjoyed it".

"Did you have a good time?"

"Fine, but saving myself for today. Had my eyebrows threaded, bought a green dress which zips up the front and had my mind read".

I forgot to mention that. On Friday night Tricia was sitting daintily and behaving herself for once when John motioned her across. After a preliminary chat, he gripped her palm and asked her to concentrate. She did as she was told; sometimes she does do as she is told.

"On your Father's side I can see rail and on your Mother's side I can see sea".

That was not bad although it was the wrong way round. My Grandfather on my Mother's side worked for British Rail in Crewe. On my Father's side my Grandfather spent years in the Royal Navy. Tricia was impressed but then John said something that worried her.

"You are hiding something from the people you love". Tricia looked at herself in the mirror. What on earth could she be hiding? The people she loves know what she does. She will have to think about that one.

It reminded me of a day at work when I was coming back from London. I was in the Gents at St Pancras at the urinal (By the way Tricia has rules on this. If she is in a gay bar or club she stands, but when she is a straight toilet she sits, like the lady she is). Anyway a guy I don't know from Adam walks in and starts a conversation.

"You're in Computing aren't you".

"Errrmmm, yes", I was a bit taken aback.

"I'm a student and was wondering about your views on JIT compilation".

So I told him. It was something I had been wrestling with the previous week.

"I think code needs to be properly tested and JIT compilation incurs high and to mind unnecessary risks"

"Thanks Iain".

My draw dropped to the floor. I checked but I did not have my name badge on. He disappeared into the station, but I knew he had read my mind. What a good job I was thinking about work at the time!

But, back to the story, if that is what this is. Having got herself ready Tricia walked into town. Her walking rules have changed. There used to be just Iain walk and Tricia walk. Iain walk gets me to where I want to go as quickly as possible. Tricia walk gets her to where she wants to go through as many people as possible. That way she may get some attention which she likes and she is safest. But she realised that meant she couldn't use the canal paths. As we know she loves walking the canals. So she made up compromise Tricia walk. She walks through Deansgate, G-Mex, Manchester Central, Knot Hill (how many names can one place have? Has the world gone mad?) and then picks up the canal. A third Iain, a third Tricia old and a third Tricia new. She misses the cobblestones which ruin her high heels, gets to her destination quicker and still meets lots of people. She does not however use the canal at all when it gets dark!

She was crossing the huge roundabout outside the flat when she got tooted by a car waiting at the lights.

"Peep, peep"

Tricia was encouraged. The car got stuck in the over-complicated traffic light system and as Tricia emerged at the other end of the roundabout she got tooted by the same car.

"Peep, peep"

Tricia smiled. She knows that if she is spotted as a t-girl there is a long hard beep on the hooter. "Peep, peep" means someone fancies her. She has got the figure of a supermodel after all. Well, that is what Tricia thinks and who could contradict reasoning like that? She lives in her own little world after all.

The shopping went well. This has now become so easy for her. Its like shelling peas. She checked out the sizes of the chic purple leather jacket she has set her mind on and there was a size twelve. She queued up with the other girls for the changing room. A perfect fit! She also found three really pretty pairs of panties which she knew she had to have. A girl can never have enough panties after all.

Mission accomplished she went to Paddys to meet Becky, then onto Megan's bistro for a meal. Then back to Paddys with Becky. The girls were getting very drunk and were about to call it a day (Tricia was by now getting confused with days) when Megan phoned. She would be along in half-an-hour. So more drink, more beer, too much beer.

Tricia wanted a dance in Naps but was worried about getting in. She was having a cigarette outside, contemplating the thought, when she was engulfed by three very attractive young ladies.

"Mama, Mama, come in with us".

And she did, silly girl! She can't remember a thing after that.

At 11:00 on Sunday morning there was a loud hammering on the door of T-Girl Towers. Tricia woke up abruptly. How did she get home last night she thought to herself.

"Trish, its me Tina. I haven't been out all weekend and there's the match today"

Tricia opened the door.

Could she take any more?

Chapter 62

America

This is a tricky one to write because so much happened over the weekend. The best thing was meeting my American friend Monica Ann again. She is getting there but I wish she'd have more patience. Anyway, and by the way, the song is dedicated to her and her fellow countrymen.

> I like the shores of America!
> Comfort is yours in America!
> Knobs on the doors in America,
> Wall-to-wall floors in America!

In which everything goes on, including a lot of transitioning chat.

Tina's handbag is a wondrous thing. Unlike Tricia's, which holds the kitchen sink in an orderly fashion, Tina's possesses all sorts of items she didn't know she had. Including, as luck would have it on the Sunday, a £20 note. Tricia keeps moaning at Tina for not buying herself a purse but Tina is quite happy in emptying the entire contents of her handbag onto the bar to ensure she has the correct change for the round.

"Look Trish, there's a condom!".

"Yes, bet its past its sell-by date".

Tricia, not anticipating Tina's good fortune in finding the money, nor her participation, had left earlier to meet Monica Ann who was back in Manchester. The girls had a long chat and re-lived former glories.

Monica was happy in England, happy in America but not at all happy in Afghanistan and who can blame her. She must keep going with what she is doing though. Tricia is supporting her as best she can with words of encouragement. She needs to see it through, then she can transition. Monica again was struggling with her trunk and Tricia offered to help, by storing it at T-Girl Towers (if Tina would allow). The girls however weren't entirely sure that was a wise course of action.

Tina appeared brandishing her newly found £20 note and a broad grin.

"Your round Trish".

"I'm not hon, God we've done that one to death, sorry".

"I've only got just enough to keep me going".

So Tricia bought the round and the girls continued to chat. Monica became tired, she had had a busy week with Amy in Yorkshire and then Manchester so left for some sleep.

"Trish, pretty please"

"What do you want now hon? Not another round".

"Can we just have a game of pool".

Tricia relented. She doesn't like playing pool much mainly because she isn't as good a player as I used to be. It doesn't help being half blind and also her hair gets in the way all the time. What happened though was amazing. The girls must have had precisely the correct amount of alcohol because they played the best pool of their lives. Hardly a shot was missed. Tina finally won but it was the result of a fluke so Tricia didn't mind. She had played as well as she could and, on the plus side, it did cut down on her drinking.

Back to Paddy's and Tina got chatting to some guys so Tricia made her excuses and went into town. She loves her little trips into Manchester now. She had to be quick because the shops shut early on Sundays but in any case Manchester United were playing in the cup so she wanted to get back in a reasonable time.

Tricia didn't buy anything but that doesn't matter any more. She had a good look round and was accepted. She returned to Paddy's to find Tina talking to Kimberley, a pre-op TS just as the football was starting. Tina always watched in New York, New York so it worked out and Tricia took over the conversation with Kimberley.

Kimberley is a lovely girl who seemed to be sailing through life as a t-girl. She had done her two years but told Tricia there were still a lot of tests she had to go through before she could full transition. Tricia made a mental note. Even after the hardest thing (although going two years dressed no longer seemed that daunting) there were still more difficult things in store.

Tina returned at half-time and settled down to join them. The game was very one-sided, United were winning easily. Graham, who was also bored with football joined with the girls and they had a very amusing couple of hours before Kimberley had to get her train to go home.

She left at nine. Tina and Tricia went to Monica's hotel to see if they could do anything with her trunk. What on earth they could have done, particularly bearing in mind the state they were in, remains a mystery but I suppose they tried. In any case they couldn't wake Monica up even after spending twenty minutes trying to find her room. No jokes please about letting sleeping dogs lie, but it was probably best all round that Monica remained aloof to the world.

They returned to the pub and who should be there in the corner? Why the limpet of course. What does the limpet do? He latches onto unsuspecting drunk girls like poor Tricia. Tricia, we know was suspecting, but by now we also know Tricia was drunk. There was no denying the limpet and while Tina was at the bar for the umpteenth time, before you could say Jack Rabbit, his tongue disappeared down her throat. A particularly rampant rabbit he was too as he pointed out to Tricia by placing her hand where her hand shouldn't be allowed to go; certainly not in Paddy's. Tricia somehow managed to escape his vice like grip after about an hour so she survived to live another tale. She noticed, on staggering out, that Tina was ensconced in a similar manner to another bloke on the other side of the bar.

Tricia staggered back to T-Girl Towers. It had been a long weekend, it had been a long day. She let herself in, tired out and without thinking locked the door. She took off her clothes, got into bed and fell into a sound sleep. Tina returned at about two o'clock in the morning. She couldn't wake the sleeping beauty at all. She tried to phone up some friends but no joy. She had to sleep on the step by the door with the dodgy hieroglyphics. Tricia knew she had messed up badly and was very apologetic. Tricia must learn to think as opposed to just drink. But Tina was to get her revenge as we will discover shortly.

Chapter 63

Baubles, Bangles and Beads

I really need to sort my earrings out. I go to all the trouble to get my ears pierced and then don't remove the studs. This is madness; it can't be that hard.

I am beginning to understand myself a little more and with that can affect the way I project myself. I am so much more relaxed and am really enjoying the weekend. The obvious song, by the way, is from Kismet.

> Hear how they jing, jing-a-ling-a,
> Baubles, bangles,
> Bright, shiny beads

Bling!

Tricia was worried about her accessories. They needed to be updated. She was particularly concerned about her earrings but also wanted to add something to her hair but she wasn't sure what. Her hair needed spicing up but, as we know, its a wig so spicing up isn't easy. She was determined to spend Friday evening sorting this lot out. I suppose in the back of her mind was her Abba outfit which she wanted to wear on Saturday night. She now has financial constraints which she needs to stick to. But she's a good girl, we know that, so will try her best. She also wanted more necklaces, rings and bracelets but how far she could go, given her budget, she wasn't sure.

Really what she wanted most was long, hooped earrings. She had tried before and had failed completely to attach them to her ears. She had to get Monica to put her studs back in. Surely it can't be that hard she thought. Other girls manage it with no difficulty at all but she is so cack-handed.

She has managed to master her necklaces and bracelets so now she must learn to do her earrings. It was all part of becoming a girl. She must not therefore drink too much and therefore shake too much the following morning. It is a challenge for her. Will she be up to it?

I decided to get to Deansgate, Manchester Central, G-Mex, Knott Hill, whatever and decided to have a beer before Tricia got ready. I had a smoke outside the Knott, an old-fashioned student pub and looked down the road. This is amazing I thought. In an hour or so's time Tricia will be walking back, as confidently and proudly as she can the opposite direction from where I am about to walk. She will look good, she will look sexy, she will be herself yet she will also be me. It suddenly strikes me what a brave girl she is. And she will be smiling all the time.

And she did. She walked so upright with such confidence, that no-one dare challenge her. And no-one did. She walked to Paddy's where 50's music was playing on the CD, the bar was quiet, the people were friendly; it was perfect. Soon she will be out in Manchester (late night shopping on Friday) looking for her baubles, bangles and beads. For now she was alone, though she did not feel alone in the pub where everybody smiled at her.

Then the mobile sprung to life. It was the limpet.

"Come round to mine, you have the address", the text read.

Tricia wanted Martin to make the effort not her do all the work. So she ignored the text, took a sip of her beer and looked around the pub. She felt so happy, she felt so free, she was on her own but with friends. She thought of a Pink Floyd song.

> *"All alone and in twos' the ones who really love you"*
> *"March up and down outside the wall".*

She actually is in heaven she feels. No mortgage worries (I sorted out those problems during the week). No credit card demands (I sorted that out too). Tricia can be who she wants, and she is. There are miles and miles and smiles and smiles to go from here.

Tricia strolled into town without a care in the world. She's done it before, she'll do it again. No grief. She bought herself some baubles, the colours matched her new jacket, and some new earrings which she will try tomorrow. She settled down to a cappuccino and a toastie. She was still happy. She looked around the shops until they shut, though didn't see anything she really wanted and she now has to really want something before she can buy it. Then back to Paddies to meet up with some friends and onto Naps. She didn't overdo it though, tomorrow is the day of the big match. Tomorrow is also the day when she will put on her new hooped earrings. She is a determined young lady.

Chapter 64

Everybody Loves Somebody

I am so much more natural as Tricia; I am being myself, not a hybrid of Iain. The fun may have gone to some extent but now everything I do has my hallmark stamped on it. From how I walk to how I conduct myself to the clothes I buy and wear, to what I want to be and do. I now have an urgent desire to get out the village, to live a different but acceptable life as myself in Manchester but I'm aware I have many friends in the village who I wish to be with as well. In short, and by the way, I am starting to love myself. Dangerous!

> Everybody loves somebody sometime
> And though my dreams were overdue
> Your love made it all worth waiting
> For someone like you

Sportswomen

The door of T-Girl Towers resounded with a loud banging (a different type than goes on inside the flat) at ten o'clock on Saturday morning.

"Trish, you awake. It's the big match and I need to get ready".

Tina had returned from her enforced absence due to financial difficulties. The big match in question was Manchester United versus Liverpool. The girls needed to be at New York New York for 12:45 when game kicked off. Saturday match days are fun. A wide awake Tricia (she was a good girl on Friday night after all) opened the door to let Tina in. She was already getting herself ready.

Tricia started the day with a match of her own. Unfortunately for her the game involved was darts and the dartboard happened to be her own ears. Getting ready was easy. It was match day so she wore her red dress with a black belt and black tights. For those who don't know red and black are the colours of Manchester United who Tricia supports. She dressed and looked delightful as always. Then came the problem. She was determined to wear her new hooped earrings and wear them she would.

The first problem was to get her studs out without losing the fiddly little clippy bits which held them in place. It took her an age, but the good news is, with Tina getting ready in the other room, she had an age. She later found out that the fiddly clippy bits were not strictly necessary since her studs would stay in without them. First mission accomplished she now had to put her hoopy ones in. The darts began. Though she was quite a good girl the previous evening, she wasn't that good and did have a bit of the shakes in the morning.

Now, I am no good at darts. I did once score 180 but went on to lose the game! What I can do though is eventually (normally too late) get the dart to go where I want it to. Tricia needed a bullseye in each ear and two bullseyes are a lot to ask. So, in front of the mirror, with glasses on, Tricia stabbed away. Her left ear became the same colour as her dress at one stage as she missed for the umpteenth time, but at least it was only a small prick. It was so frustrating. Eventually she hit the bullseye. Her right ear seemed easier (why is it that its always easier on the right side?) and she managed it pretty quickly with far less stabbing going on and no blood. She couldn't beat Phil Taylor but she would probably distract him for a while.

There was still forty minutes left before they needed to go she did a couple of Sodukus while waiting for Tina to finish. She leaves Tina to her own devices; if she disturbs Tina for some reason the process seems to take ten times longer. Finally she got the nod from next door. The nod from next door coming from Tina's nether regions as she was wearing hold-ups which wouldn't hold up. This is why Tricia wears tights. Hold-ups are far too much trouble.

Match day Saturday in Manchester is fun, well for Tricia anyway. T-Girl Towers is only two miles away from Old Trafford so the girls have to brave the queuing football traffic when crossing the road to get their cab. Tina, wearing her black nothing to the imagination skirt and hold-ups which didn't hold up caused a complete stir to which Tricia was included. It took the cars and cabs no time to realise that the two demure young ladies trying to cross the road were in fact transgendered. A cacophony of car horns filled the South Manchester air. This was not peep, peep; but toot with a vengeance. Tricia was having a great time and waving to everybody but Tina wasn't so sure. They eventually crossed the road, ignoring the ribald comments and immediately got a taxi. Another advantage of match days is that there are taxis everywhere. Two young girls, Manchester United supporters of course, were walking past as they boarded the cab, smiling and laughing. They give Tricia the thumbs up. It is great being a t-girl she thought, not just for herself but for all around. It makes people happy. Tina couldn't see what all the fuss was about.

Well, Manchester United didn't win. They were destroyed by a much more hungry Liverpool side. Tricia suddenly realised that it was only the second time she had seen them lose while watching them in Manchester. She's been coming up now over a year. That's a pretty good record Mr Ferguson.

The loss didn't matter though. Tricia realised how happy she was, how much better she felt in her own skin and how more natural she was as Tricia. She went to the ladies to top up her make-up and just beamed at herself. She wasn't frightened any more, she was fine with conflict, she could get on with being herself. She was to have problems later in the day but lets not worry about those now. She was one happy t-girl and felt, maybe for the first time, that she was making great steps to becoming a real girl.

Chapter 65

Mein Herr

I made a decision this weekend which will likely affect things. I am not going back with the first bloke that snogs me or pinches my bum. I am Tricia, I am proud of being Tricia so I am not going to get myself used. That makes the song easy by the way.

> And though I used to care,
> I need the open air.
> You're better off without me,
> Mein Herr.

Decision Time

The girls returned to Paddy's after the match but Tricia knew what she wanted to do. The new improved Tricia, the Tricia with added sugar wanted to hit town. So, her earrings jangling away in the breeze, she wasn't used to that, that is precisely what she did. There was nothing she particularly wanted to buy but it was always fun having a look round. Se got herself a toastie, got told off for taking a picture, tried on a couple of dresses, passed with little trouble (though people knew) and returned to Paddys relaxed and refreshed to meet with Tina again who was far too refreshed and relaxed.

"Trish, I've drunk too much, I've got to go back and have a kip".

"That's ok hon but leave the door unlocked. I want to have a play with my Abba outfit".

So it came to pass that Tina went home, locked the door and went to sleep.

So it came to pass that Tricia, after a couple – and only a couple of beers, marched through Manchester determined to change into the dancing queen.

So it came to pass that Tricia got back to a locked flat and, try as she might, could not wake up the only sleeping princess who could open the door. How she wishes she was a handsome prince with a loud voice! Not really. She shrugged her shoulders and walked back to Paddys. At least she had a break from drinking.

Now, those of you who are following this will realise that Tricia isn't as green as she's cabbage looking. She had on, as we know, her Manchester United kit, her utilitarian red dress and tights with leggings. Her legs were shaven. She merely had to take off her leggings, stash them in her black handbag which holds the kitchen sink and which she had with her, and she could still look dead sexy. So she did, she is a surprisingly resourceful young lady. She changed in a flash without flashing and got into Naps with no problem and was immediately surrounded by, to put it politely, a number of not particularly attractive men. Tricia then made a momentous decision. She was going to be the one who chases now, but she can wait until the right man, woman, t-girl, whatever (she is of course bi-sexual) comes along. There are, after all, plenty of fish in the sea. Men are two-a-penny and want everything now. Tricia doesn't, she had just got into Naps for goodness sake, why would she want to give one of them a blow now. So she fluttered her eyelashes, jangled her earrings and went upstairs for a dance. She will re-evaluate the position later but for now she is no longer a toy for men to play with. She enjoyed her dance and left relatively early on her own. That did not worry her. This time she left the door unbolted and Tina, who did eventually manage to wake, returned much later with Steve, who had previously been with both girls. That too made Tricia think. She is more confident, relaxed and happier now, she just needs to be more in control. She is still becoming who she wants to be, but still needs more time.

On Sunday Tricia went to Paddies with the idea of again going into town. But Megan and Becky turned up and they had a wonderful afternoon chatting amongst themselves and with another girl called Amandine who had a girlfriend living abroad. They all hope Holly will return from America but that is dubious. Armandine, please don't bank on it. You know what happens with banks. Tricia will get Monica to chant for Armandine too.

Tricia left early for a Chinese buffet. The restaurant was empty, as was the village really. The credit crunch is affecting everybody. There are girls she hasn't seen in ages and that is sad. She must keep developing herself though, she must keep finding her independence. She still loves being Tricia, maybe more so now than ever before.

Chapter 66

Pack up your Troubles

Poor Iain suffered a terrible week at home. He sweated buckets, there was catarrh floating through him, he coughed and he shuddered. I have heard that when you are on girl pills, there is point where you turn. Where the amount of estragon starts to exceed the amount of testosterone. I wonder whether this is what was happening now. At the end of the week, to balance things up, he heard that his daughter had gone into labour. So this weekend he could become a grandfather (does that make me a grandmother? There is no way my skirts are getting longer!). If his daughter can keep her legs shut until Sunday, the baby will share the same birthday as Iain's Mother. Life is full of co-incidences.

> Pack up your troubles in your black handbag
> And smile, smile, smile.
> While you've a Lucifer to light your fag
> Smile girl, that's the style

Troubles at home, troubles at work, troubles with jewellery

Tina texted some not so valuable information:

"Hi Trish, Running late, Graham shagged me all night. Pick up some milk if you can. Will let you know of progress".

Tricia knew Tina would be late, she always is, so a useful text would read:

"Hi Trish, am on time, get into gear and quick"

But Tricia always gets into her gear quick. At least she got the milk. I got a message from work.

"Important meeting Monday morning. No bling!"

No bling? If only they knew what I was about to put on. But there are issues in both our lives that are distracting Tricia from the vital activity of having fun.

- Mortgage and credit cards recently sorted out but I will still be struggling in three months

- Daughter number one about to drop

- Daughter number two just split up with first boyfriend and is struggling

- Daughter number three with new boyfriend very happy, but showing no interest in college and has started drinking and smoking

- Problems at work

- Tumble drier not working properly

- Sky television not working properly

- Front door lock broken

- Curtains needed in both twins' rooms

- Results of my blood test due on Wednesday

- Mother's birthday on Sunday

- Mother not getting on with son-in-law

How much can one person put up with? How much weight can one person carry on her shoulders (quite a lot actually, you should try picking up Tricia's black handbag). Some of these things are hugely emotional and I know Tricia struggles with them immensely, as do I.

But enough of all that. With her bangles bought and her earrings in, Tricia was in a mood to experiment. She had loads of make-up which she hadn't used for ages. Her look seemed to have settle down to white and brown mascara, no eyeliner, stable lipstick and pink blush. She wanted to try out different colours, different blends on herself so spent the weekend trying different things out. She tried wearing her belt lower, she put clips into her hair, she marched around town looking for simple, inexpensive things to complement her clothes. She bought some new dangly earrings and some new hair clips, knowing that she needs to match them with her girly pink biker jacket and her purple check jacket for when it gets warmer. She also found a really pretty blue dress which she just had to buy. She was to wear it later with leggings but was looking forward to the summer, when she could wear it with sheer tights. She will look so girly.

In her reserve jewellery bag she found some necklaces and chains see hadn't worn for ages, and a really pretty ankle chain which she had forgotten all about. The trouble was .....

By now you know that the thing Tricia hates most about being a girl is Nair. Well, a close second to Nair are wires, I don't like wires either. Why do they always cross themselves? Why does it take an age to unravel them. Tricia opened her jewellery box and removed a whole clump of knotted mess. She sighed. I would have given up and thrown them all away but Tricia is made of sterner stuff. In any case she had plenty of time; Tina had still to get ready.

For the next half hour she struggled and sweated trying to unravel the unholy mess into things that were wearable. Did she do it? You know she did! Shaking hands didn't help but by the end she had rescued five necklaces, a choker, loads of bangles and her ankle chain. She put it on immediately, it looked dead sexy. Tricia was happy and happy to go out. Tina was finally ready. Tricia left the untangled jewellery separate on her bed. She would decide what to do with it later to stop it knotting again.

Tricia and Tina went out again into the big wide world with a smile on their painted lips and a song in their hearts..... "Pack up your troubles".

Chapter 67

One Hundred Acre Wood

This was a lovely gentle gentle day which only goes to show that you don't always have to have slap and tickle to enjoy yourself. However I am reading a book called Mrs Clapps Molly House in my spare time (and I have plenty of that while waiting for Tina) and the slap and tickle that went on in the past was far more debauched than I ever get up to!. The book its highly recommended though. Oh, and I dressed in my purple gear so, by the way, I guess I must be Piglet. In which case the Willy nilly silly old bear must be Tina.

> She's Winnie the Pooh
> Winnie the Pooh
> Willy nilly silly old bear

I wonder what's going to happen exciting today?

Deep in the heart of the four acre village there was a place known to everyone as paradise. It was where it all began. It was not a garden but a shop which served particularly good honey. Tigger had recently heard about it and wanted to explore it for herself, particularly since her friend, Winnie the Pooh, was fast asleep in bed. So Tigger arranged to meet Piglet in Paradise at two.

Piglet knew that Paradise lay on the other side of the man made river which ran through the middle of the four acre village and was looking forward to clip clopping across the bridge in her five inch trotters. She was also looking forward to meeting Tigger. She had heard about her legendary boing and after all, spring was on its way wasn't it? The weather was certainly warmer and brighter, as was Piglet.

Piglet decided to dress in a conservative manner so, as Piglets do, she dressed as purple as she possibly could.

"Purple piglet, no surprise"

"The lean on her will turn mens' eyes"

So Piglet crossed the bridge and entered Paradise where Tigger and Owl were already having a chat with Eeyore. Eeyore, Piglet was to find out, used to wear a dog collar but grew out of it as her life and body developed.

The honey was indeed excellent and the mead even better as the re-united friends chatted their way through the afternoon. They later were to be joined by Baa One and Baa Two. They ought really have moved from paradise and drank in Baa Baa but then some things are not to be. Baa One and Baa Two used to be rams but had a while back converted to ewes. After finishing the delicious honey the replete friends crossed back over the man-made river and continued their conversation in a re-opening in the village. The honey wasn't quite as good but was easier to find. Nobody would get stung here.

A happy Piglet, a merry Piglet, a full Piglet went back to the (public) house she called home and had fun watching a game played between fifteen dragons and fifteen leprechauns with a funny shaped ball.

Piglet later met up with Christopher Robin and more of her friends. Christopher Robin lent her a book entitled "Mrs Clapps Molly House". Piglet, who was well read and often read was later to discover precisely what a Molly was, and what went off at Mrs Clapps House. Actually pretty much everything came off at Mrs Clapps House.

After such a busy day Piglet suddenly felt tired and realised that it was time to return to her own abode away from the four acre village on the eighth branch of a tall oak tree. There she fell fast and happily asleep.

Chapter 68

The Party's Over

Would you Adam and Eve it? Three days earlier Iain was told he hadn't got cancer. It was Easter weekend so I could spend a long time celebrating. I even took the Thursday off work so I could be myself in Manchester for longer. Then what happens? And, by the way, the party is definitely over for a while.

> Now you must wake up, all dreams must end.
> Take off your make up, The Party's Over.
> It's all over, my friend.

She Fell Over*

Tricia was going to enjoy extended time in Manchester but in the end had to leave early. It was no fault of her own though, was it? The trouble is her walking boots are falling apart and she can't find another pair in her size. She thinks it was the boots which caused the problem, not the booze but isn't totally sure. Yes, she had drunk a lot of beers but that was over a long period of time and she didn't feel particularly drunk. Anyway, stuff like that happens and she had just heard she hadn't got cancer. Cancer or a few bruises, what would you prefer?

But, let's begin at the beginning for once. It was Easter so no work on Good Friday or Easter Monday. I took Thursday off as well so Tricia could be up for Wednesday night. Wednesday night is girls night in the village and was it just! It was just like Sparkle revisited. At one stage in Paddy's there must have been more than twenty girls. Paddy's was almost no-man's land! Naps was even busier.

Tricia was going to enjoy this Easter and it started really well. In Paddy's she noticed Georgina talking to a girl who looked a bit like Tina Turner. Tricia joined in the conversation and, at last, met Morticia. If you roll back many many chapters, back to the Ladyboys and show business, where Mark discussed being a lapsed t-girl, and Tricia didn't understand. Well, Morticia is Mark, clearly lapsed no longer and the transformation was amazing. Tricia is sure that Mark will forgive her when she says that he just looks normal, but as Morticia she looks brilliant.

Georgina was chatting with Dave by now and later joined Tricia at the back for a cigarette.

"There is no way I am taking anyone that drunk back to the flat. I've got the neighbours to think about".

Tricia nodded her head sagely.

About an hour later Tricia was having another cigarette. This time at the front of the pub, when a mini-cab pulled up. This was shortly followed by Dave and .... Georgina looking very surreptitious. Tricia shrugged her shoulders. Each to their own she thought.

She went to Naps with Morticia and Glenda, tried to get some dancing lessons going with the girls but failed miserably because everybody had had far too much to drink. She went downstairs and sat at the bar. An admirer started puffing out his chest and showing off his muscles for her benefit. She resisted. She is jingly-jangly Tricia now.

Walking home through Manchester in the early hours, a coloured guy passed her the other way.

"Alright darling?" Tricia smiled back.

"How much?"

Tricia wouldn't have minded but she was wearing trousers and wasn't dressed like a prostitute at all. She did notice however that there weren't hundreds of attractive girls like her walking through Manchester at two o'clock on a Thursday morning!

All was well though and Tricia was happy. Wake up tomorrow, blue dress and leggings, nothing too flash, a couple of beers and then her eyebrows needed doing again. She would get them threaded. It lasts longer than waxing. So she did. She met Georgina in the pub who assured her that nothing had happened the previous night, but the earth had moved in the morning. Tricia wasn't concerned about such things, let people be is her motto, but she was pleased Georgina had a good time and pleased for Georgina that it was going to happen again that afternoon.

Eyebrows suitably threaded she walked around the shops, had a coffee, no worries, then returned to Paddy's where she met Gavin again. Now Gavin is a very attractive and well spoken guy. Its just ......

"Can I kiss you darling".

Tricia kissed Gavin but noticed that his eyeballs weren't entirely where they should be.

"You are the most beautiful girl in the world".

Fortunately even Tricia wasn't that gullible and she alerted Paul behind the bar who gently escorted Gavin off the premises. Where was Stacy when you needed her?

So off Tricia trotted to the straight pub where Manchester City were on television playing in Europe. Pretty pretty and pretty much the only girl in the place she had a great time. City fans are more dangerous and less cosmopolitan than United fans which all adds to the tension.

"If City equalise I promise I'll give you kiss".

His mates roared with laughter.

"Ooooh honey, that adds some spice to the game". Tricia winked. City weren't however to equalise and lost badly, as was Tricia.

Quite happy and looking forward to a ruby to finish off the day she walked through the car park back into the village. She had done this one hundred times before but she didn't see the kerb. She crashed into the concrete of the car park. Her right hand and shoulder were clutching her handbag so didn't break her fall. Disaster!

The following day she woke and saw the extent of her injuries. She couldn't carry on, she had to go home. But a funny thing happened. She went back in drab protecting her injuries as best she could with her Victoria Beckham sunglasses. She was called Bono by some youths but, as we know, she has been called much worse. It was only later I realised that men like to show off their scars like war wounds. Its only girls who try to disguise them.

* She fell over is a derogatory comment made by football fans when a player from the opposing side gets badly injured.

Chapter 69

So Long and Thanks for all the Fish

God it was good to get back and be myself again. Everybody was so friendly and pleased to see me. They all checked my face for scars but they had pretty much healed and my concealer worked wonders this time. I love YSL La Touche Eclat, it's my one make-up must. I also found another use for my lovely black handbag. I am beginning to feel lost without it. By the way, I thought the radio series was the best of them all, apart from the book itself of course..

> You may not share our intellect
> Which might explain your disrespect
> For all the natural wonders that
> grow around you

In which Tricia returns, meets friends old and new, gets locked out and has difficulty with skyscraper heels.

It was to be three long weekends before Tricia's next trip to Manchester following her trip. The good news was that Tricia's face had fully recovered and once again she looked like a siren from the silver screen. Or just a girl requiring a screen and a siren depending on your point of view. Tricia was determined to dress provocatively for at least one day so would need to keep her point out of view, neatly tucked away.

It transpired that Tricia wasn't the only one to have a fall. Tina was leaving Georgina's on her bike when she fell off. This was to affect the sexual positions she could assume but not her sexual appetite. So it was a very unassuming Tina who went round to Graham's for her now regular

Friday night. Tricia was therefore on her own but that didn't bother her. Even though she was late in to Manchester the sun was shining and she had until eight fifteen before the light went. This is far better than the miserable winter nights she thought to herself as she zipped up her sexy green dress. Three weeks hadn't affected her make up skills and she carried on experimenting, putting a clasp rather than a clip in her hair. She was ready in a jiffy and strode in through the centre of Manchester with a purpose.

When she got to the pub, who should be there but Mark (not Morticia) and Georgina so she was with friends straight away. Not that that worries her unduly. She can easily make new friends if she needs to. What was nice was that everybody said they had missed her. The gays behind the bar, the gays the other side of the bar all checked her face had cleared. She was indeed surrounded by friends and this was a recurring theme throughout the weekend as she met more and more people she knew.

It was in fairness to be a fairly uneventful night; but that suited the now un-suited Tricia. The new jingly-jangly, dingy-dangly (all adjectives relate to her earrings and nothing else) Tricia. The new improved, confident Tricia. There were some guys who took an interest in her. Indeed her backside got pinched as soon as she got into Naps, and she got chatting to a rugby league supporter from Salford. He was very nice; but no up and under this time. It was far too early, and anyway Tricia hadn't danced for the last three weeks.

She left early, around two, after all tomorrow was to be a busy day. Tomorrow Tina would be back early, so she marched home quite happy. When she got there she encountered a nutty problem for a girl with nuts. They had changed the programming on the entrance into T-Girl Towers so when Tricia waved her key fob delicately at the door like the good fairy she sometimes is, nothing happened. She tried again and again but the door refused to budge. There is only one thing for it, she mused. She would have to go to the office and speak to the overnight caretaker. Was she frightened? Of course not, the overnight caretaker had seen her many times before in varying states of drunkenness.

"Can you help me, the door won't open?"

"They've re-programmed it"

"Well?"

"That's why the door won't open"

Tricia wondered whether the overnight caretaker had any intelligence or indeed was worried about care at all.

"I know that, but I can't sleep in the street can I? I'd be beaten to smithereens when the sun came up".

"Sun, in Manchester?"

"Surely you must have a fob that works"

"Yes, but I've only got one"

"Well can you come with me, open the door, then you can come back here"

"I can't leave the office unattended"

"Well, can I borrow the fob?"

"Yes, but you must bring it back".

Now there was a challenge. If she brought it back she would be locked out again but she took the key anyway and put her thinking cap on over her wig, as opposed to her wig cap under it.

In the Hitch-hikers Guide to the Galaxy it was stated that the most important piece of equipment you need to travel with is a towel. Tricia lit up, the thinking cap lit up. In Tricia's guide to the suburbs of Greater Manchester, it states that the most important piece of equipment you need to travel with is a black handbag which can and often does contain the kitchen sink.

She waved her, by now magic wand and the door creaked open. She quickly took her purse out of her handbag (clever girl) and jammed it, the handbag, in the door. She rushed back to the caretakers office and returned the fob.

"Its all right love the cameras are watching your bag"

She hurried back to the door and using all her strength (which wasn't much) dragged it open, slung her bag back over her shoulder and sneaked in. She was a clever girl, even after fifteen pints!

There was a rat-tut-tutting at the door at around ten in the morning. It could only be Tina.

"Trish, you awake, can you let me in?"

Tricia was, but she was busy playing with her Sindiy doll so was in her own little world. A world where nobody can or should enter.

"Damn" She cursed to herself.

"Yes hon, just coming"

But sadly she didn't.

What we don't do at this point is discuss the difficulties Tina found in trying to get into a decent position to have sex with Graham. What can be relayed however was that Tina was kept up pretty much the whole night. The two, it appears, have undiminished sexual appetites and are therefore likely well suited to each other, But, thinks Tricia, "it won't last". We shall see.

Tricia really decided to go mad with her clothes and make-up and ended up more purple than she had ever been before. Purple however is the colour of the season. Tricia knows these things. When she left the flat with Tina, it was difficult to ascertain who it was who had fallen off the bike. Tricia, you see, had decided to wear her sexy high heeled shoes. Wearing them was one thing; walking in them was another thing altogether.

"Trish, walk elegantly, you look like a deep sea diver emerging from the depths"

"I've never seen a deep sea diver dressed like this. I know hon, but it will take time. Anyway, aren't we about to enter the depths according to some people".

A guy arriving at the flats keeled over laughing at Tricia's pathetic attempts to walk like a lady. She is though, we know, a determined girl and figured that if other girls could walk in shoes so high then so could she. She did in fact get much better as the day wore on. By the time the shadows of the setting sun matched the shadows under her eyes she was actually walking like a bloke in high heels. But then I suppose, that's precisely what she was. It will take time but she will persevere with the shoes. She always does. We know.

Chapter 70

Blue Moon

A lovely couple of days even without Tina. I did so much and felt, probably for the first time, really comfortable walking around town. I think my dress sense is coming on. It was a brill idea to use my leggings and tights as camouflage for my sexy blue dress. I didn't think I could possibly wear anything so short but it only goes to prove that if your in the mood you can wear anything... or nothing. By the way, this is a song most often sung by Manchester City supporters and I support Manchester United; so I shouldn't really use it. But it works, sort of.

> Blue Moon
> Now I'm no longer alone
> Without a dream in my heart
> Without a love of my own

In which Tricia goes back to basics, gets wet (though it wasn't raining in Manchester for once), meets a virgin in the gay village! And exposes rather more of her anatomy than she really ought.

Tricia texted Tina to see whether she was having her normal Friday night shag with Graham. She got the following reply.

"Sadly not Trish, at Scarborough avoiding niece's fancy dress 21st so won't be around this weekend"

For the first weekend of the year therefore, Tina would not be in fancy dress. How very strange. Tricia thought that she should have gone in any case. She could have gone dressed as a bloke. Tina is Godparent to her niece and her responsibility ceases now her niece is 21. The poor girl! How on earth could someone like Tina install morals and responsibilities? I bet she's sex mad.

Tricia loves it now the clocks have gone back. No need to rush from work at half three any more. She can tidy up properly and leave work ship-shape and Bristol fashion ready for her return on Monday morning. She could also take her time dressing and putting on her make-up without the use of candlelight. It was late but still light as she strolled through Manchester without a care in the world, heading for, guess where.

There she met the girls from Huyton who come up every couple of months or so. Mother, Grandmother, Daughter and Mother's sister. A real family affair and great fun to talk to.

"Trish, why have you changed your wig?"

It was about two months ago when Tricia got her new wig. It wasn't working, Tricia knew. It was also cheap (unlike the new Tricia) so was falling apart. Tricia promised to go back to her old wig straight away. Straight and dark, though undoubtedly old-fashioned. It was however Tricia, and in her heart of hearts she knew it. When this wig gives up the ghost she will need to buy a similar, similarly expensive one.

Tricia also met Susie, which is a particularly unfortunate name if you happen to be a t-girl with braces in your teeth and a pronounced lisp.

"Hi hon, what's your name?"

"Thuthee"

Tricia's hand immediately dived into her black handbag which holds the kitchen sink to rummage around for her girly umbrella.

Actually, Tricia herself is trying to develop a lithp too. It makes her voice sound more feminine and, with her tongue gently protruding from her painted lips, looks dead sexy. But not quite tho pronounced a lithp as Thuthee.

On the Saturday Tricia wanted to début her sexy blue dress, but how? She knew she wouldn't get back home to change and the dress was far too sexy for the daytime when she wanted to go round town. A voice came into her head. 'Tone it down Trish'. So she put on her sexy fishnet tights (on the way out), her black leggings (on the way out) and her girly pink biker jacket. She wasn't sure how impressed Tone was but it worked for her, and she walked into town with an added wiggle in her hips knowing she looked dead sexy.

Now, as we know, most of her wardrobe was on the way out, one item though, her boots, she shouldn't have worn at all; in fact she should have thrown them straight in the dustbin. They look tatty, have holes everywhere and the kitten heels disappeared long ago. She also suspects they may have been partially responsible for her fall a month or so ago. She was having a break from shopping under the big wheel when she got molested by an elderly lady and her two sons who were in their twenties.

"Honey you look great but how can you walk around town with holes in your shoes?"

Tricia was despondent. She didn't realise that holes showed. They were holes after all. She was also told off about blobs of eye-liner looking messy. Yes, Tricia has taken to wearing eye-liner again and is getting better at it, but clearly needs more practice. She will learn, we know she will.

"Are those real boobs?" Said the lady

Tricia quickly remembered and offered her left one for inspection.

"Very life-like"

The boys had a feel too and admitted that she didn't look half bad for a t-girl. That was good enough for Tricia who knew she still had a distance to travel.

It was a somewhat smaller distance to Long Tall Sally where Tricia gets her footwear. Sadly she couldn't find any she liked which she could walk a distance in. There were no boots at all, wrong time of the year, and no shoes which screamed out Tricia. She kept her powder dry though she would return in a month or so. Until then she would have to make do. She wasn't sure how though.

Back in Paddy's Tricia bumped into Benjamin who was talking to Tricia's favourite rent boy James and his 'date' for the evening. His 'date' was already plied with drinks. He not only had an open wallet but he was also half asleep. That meant a couple of hours of free drinks for Tricia and Ben.

"Don't worry" said James, "He earns a fortune, I know, and if I can get him drunk enough I won't have to perform".

It was Ben's first time with a t-girl and he wasn't sure. He was very nice though and Tricia took him as far as she could. They had an extremely long snog together which they both enjoyed. Ultimately though the guilt in Ben won. He had a wife and children to get back to. Tricia suspects he will return but it will take a while. She will look out for him.

"I kissed a girl I liked it"

"It tastes of stale tobacco"

Later she met Steph, or mad Steven as he was known in the pub.

"I really want to dress like you Trish, I won't look so good I know but I am determined to try".

"Ok hon, underdress next week and we'll try some make-up.

"What's underdress?"

Tricia explained manfully, though that isn't strictly true.

At the end of the evening she went into the ladies and took off her fishnets and her leggings. Crikey, she thought, this dress is a bit short, in fact its far too short. She disregarded her instincts, shrugged her shoulders and marched into Naps where she was a hit with all. She found many many dancing partners and prospective partners but as we know, Tricia is not prospecting at the moment unless someone really catches her attention. None did but it was a very happy young lady who swanned back through the City in the early morning in her sexy blue dress. She checked when she got in. Phew, she still had her pretty yellow thongs on but they didn't cover much. When she bent over she was effectively mooning to everyone behind her; maybe that's why she so popular. Next time, she thought, I'll have to remember that I have two more cheeks to powder.

Chapter 71

Hello Young Lovers

Georgina and Dave, is that going to work? At the moment they are doing well and both are giving each other the necessary room. I hope it will last but suspect it likely won't. Georgina seems very happy at the moment. Sadly I am seeing much less of Tina who is skint. She is now only out on Saturdays. On Fridays she has her weekly fun at Graham's and Sundays she goes back home. Never mind, it doesn't stop me enjoying myself! By the way, for Georgina and Dave, not so sure about the young though.

> Hello young lovers, whoever you are,
> I hope your troubles are few.
> All my good wishes go with you tonight,
> I've been in love like you.

In which there is trouble on the dance floor (again), Steph makes her début and Tricia fails to avoid the limpet. Is it time for her to buy a hat?

After waiting interminably for Tina to get ready (actually she is quicker than she used to be) the girls arrived in Paddy's to find a drink waiting for them from Dave. It appeared that Dave and Georgina were now officially an item. What particular item I will leave to your imagination but they were certainly meeting each other on a regular basis. A schoolgirl and a Grandad, the perfect combination. But hang on, doesn't Tricia like to dress as a schoolgirl and isn't she a Grandad too. Don't go there Tricia too complicated.

It was Birchplace weekend so there were a few girls up, or down, depending on where they came from (think about it). Tricia has become good friends with Rita who is actually a councillor on transgendered issues in Aberdeen; but also a lovely warm person. So for a long Saturday afternoon Tricia was regaled with stories from Rita's past. About the girl who looked and sounded so much like Cher that she was called Cher. About the girl who took so many hormones she never knew if she was up or down or up and down. Fortunately Tricia doesn't have such issues. She has time, but what will time do for her? She doesn't know yet.

She left Paddies and met Clare who was Tigger but looking great as Clare and Jennifer in Velvet. Jennifer is recently post-op and about to fly to Dubai. Scary stuff, but Tricia learnt from Georgina that there are no travelling problems or issues in Dubai provided you have documentary proof that you are transsexual. Tricia hopes Jennifer has a lovely time, she was a lovely attractive girl and they will meet up again at Sparkle which is only a couple of months away YAY, YAY, YAY. Maid Michelle is coming up too. Bet we won't get drunk?

There was a lot of trouble this weekend from straights. Tricia thinks it is fine if she is outside the village but when in the gay area people should accept us and respect us for what we are, not be downright derogatory. It came to a head on the dance floor at Naps where a guy and his girlfriend were taking the piss. Not of Tricia, we know she looks feline and dead sexy, but of a girl who was just starting out and didn't have much confidence. Tricia saw what to do and started dancing dead sexily with them, thrusting her backside into them whenever she could. She had a few quite words and was not going to be defeated. She danced them off the dance floor then went to talk to the girl.

"We are just different but we are open, free, honest and genuine" she said.

"But don't knock people's confidence" Tricia replied.

"I know, I can see that but you must see that some of them look ridiculous".

"Surely that is not our concern. Let make them feel comfortable and they will get better".

"I suppose so. But my boyfriend is a bit of a bigot"

"Train him then. He's not much of a catch like that".

"I know, but it's not easy".

The two girls smiled at each other and kissed. Maybe Tricia has changed two people. Maybe not.

The following day the sun was shining. Tricia had a mosey around town, bought some earrings to go with her green dress which zips and unzips at the front; its brilliant now her ears are pierced and she can actually put the earrings in.

Inevitably she ended up at Paddy's where there was more trouble. This time it involved a six foot four inch t-girl who claimed to be dressed for the first time. Tricia wasn't so sure because she looked brilliant. It's impossible to pass when you are that tall without heels and she took a lot of abuse from a drunken Irishman. Not for the first or last time, Paul stepped in from behind the bar and ejected the Irishman who threw his glass at the door.

Tricia went outside for a cigarette and walked down the street a little to take advantage of the sunshine. She was puffing away happily when a BMW pulled up in front of her. The driver looked at her, smiled, and beckoned her in. Tricia smiled but shook her head. She did wonder though how much she could have earned.

When she got back to the pub the rumours had started that Tricia was going to make up Steven later. Steven had told Georgina, silly boy. She was advised not to bother. Just then who should turn up but mad Steven looking vaguely effeminate but wearing the same red biker jacket he always does.

"You must admit I have made the effort Tricia, and I have some make-up in my Tesco bag"

"Hmm" Tricia studied the contents of said bag. Three foundations – all half used and some mascara. No blush, nothing for the eyes and no lippy.

"Never mind hon, I have brought a spare brush and sponge so you can use mine". Tricia steered Steph into the ladies away from prying eyes and handed Steph her foundation and a sponge. Fine. Then her concealer; fine, but it couldn't really conceal anything. Then her eye pencil. Disaster. Steph looked more like an American Quarterback than an American Beauty as the eye-liner was applied at least three inches below Steph's eyes. Tricia shook her head. At least she had brought some make-up remover. She took over to do Steph's eyes but let Steph do her own blush and lippy. Not bad thought Tricia, considering the material.

"But you really need a wig Steph, never mind I've got some spare at the flat. I'll bring one next time".

Steph got a round of applause alongside a few giggles when she returned to the bar. But there is time!

Tricia was about to leave when who should turn up. The limpet! Damn thought Tricia and for the next hour she could hardly breathe as the limpet's tongue forced itself deeper and deeper into her mouth. Oh well, thought Tricia, at least I wont get drunk tonight. Tricia was thankful for small mercies.

Chapter 72

Ascot Gavotte

I love the walk through the canal but Tina isn't so sure. The funny thing is that when I walk it alone I get no comments at all. When I go with Tina however all hell seems to break loose. Maybe its because she dresses so more provocatively than me. Still, its still fun, and I like fun. By the way, this song was a synch.

> Ev'ry duke and earl and peer is here
> Ev'ryone who should be here is here.
> What a smashing, positively dashing
> Spectacle: the Ascot op'ning day.

The Grand National

In the locker room, where they ought to be kept, the weight of the fillies was checked. They both came in under so were handicapped by being given extremely high-heeled shoes to wear. The mares put them on without complaint; they loved wearing high heels, and descended in the lift to the paddock. They were ready, they were pretty, they were honed to perfection, and they were fancied? Perspiring slightly they were the picture of physical health. The trouble was that their odds increased when they left the safety of the tower block.

The paddock consisted of a square of grass outside the flat. They paraded with elegance and beauty (ha-ha) across the greensward while preparing themselves for the first fence. T-girl Tricia sported purple, gold and white colours. Brazen Tina's silks were black and white, at least that is what Tina said. They caused quite a flutter, but it was only their eyelashes.

The road fence was a major challenge. It was a dual-carriageway. The fillies often get problems there. If they get spotted there would be a cacophony of car horns tooting at them. This time they safely crossed and went downhill to join the water. The going here was poor since it consisted of cobblestones and a couple of banks. It was not easy in such high heeled hooves but they kept going, up and over the bridge which links up to the main canal and the next fence.

The water jump consists of walking alongside a bar, Dukes 92 which has a sprinkler over the canal path to clear the excesses from the previous night. Surprisingly the fillies nearly always clear this fence with no difficulties. Maybe it's because their heels are so high. Then there is the long haul under the Deansgate tunnel before the next big test.

The yearlings disappear into darkness but when they re-appear there is the challenge of ten bars in a row which they have to walk below. In the sunshine the other side of the tunnel, the revellers outside have their eyes peeled on the track. The trick here is not to get noticed until at least the sixth bar. If they get noticed immediately, by the time they reach the tenth bar the jeering and howls of abuse are deafening; and they can't gallop away because of their high heels. Safely over that fence there is another tunnel to offer them some relief before they pass the old Hycienda, where Boy George famously played before hitting the biggest challenge of all, the Beechers Brook of this course, the Rain Bar.

The grass bank outside the Rain Bar faces the canal path giving the racegoers an opportunity to pick up the mares early and watch their progress for a good two hundred yards. Brazen Tina normally falls at this fence but, for once, they get through only slightly scathed. Fortunately Canal Turn follows and they are out of view again. Then there is an easy part of the course, although they need to be careful when passing under Oxford Road, they can drop a clanger there.

At the other side of that tunnel is the Chair, actually a bench, so they sit down and light up. Their calves and thighs are aching now after walking in such high heels. You see, they are such pictures of health!

Moving on again they have one more lock (it could have been called

Devon's Lock but unfortunately wasn't) and one more fence (tunnel) originally called Valentine's Brook but now known as Tricia's Gobble before the home straight and the cheers and applause of the fanciers in Canal Street can be heard. The course bends left then right before the end is in sight.

"Normal Dears", says Steve behind the bar. Bar Paddys Goose.

Chapter 73

The Brindisi

Its not my fault I promise. Whenever I get ready to leave the pub someone walks in who I know, we get talking, and then someone else joins in, then, before I know it, its evening.

I like to start the days fun with a couple of drinks to settle me in but that now hardly ever happens, it ends up more like a gallon than a couple of drinks. Maybe I should change pubs? No. This is my pub, this is my home from home, this is my base and these are my friends. I just need to think of some sensible exit plans. I will.

By the way I can't believe I haven't used this one before. It is of course the Brindisi, the drinking song from La Traviata, and I certainly do plenty of that.

> Be carefree - for wine and song,
> With laughter, embellish the night.
> The new day, breaking, will find us still
> In this happy paradise.

They all get drunk together

Tricia arrived in Manchester after a calm, relaxing week, plenty of sleep and completely ready for the rigours ahead. Wrong. Tricia arrived in Manchester after a hugely stressful week with hardly any sleep. Work was a constant worry; her teenage daughters were fighting with each other and her finances were in a mess. Life is hard for me but Tricia was up for fun (isn't she always) There would be no Tina on Friday night again. She was going round to Graham's to be kept up all night. At least it will save her money. So poor Tricia was on her own again. No, not poor Tricia at all and she wasn't on her own either. She never is.

After a minute in Paddy's she bumped into Raymonde. Raymonde with an 'e' and the 'e' is important because it makes Raymonde feminine. Anyway, as we know, Tricia knows all about 'e's. Raymonde met Tricia when Piglet met Tigger so they knew each other well. If only Tricia could remember. Then she saw the light. Raymonde was not in her own skin then, so she presumably was Raymond. The two had a great evening together, ending up in Naps but they did a few of the bars in Canal Street for a change. Well, a change for Tricia anyway.

Tricia didn't stay in Naps too late. It was going to be a busy Saturday. Manchester United could win the championship and it was a 12:30 kick off so Tina was expected at 10:00 to give herself enough time to change and get to the village. What was to follow was, sadly, a fairly normal Saturday in Tricia's life. A pint before the match, pints during the match, a game of pool with a few pints afterwards. Back to Paddy's and guess what; a few more pints. Two things about Tina and Tricia; they have both stamina and stupidity in equal measures. Tricia vaguely remembered that United did indeed win the game and the championship.

Tricia staggered home and set her alarm for nine o'clock to wake her up in time to get ready for Naps. Tina got the taxi home and set her alarms (all three) to get her up at eight thirty so she would wake up in time for Naps. The lack of synchronisation must have been important. Tina burst into Tricia's room at one o'clock in the morning.

"You didn't wake us up; its too late for Naps now".

It was, of course, Tricia's fault. The fact of the matter was though, as Tricia well knew, that a neutron bomb wouldn't have woken them up. She gestured Tina to bog off before going back to sleep.

All of which meant they could get up bright and early on Sunday morning. Well earlyish and watch the BUPA marathon runners through the windows of the flat as they got ready. It was race day in Manchester. Goodness knows how many starts there were. Tricia counted at least ten waves of runners, each one seeming to go on forever. There was of course one person who was not racing but did eventually get ready.

Dressed to kill, if not to run, the girls traversed the marathon course on the other side of the road. For once the cheering was not aimed at them. But if only the marathon supporters knew?

In Paddy's they straight away bump into Tom, who straight away accuses Tina of blowing him on Friday night. Sadly Tom isn't all there and Tricia was able to confirm that nothing of the sort went on on Friday night; well not with Tom anyway. Tom then explained that he got a text telling him he was mixing with dangerous company. Dangerous company? Tricia? Hardly the Mafia. But then Tricia knows that Tom doesn't know how to pick up texts. She tried to teach him but gave up. It was just another of his flights of fancy which, for once, wasn't either Tina or Tricia.

Fortunately it was about this time when Georgina and Becky arrived to take the pressure off. Tom doesn't get on with Georgina so went to the bookies where, Tricia hopes, he won. She is a charitable young lady. The girls had a long chat before Tricia made a momentous decision. She was going to walk around town. She had, after all, spent her entire weekend thus far in pubs and nightclubs. Anyway, she had some shopping to do.

First stop, to get some perfume. She had run out. She was going to change from Victoria Beckham since she was now jingly-jangly Tricia who experimented. She eventually plumped for Rock Princess by Vera Wang which she thought was very apt. She had also run out of foundation so went to the Lancombe counter in boots where the girl was very helpful. They tried a few different ones before plumping on a slightly lighter shade which seemed to go best with Tricia's complexion.

She went for a coffee and a toastie (she still watches her weight which is showing no signs of increasing, surprise, surprise) before returning to Paddy's in a very relaxed frame of mind. On her way back through Piccadilly Gardens she was wolf-whistled from behind by one of a gang of guys. She turned round.

"See, told you she's a tranny"

You can fool some of the people some of the time but not all of the people all of the time.

Back at the pub Tricia re-unites with Tina and they meet Sonja and Tracy who Tricia vaguely remembers from a previous drinking bout. They have a wonderful night and end up getting everyone to join in dancing with them. Dancing in Paddy's, whatever next!

Chapter 74

If I Only had a Brain

Iain is very cross with me but I don't think he should be. It's what I think, and Tina agrees with me. Kimberley is going through her sex change with straw on her head and, I really wonder, straw in her head too. Kim, ditch the rug and get a new one. Pretty please, just for Tricia. Get yourself sorted out because I don't think you are going the whole way as you are and I desperately want you to. You see, I'm not such a bad girl! By the way, isn't this song soo happy. But you know what they say.

"Show me a happy man and I'll show you a fool".

> I would not be just a nuffin'
> My head all full of stuffin'
> My heart all full of pain

Trouble and abuse.

For once Tricia missed a Friday night. I had to do an interview, on film with my daughter, about the difficulties of raising twins; and there are many. My other twin daughter wanted to do 'the difficulties of being transgendered' but wasn't selected. Maybe the world isn't quite ready for us yet; maybe this was too controversial. Or maybe her pitch wasn't quite good enough. Who knows? Anyway Tricia was straining at the leash to get up to Manchester and get out. She eventually managed it mid afternoon on Saturday. Plenty of time to get ready.

While she was getting ready, sexy blue dress with the zips again, she got a text from the limpet.

"Where were you last night"

Is Tricia the only person who uses punctuation, who knows what a question mark means? English is a dying art she thinks. But the good news was that she had at least avoided him again. The limpet only comes out once a weekend. A close call.

Tricia looked and felt great. She was meeting up with Tina and walked the canal without comment. Even better when she walked through Canal Street she got cheers and wolf-whistles from a gang of guys out on a stag party. She doesn't think they were being ironic. She doesn't think they knew what ironic meant.

Tina was talking to Kimberley who was up again. Kimberley disappeared to the ladies.

"Trish, I'm not sure she's all there you know" said Tina.

"How do you mean hon?"

"Well, how can you be going through the transition with a wig like that. She looks like a scarecrow".

Tricia giggled.

"Don't be uncharitable Tina, but I do agree with you".

Tricia, the good girl that she is, and the brave girl that she is, took Kimberley to one side and explained what she felt. Kimberley didn't object. In fact she had apparently taken loads of abuse in town earlier. Tricia thought............ she doesn't really get any abuse at all herself. Maybe she had a point about the wig after all. Kimberley promised to think about it. So all was well which ended well.

To Napoleons and surprise, surprise, Tina pulls.

"He's great Trish. He's called Scotch David and he's sophisticated and a good looker".

"If he's sophisticated, what on earth is he doing with you?" Tricia was as ever honest. She went upstairs to dance.

About half-an-hour later there was a huge commotion downstairs. A few moments later Tina pulled Tricia off the dance floor.

"Trish, Trish, I need you outside"

"What?"

"Don't argue just come outside"

So Tricia went outside the club to see what all the fuss was about and saw a small man being talked at by a larger policewoman.

"Trish, you do know there's nothing wrong with Scotch David don't you" said Tina.

"Can't say I do hon, I've never met him before in my life"

It transpired that Scotch David had been caught stealing by another t-girl the previous week. She noticed him in Naps and reported him. Tina's protestations got her nowhere and Scotch David was escorted by a very patient policewoman into a Panda car looking very sheepish. Apparently video evidence was going to be called. Another case solved. Another stroke of luck for Tina.

Ironically Tina was struggling for money herself. Following the Saturday night she only had £20 in the world to her name, and £40 was the minimum for a Sunday.

"Never mind Trish, I'll just have to cadge off a few blokes".

Tricia as always was ready long before Tina. She had an idea. She would go to visit Megan at the Binary Bar. She felt so comfortable walking around that it wasn't a problem. What was a problem was which shoes to wear. Yesterday was easy, gold dancing slippers, but she didn't want to wear them again today. Tricia had another idea. Floaty white dress she has never worn before. If she wore that she could then wear her strappy white sandals and her footwear problem was over. The sun was out after all. Her white handbag could be re-introduced as could her white jacket. What a clever girl!

Tricia bought her floaty white dress on impulse. She didn't really think it was her. When she walked out of the flat and crossed the grass she immediately changed her mind. The wind gently rustled the skirt and she felt fantastic in it. She bought a paper and went to the Binary Bar. She asked behind the bar for Megan, but Megan had left, only last week. Tricia bought a beer and texted Megan to find out what had happened..

"Yeah, I start on Tuesday at Ithaca in the City. Big time this time".

Tricia wishes Megan luck as always, not that she needs it. Tricia was the only customer at the Binary Bar and it was Sunday lunchtime, so decided Megan had made a good decision.

Tina was to make a good decision too. With only £20 left they would walk in, not take a taxi. Tina even agreed to follow Tricia's route, down the dual carriageway to Deansgate then pick up the canal. All was going swimmingly until the girls reached Bechers Brook. They got spotted early and received a cacophony of abuse.

"Get your tits out ha-ha-ha".

Tricia cursed to herself. This does not happen when she walks alone.

Even worse was to happen when they got to the pub. Tom was in and gave Tina even more abuse. He was going to knock her block off. Tina went for a cigarette, Tricia calmed Tom down; it was all fantasy again but at least common sense prevailed.

Tricia went for a cigarette and when she returned she found Tina with a bloke. She guessed the cadging had started. She motioned Tom to join her at another table on the other side of the pub. About half an hour later Tina joined them.

"Trish, I've pulled a dud. He won't buy me a drink. After all that snogging as well".

"Never mind hon, its the last game of the season. Lets go to New York New York and watch the game. Tricia wasn't really interested as United had already won the title but noticed a lot of noise next door on the dance floor. She asked Sylvia behind the bar what was going on.

"Its Peggy, the drag Queen. I wouldn't go in there if I were you, you'll get murdered".

"Then that, Sylvia, is precisely what I will do. You coming along Tina?"

"No way! I'm watching the game".

Tricia suspected that wasn't the only reason however she confidently walked next door alone. Immediately she became the target. Now, she knows she's got chicken legs but they are not called Benson and Hedges. For a good three minutes the abuse rained down on Tricia. But at the end Peggy gave Tricia a wink and blew her a kiss. Tricia blew a kiss back. The audience thought it was hilarious. Everybody had fun.

Tricia went back to Paddy's without Tina. Tina was spent up; so much for the cadging. There she met Julie who she knew. What she didn't know was that Julie was banned. After a bit of a scuffle with Paul, Julie eventually found her way to the exit.

"She's just trouble" said Marie behind the bar.

"She seemed ok to me?" Tricia tried to defend her.

"Trust me" said Marie.

"I trust you. Time I went home anyway, it's been a long weekend".

So Tricia, still loving the feel of her sundress, picked up a sandwich at Sainsbury's and went home for an early night. Work tomorrow. Damn and she's had such fun. Why can't she do this every day of her life?

Scary thoughts Tricia.

Chapter 75

The Great Pretender

I could murder that Tina sometimes. She does some right silly things and now she has fallen out with Georgina. She fell out with me at the start of the year too. I think a lot of it is in her mind and her attitude sometimes doesn't help. There is, by the way, a lot of pretence about what she does; and I suppose a lot of pretence about what I do. But then who's pretending? Is it Iain or is it me?

Queen at last. How on earth can you have a book about queens without Queen. That's my excuse anyway.

> Oh yes, I'm the great pretender
> Just laughing and gay like a clown
> I seem to be what I'm not you see
> I'm wearing my heart like a crown

In which Tina and Georgina fall out. Tricia becomes a cover model, Tina becomes a Domme and Tricia and Georgina do some sunbathing.

Tricia heard some bad news during the week, and she doesn't like bad news. Tina had fallen out with Georgina. Tricia knew it was inevitable because they are both so different. So Tricia went up to Manchester with just one thought on her mind. To get them back together again. Tina had been walking with Georgina during the week and they returned to Georgina's house. Just before they got there apparently Tina started flaunting her backside. Tina claimed Georgina had done the same in the past but Tricia couldn't comment because she had never seen Georgina do it. Tricia knows Georgina is wary of her neighbours who do accept her as Georgina. Tricia

317

just wanted to bang their heads together. By the end of the weekend they were talking, but only just. Time will likely heal but Tina needs to stay away from Georgina's house for a while.

This weekend Tricia was determined to try for another first. She was going to do it last weekend but hadn't prepared thoroughly enough. Tricia's cunning plan was to go sunbathing in the park next to Canal Street, Sackville Gardens. Yes, sunbathing in public in a bikini. Whatever next?

The previous weekend she had her bikini on under her floaty white sun dress. She thought there was a public convenience in the park where she could take the dress off. There wasn't. To take off her floaty white sun dress would mean that initially she would have to take her wig off; and she didn't want to do that in the park, in public. She didn't want to strip to her bikini in Paddy's either; so she shrugged her shoulders and decided it could wait for a week. She put her thinking cap on over her wig. What could she possibly wear that is dead easy to get on and off again? She also wanted to buy a nice girly beach bag and a fluffy towel. On Friday night Georgina agreed to sunbathe with her so she had Saturday to sort it out.

Friday in fact was a relatively quite night but Saturday was something else. The girls wanted to do some shopping so walked in again (from this you may surmise that Tina was skint). They survived Bechers Brook this time and were nearly at the pub when they bumped into John. While they were talking two buses accelerated past them causing a breeze. Tricia, wearing her little purple skirt, immediately put her hands down to protect her innocence (?). Tina, and it was on the other hand, did the complete opposite and her little white skirt rode up giving the whole street a glimpse of what was underneath.

"I felt like Marilyn Munroe Trish, and you have to admit my undies are dead sexy".

"Marilyn Munroe? I see absolutely no resemblance but yes hon your undies are very sexy but no hon your stockings and suspenders don't match. You should have asked Trinny for advice".

It transpired that John had been given a gift which he wished to sell on. He met the girls in the pub later and opened up his plastic Tesco bag. Inside was a black leather cap. Tina immediately showed interest and tried it on; Tricia immediately knew it wasn't for her.

"What do you think Trish, looks great doesn't it".

"Looks good on you but it's not for me. I'm far too sweet".

"John, I'll give you a tenner for it". Tina may have been skint but some things are irresistible it appears.

"Don't worry Tina, it was given to me, a fiver will do". John, at least, was being fair.

Money exchanged hands and John went to the bar.

"That's it Trish" said Tina triumphantly, "the missing piece in the jigsaw".

"The missing piece in what jigsaw?"

"Yes. I am going to become a Domme".

"But Tina. You can't just become a Domme like that, with a hat. It needs to be in you, you need to practice".

"I'd be a good Domme, don't you think?"

It was Tricia's round.

"Usual for me please Steve and a white wine and lemonade for the new Domme".

"New Domme? Ha-ha-ha-ha-ha-ha".

Tina looked daggers at Steve. Quite suitable for a Domme, Tricia thought.

After that pint the girls decided to go into town. This was a rare and sensible move by them and would stop them getting totally smashed again. We know what Tricia wanted; sunbathing stuff, but Tricia was intrigued about Tina's shopping list.

"Let me see. Some black skin-tight leather trousers, a crop, some handcuffs?"

"I am just preparing for now Tricia dear, so just some make-up. Remember though, there's a girl not a million miles from here who I can practice on, so careful what you say".

Tricia dropped her best curtsey. "Yes Ma'am".

Tina got her make-up, Tricia got her beach bag, but no towel. They were walking back through the Arndale when they noticed a photo shoot going on. It was open to anybody and whoever won could become a cover girl in a Sunday magazine. Tricia thought hard. Her rules are simple. Always say yes unless she can see danger. That way fun things happen. She listened. No dum, dum, dum, dum. Just then they got approached by the organiser of the shoot.

"It would be great if you two could join in".

"Yes please" said Tricia.

"I'm going for a fag" said Tina.

So Tricia lined up behind a couple of (rather more) attractive girls and waited her turn in front of a reasonable audience. Four pictures were taken. Tricia tried some poses which had been practising for a while now, and she got a round of applause and some whistles at the end. Everybody was lovely, everybody was happy, it was fun!

Tricia had an early night on Saturday in preparation for sunbathing the following day. My, she is becoming sensible. She still didn't wake up until mid morning though. She put on her bikini then her make-up, before zipping up her green dress. This will be so easy to get on and off she thought. No Tina to worry about today. She was spent up again. So Tricia put a towel and her handbag into her new beach bag and marched through town to meet Georgina and, after a couple of swift pints, some serious sunbathing.

As you know however things don't very often go to plan in Tricia's life. In Paddy's she not only met up with Georgina, but with Thuthee and Rita too, and the girls had a gossip which lasted rather longer than a couple of pints. Great fun but it was half three before Georgina and Tricia hit the park.

It has to be admitted that Tricia caused a bit of a stir when they arrived because Sindiy refused to behave herself and Tricia had to re-tuck. But safely and gracefully lying down gave her a chance to talk to Georgina. It seems that things are not going entirely smoothly in her relationship with Dave. Tricia could see the problem. It appeared Georgina both wanted 100% commitment but also wanted some space to herself. Not an easy mix. Tricia expressed her concern but left it at that. She knew Georgina would sort it out. As for Tina and Georgina? Well, Tina is still not going to be invited back for a while.

One hour was long enough. It was proving the point that counted, but people didn't seem to notice the point so that was ok. Then back to Paddy's where a couple of rent boys came in and made some interesting comments.

"Trish, what have you been up to? I can see friction burns on your knees".

"I promise nothing. I'm jingly jangly Tricia now. I fell over six weeks ago and it still hasn't recovered". Tricia wasn't entirely sure she was believed but we know it was the truth.

"Trish, why don't you go the whole way? you'll look so much better"

For the first time in Tricia's life she didn't immediately say no. That is very, very scary!

Chapter 76

I Want to be Loved by You

It is Iain's birthday. I had my first birthday a couple of months, so this chapter is a mixture of what is in both of our minds and is somewhat different that the other chapters. Tamsin Heath is about to appear. Why may she be important?

By the way let's do some Marilyn Munroe. There is no t-girl that doesn't love Marilyn Munroe. I could of course have chosen "Happy Birthday Mr President" but instead something from "Some Like it Hot". The first film I saw with men who dressed as women. I was engrossed but was too young to understand the humour. I did wish though.

> I couldn't aspire
> to anything higher
> and to feel the desire
> to make you my own.

The Birthday Girl

Now this is interesting. A window of opportunity (how I hate that expression) opened up for Tricia late on Friday. I was prepared to stay at home at the weekend since the following weekend was Iain's birthday. However twin one decided to stay with boyfriend and twin two made a last minute decision to visit her Mother in Leeds. Tricia could have escaped the cage. She and I fought and thought but for once I won. There are bigger and scarier things ahead. We both need a rest, need to relax; we can't keep going at one hundred miles an hour. There are also things I need to sort out at home. Tricia listened and finally agreed. She was thinking of one thing in particular:

When my eldest daughter was small, aged around two and three, she had a certain characteristic. Before she ran or did any physical activity she used to draw herself in, concentrate intently, then go for it. It only took a second or so but you could see the determination on her face. That is what Tricia needed to do. There is hopefully much more fun on the horizon but she needs to focus and concentrate herself now. Good girl Tricia and it did pay dividends. Twin two had to return early from Leeds and I was at home for her. We were both really pleased.

It is now Friday night one week later. It is my birthday and I am in a euphoric mood. I am sitting in the pub, the Knotts Bar and I can't wait to change, to be Tricia, to be who I have always wanted to be but never dared. What happens tonight doesn't matter; what is superb is the way I am thinking now. I am so deep inside myself. I've never felt like this before. Soon I will go out proudly and show myself off to the world; soon I will be my real self. I thought earlier in the year that things had worn off, but they haven't at all. They are even stronger now. I am even stronger now. I'm meeting Becky at five in Paddy's. YAY!

I am now dressed to kill and am in Paddy's. I'm getting the eye from a guy but he's got no chance. Walking through Manchester wasn't a problem. I walked tall, I walked proudly; I was Tricia. I got a few beeps at the big roundabout but they were kind beeps. I looked sexy, I looked provocative, I probably looked transgendered but who actually cares. I don't. It causes fun, it causes a laugh, it lightens people's day. It is now though very, very serious what I do and how I do it. It matters so much to me. That, in itself, is frightening.

My birthday is over but I enjoyed it immensely. It was spent with my best friends, my closest friends; Megan, Becky and Tina amongst others. I'm at Megan and Becky's flat writing this at 11:00 on Saturday morning. I'm very, very hungover. What is interesting is what is in my mind. I want a man. I want someone to kiss and cuddle up to, someone to give myself to. Someone who can go as deep down inside me as I can myself. Someone who can fulfil me, who can satisfy me. Maybe tonight I will find someone. Since becoming jingly-jangly Tricia this is the first time I have felt this way. Though I love dressing Sindiy, she is not enough for once. I suppose I am now officially a horny bitch. I want, no I need, someone to make my own; to kiss and to caress, to grow deep inside me causing me pain, but so much pleasure too. I want to feel needed, I want to feel happy. Happy is good. Happy is fun. Tricia likes fun....

Oh, I haven't told you, I have another name, a pen name. Am I Iain? Am I Tricia? Am I Tamsin? Tamsin Heath is my pen name. Why I chose that I don't know but I don't care and now it's done. Tammy may release Tricia but we shall see. If you see her anywhere you'll now know it's me, Tricia, and I'll always be Tricia because I love being Tricia and being called Tricia. Tammy will hide my identity which I don't. That is why she is so important. Good luck Tamsin, go for it girl, its what we all want.

But we know what Tricia wants now. Megan and Becky got her a birthday card. On the front it had a fifties girl with a fifties guy. "She had every intention of making the same mistake twice". Is that really Tricia? Is Tricia such a tart? Yes, sometimes it probably is exactly me, most of the time it probably isn't. I have to learn to live with it. They also got it right with the present. A new notepad; even more chapters; sorry.

I am now back in the pub. Thank you Becky for driving me in. It is half past one. I am waiting for Tina; in fact the book ought to be called "waiting for Tina" because it happens so often. I am shattered and not really enjoying my pint. I'm still as horny as hell though. If anyone approaches me they've got a good chance. Hang on though; I have to be a bit choosy. I'm jingly-jangly Tricia now after all.

Its now ten o'clock at night and I am back in the flat. I was asleep until Tina poured a pint of water over me. I am still as horny as hell. Get up Trish, get out, have fun. Sexy yellow dress will work and don't worry too much about your make-up. Just be yourself girl, that is what you are quickly becoming and you love it! Will she find another horny guy just like her tonight? Who knows, who cares, what is for sure is that you won't find the answer here.

Its Sunday lunchtime and Tricia is back at the pub. A few beers then into town then to New York, New York then back here for the Sunday crew. This morning Tricia was thinking even more dangerous thoughts. She was thinking of a life without her dolly, without Sindiy. Could she manage it? Could I live without after fifty years with her? For the first time in her life Tricia thought it was feasible. In the pub are Mark, not Morticia, Glenda, Georgina, Saskia and Andrea. Yes, the lunatics have taken over the pub. Saskia tries on my shoes, my white sandals. How can you tell the difference between a girl and a t-girl? You look at the sole of their shoes. Saskia found the label on the sole of my right sandal. I must do better.

After a lovely trip around town; I bought some more perfume, Showtime by Kylie Minogue, very sweet, very feminine, I went to New York New York to watch the drag act. I think in all honesty I could have done better. But then I am not a drag queen. Back in Paddy's I meet up with Mary, Les, Al, Peter et al and have a wonderful night. The Sunday evening club is fun. Got bought a few beers from a bearded Irishman who wanted to be a girl like me. I think, firstly, we need a razor!

It's reached Monday morning. I've another day off work so could dress again. But no, I've done too much already. Its simply not in me to do another day. I am quite old, although I don't feel it. As if to prove a point Sindiy just would not behave herself and was craving attention all morning. There is only one thing that will stop that. There is only one thing that will make me whole, or hole. You know I may just do it. I so love being Tricia.

Chapter 77

The Flower Song

By the way, this is one of my favourite Arias, The Flower song from Carmen by Bizet. It was easy to pick (get it?). You see, it is going to become my trademark. The trouble was that until the weekend I only had one flower to put in my hair. I soon put that right though. Now I am going to wear a flower in my hair wherever I go. So San Fransisco! So pretty, so girly, and so me. So there!

> The flower which you threw to me
> in my prison stayed with me.
> Withered and dry, this flower
> kept all the while it's sweet fragrance;

Tricia is bum

Tricia couldn't wait for the weekend. She is so happy being herself she could cry; but they would be tears of joy not hurt. I gave her instructions to watch the spending. She sort of listened but as we know she is a very independent young lady. It's probably because of that she again had the time of her life.

For once Tina was to join her on the Friday night. She had a little money and managed to postpone her regular night with Graham until Sunday.

"Trish, I'm going to pull tonight, I can feel it".

"Aaah Tina, but what precisely will you be pulling".

Tricia didn't worry about such things. She wanted a laugh and to be happy. Quite often men got in the way. The girls got a cab to the village; no walking in heels that high and were enjoying their first drink when Tina sighed. Tina's normal sigh in ecstasy, lying on the bed with her legs around some man's neck. This sigh however was one of dismay.

"Look at those two girls over there Trish, they're not even trying and don't they look miserable".

Tricia glanced sideways but was more stoic. Two girls were sitting, badly dressed and made up with legs akimbo. They did look miserable.

"Blimey Tina, you can see what they had for dinner". This was an expression used by my Father when inelegant ladies didn't sit properly. Tricia got up to buy the drinks and smiled at the miscreants. No response. Tricia brought back the drinks and smiled again. Still no response. Tricia asked if they were enjoying themselves and got her head snapped off. Some people, she thought, don't want to be helped. So she didn't bother suggesting a shave.

Tina went out for a cigarette and was swiftly replaced by a tall bloke with shifty eyes. The shifty eyes looked at Tricia. Tricia smiled. She had seen it all before. The shifty eyes returned to the problem in hand. With the other hand guarding the aforementioned problem, the shifty eyes swiftly became less shifty; then they got up and left. Tricia gracefully placed her own hand over her mouth and giggled.

Tina and Tricia decamped (never) to Naps where they met Mark, not Morticia and Glenda. Sadly the club was quiet, most likely because Sparkle was just around the corner, and Tricia had the dance floor to herself but she didn't mind. She took it over for about an hour dancing with a number of different people. Tina meanwhile was doing her forlorn, distressed, abandoned act downstairs to the two nonagenarians that would listen. Tricia decided to cut her losses and go; though losses isn't fair and cut she is still thinking about. She was dead happy and looking forward to Saturday.

She was walking back to the flat, opposite Oxford Road when she was accosted by a bunch of teenagers.

"Hey you're bum, say I'm bum"

"But I'm not bum I'm Tricia"

"You are bum, and I love your skirt. I've got the same one in black"

"I'm not bum", Tricia was adamant.

"But bum is cool"

Just then one of the guys gave Tricia a peck on the cheek.

"I shake my lettuce to you"

Tricia was getting very confused but everyone was being so friendly towards her.

"Alright then, I'm bum", Tricia smiled.

"Hooray"

"You are"

They went their separate ways waving to each other as the gang disappeared around the corner. What on earth was all that about? Tricia doesn't understand modern slang but it seems like fun, and as we know, Tricia likes fun.

Both girls were out again on the Saturday. It is probably fair to say that they were both further out than at any time of their lives.

"I've found it!" said Tricia

"I didn't know you'd lost anything" said Tina who was frantically searching for her lighter.

"Look in your handbag hon. No, I've found my defining characteristic".

"Your defining characteristic?"

"Yes, my trademark".

"And..."

"The flower in my hair. Everybody likes it and it's girly, just like me. Wherever I go I'm going to wear a flower".

"But you've only got one flower, you told me last night. Soon it will droop and that would make a change".

"Maybe it could borrow some of your Viagra. No, I'm jingly, jangly Tricia with a flower now, and I can easily buy more".

"I've found it!" said Tina, whose lighter was in her handbag after all.

Dressed to kill and feeling sexy the girls got into the lift and checked themselves out in the big, stained mirror as it descended.

"Ding". The lift stopped on the fourth floor where a little Caribbean boy and his parents were waiting. The little boy looked at the two big girls and hesitated.

"Go on" said the Father.

"Its alright, we don't bite" said Tricia.

The little boy slowly walked in and stood next to Tricia as the doors closed. They both began to giggle.

Saturday turned out to be a typical Saturday, which meant Tricia failed in her quest to buy more flowers, failing to leave the sanctuary of the village. First they met a lovely, intelligent man called John in the pub. Then Georgina came in. While there were still sores to be healed, they were healing. Then Tricia thrashed Tina at pool in New York, New York where they bumped into a pissed Scotsman who was watching the rugby.

"You two must be the ugliest girls in the world". He wouldn't shut up.

Now Tricia knows two things for sure. She definitely isn't the prettiest girl in the world but, by the same token, there is no way she can be described as the ugliest girl in the world. The Scotsman was told to shut up and bugger off by the regulars who always look after Tina and Tricia.

Back in the pub and Tricia was slowly losing the plot. They were talking to a brother and sister, she gay, he an admirer and to Thuthee. Other girls joined in. Tricia decided to cut her losses again and go home for an early night. She was both drunk and tired. Tina decided to take a wakey wakey tablet and persevere.

Sunday arrived and following her early night, Tricia was ready for it. No Tina, we can guess what she was up to. So Tricia marched back to where she imbibed and had a long happy afternoon with Georgina, Tim, Julia, Mark and Glenda. She was however a sensible girl and had planned her exit strategy.

"I'm going into town to buy some flowers for my hair, see you in an hour or so".

She was just walking into Piccadilly Gardens when some black girls shouted at her.

"Whaaay sexy". They smiled and Tricia smiled back.

About fifty yards down the road some black guys shouted at her.

"Whaaay cool". They smiled and Tricia smiled back.

Tricia thinks there is something different, something special in the attitude of Caribbean people. They are so much more chilled it seems than any other race, and because of that they enjoy life so much more. She had noticed this before. She smiled again. She can think of one other group of people this may apply to. Young, English teenagers. Maybe there is hope. Or is it just that the social conditioning hasn't yet kicked in?

Tricia bought six new flowers to go in her hair and was happily drinking her cappuccino and eating her toasty when she looked down to a horrible sight. Sindiy had lost her moorings and could clearly be seen poking out from under her extremely short white skirt. Fortunately the table at the cafe offered some protection but Tricia hastily ate up and re-adjusted herself in the ladies before going back to the pub. Careful girl, you'll get arrested at this rate.

Back at the pub Julie made an important statement.

"Tricia dear, you will only know what to do if you come and live in Manchester full time. It has changed our lives".

Tricia thought deeply.

Manchester was indeed included; but that was longer term. For now though Sparkle was in two weeks and she wanted a good run up into it. So why not stay at home next weekend and take some time off work just before Sparkle. That would give her time to try to get Tamsin out into an unsuspecting world. Tamsin may be the key, or she may not; but Tricia knows one thing. Trying to get Tamsin out will be fun, even if it doesn't work. And what does Tricia like?

Chapter 78

House of Fun

By the way, I used to love a television comedy show called the Young Ones, where this song comes from. The House of Fun is of course Paddys Goose. I feel such a girly girl at the moment wearing my flowers. It was Sparkle weekend again and although I sparkled all the all the time I have to admit it was mainly in the pub. I had a great weekend though. So many friends old and new were there. Particular thanks to Michelle and Jackie who I spent Sunday afternoon with in the pub with while we were momentously saving the test match. We were too drunk to notice. But it made Iain smile.

Welcome to the House of Fun
Now I've come of age
Welcome to the House of Fun

Sparkle Two

Was it really that time of year again? Has a year already passed since Sparkle? Doesn't time fly when you're enjoying yourself and Tricia was certainly doing that? It was indeed time for Manchester to be inundated with the transgendered and for once Tricia wouldn't be the only t-girl in the Arndale Centre. That is if she managed to get that far. Recently she had been finding it difficult to get out of the front door of Paddys Goose.

Having missed the previous weekend, Tricia went on Wednesday evening for a change. Wednesday night in the village is of course t-girl night; although with Sparkle imminent it wasn't quite as busy as normal.

Tricia was enjoying a cigarette at the front of the pub when an attractive young girl joined her.

"Have you seen a fit bloke out here?"

"No, I can't say I have". Tricia would certainly have noticed a fit bloke.

"I was talking to him in the pub earlier. My friends said he came out here but your the only person out here and you are certainly not a fit bloke".

"How do you know?" Tricia never did find out whether the girl found her fit bloke.

"Crikey, your down here early" said Lee behind the bar.

"Yes, and I'm here until Sunday. It's Sparkle you know"

"I was aware Trish. We'd better order another barrel of Unicorn then".

Tricia met Jacqui who only got out occasionally and looked really good, except her wig was all over the place.

"Honey, you look wonderful, but what is that thing on your head? Is it alive?"

"I just can't get it right? I've been trying for hours".

"Lets go into the Ladies and I'll see what I can do".

Tricia, now vastly experienced at wig styling worked her magic. Using her dexterous wrists (don't ask how she got them but remember I used to bowl leg spin) she shook and shook the cheap rug until it showed some semblance of order. She then brushed it carefully before placing it back on Jacqui's head. She showed Jacqui how to adjust it from the temples and then gently styled it using her fingers. Jacqui looked in the mirror and smiled. Tricia was a clever girl. Tricia and Jacqui went off to Naps and strutted their stuff before Tricia settled Jacqui down with an admirer she had known from the past. Jacqui is going to have an interesting night ahead of her she thought.

The following day Tricia decided to wear her secretary's outfit as everybody would be working while Tricia was having fun. So check blouse, black knee length pencil skirt and jacket. Still dead sexy. She was walking through

Canal Street when she passed a gang of young lads. She got a wolf-whistle followed by;

"That just isn't right".

Tricia smiled at the guys. Tricia smiled to herself.

As we know, Tricia is now good girl so she listened to me and only spent a little money on some hooped earrings and some more flowers for her hair. She did see, and tried on, a lovely pink dress but decided that although it was decidedly feminine, it was not girly enough for her.

Back at the pub and the girls are beginning to gather for the weekend. Tricia bumped into Paula whose ample charms have already been documented, and Rita.

"What's this about you falling down a manhole? I didn't think men had them".

Paula had been alerted of Tricia's accident a month or so ago.

"I suppose we will have to see". The chop was still on Tricia's mind but it is good that she has to wait. She behaved herself for once and went back to t-Girl Towers early. She did enquire about Tina's lost coat (why does she always lose things)? But with no joy. Anyway, thought Tricia, Tina needs a new coat. It was probably snaffled at Naps. Both girls are wary of what goes on in Naps.

Now, the trouble with Sparkle is that you get to meet many, many old acquaintances. Tricia left for the pub early on Saturday and when she arrived Georgina, Saski, Debbie, Paula and Rachel were already there. Tricia decided, since it was Sparkle, to wear her tiny pink ra-ra skirt and a little top that showed off her toned stomach. It was the first time she had the confidence to show off a bare midriff, apart from sunbathing in her bikini that is. She certainly did sparkle but different girls kept coming into the pub so it wasn't until late in the afternoon before she ventured out of the pub. She went into the ladies and freshened up her make-up. She strode confidently into the outside air, ignoring the comments being shouted by the girls at her table.

What Tricia didn't realise, what the girls were trying to tell her, was that she was suffering from what is known as wardrobe malfunction. Her little ra-ra skirt was tucked inside her panties at the back. Fortunately for Tricia she was wearing matching pink frilly panties so at least she was colour co-ordinated. She wandered around Sackville Gardens looking at the displays before returning to the pub and being informed of her problem.

"Oops" Tricia blushed the same colour of her panties and pulled her skirt out.

"But nobody said anything".

"They must have been enjoying the view" said Rita with a smile.

The rest of Saturday passed Tricia by. She can however remember being in Naps with a tableful of girls and hoped she behaved herself. Apparently she did. Appearances, Tricia now knows, is everything.

Sunday arrived and Tricia was up for more. Again she left Tina, who was at least an hour behind her, at the flat. She was sitting on a barstool talking to Georgina when John walked in.

"Hi Trish, you left you knickers in my flat".

"I most certainly did not, they were on display for all to see yesterday afternoon". Tricia checked, she was wearing her yellow knickers today.

"Will you give me a pair of your knickers?"

"Do you want to wear them?"

"No but they would remind me of you".

"Clean or dirty?"

"I'll leave that to you".

"Ok hon, I'll see what I can do, and Marty, what are you doing in my handbag?"

"You promised me some toffee bon-bons. I was just seeing if you've got them.

"Well I did get some, but I've eaten them all so you'll have to wait. Hands out". Tricia slapped Marty on the wrists. Tricia is getting to know and be appreciated by more and more people.

Tom walked in and a recollection from last night in Naps came to Tricia. Tom had pulled a transvestite who didn't bother about make-up or wig. So from the neck up he was a bloke and from the neck down a girl; a sort of semi-transvestite. Tricia doesn't mind. Each to themselves she thinks and Tom seemed to have had a good night.

Georgina, Tina, Mark, Glenda, Paula, Michelle, Jackie, Steph, Thuthie, Debbie, Julia, Tim, John, Kevin, Angela, Saski etc etc all crossed Tricia's path on the Sunday in the pub. She remembers little except two lovely comments from Tim.

"There isn't a bad bone in your body" and

"You looked elegant as usual, even if your skirt was tucked into your knickers". Elegant, Tricia had never thought of that before but liked it a lot.

As she elegantly downed her fifteenth pint of beer for the day, the fact that England were far from elegantly saving the test match passed her by. As did the fact that Tina was sitting in the corner quietly (for once) talking to a big guy wearing a Stetson. She was later to find out. Tina brought him back to T-Girl Towers that night, that his name was Tex. Now where was that going?

Chapter 79

Let's Fall in Love

I am becoming even more confident and relaxed in the outside world. I am truly Tricia, I am truly she. I don't think Tina is but nevertheless this chapter is dedicated to her, and the day she got engaged. Her relationship with Tex had certainly blossomed since last week so, and by the way, let's do it. Lets fall in love. And why not?

> Birds do it, bees do it
> Even educated fleas do it
> Let's do it, let's fall in love

Is marriage on the cards?

Tina Tresvain, and for some reason Tricia found out that her full name is actually Tina Trescothick Tresvain (I thought he had opened the batting for Somerset and England but may be wrong) was out on a Friday night. Graham seemed to be overlooked. She was instead to meet up with Tex in Naps and guess what was on the cards. I'm sure you have. But sex is always on the cards as far as Tina Trescothick Tresvain is concerned. Sex with Tex sounds good.

So, and looking gorgeous as always, Tina and Tricia get a cab to Paddy's early on Friday night. Both girls immediately noticed a strange atmosphere in the village. Maybe their feminine intuition was developing. It seemed a darker and far more serious place than for Sparkle the previous weekend. They weren't over-concerned, after all there were police patrolling the village all the time and CCTV cameras everywhere. There did seem to be anger in the air though. It's funny how sometimes you can smell it. DUM DUM DUM DUM.

Tina had to go to the bank and while she was gone Tricia went out for a cigarette. Happily puffing (careful) away, a gang of black guys approached and surrounded her. They circled around her. She wasn't scared because she could have dived in the pub if she needed to. She might have had to ditch the heels though. She smiled at the gang. One said, "OK she's cool" and they walked off. One turned round and winked at her. She winked back. She thinks they just wanted to check her out but it was frightening nevertheless.

Tina returned from the bank.

"That was horrendous Trish, I got all sorts of comments".

"Did anything bad happen though?"

"No, I was just followed back into the village with a load of guys shouting at me".

"Well, at least you didn't react".

"There were half a dozen of them at least. No way I was going to take them on".

"You should have just smiled at them to show them how comfortable you were".

"Comfortable, I was shaking like a leaf!".

"Never mind, your here now, safe and sound and your boyfriend is coming later; almost certainly I'd say".

"I hope so".

Life can be difficult for girls like these sometimes.

Paul arrived for his stint behind the bar and got talking to the girls.

"Do you know what happened last Sunday night after Sparkle?".

"No". Tricia looked embarrassed.

"No", Tina looked embarrassed.

It transpired that Tina was found by Paul in the ladies, fast asleep, at half past midnight; an hour after the pub had shut. Everybody else had gone home.

"Was there a man in there with her?" Tricia was simply relieved that it wasn't her.

"She was on her own, but she had a smile on her face".

Tex, thought Tricia.

"Trish; you and I went to Naps and got let in. I had to meet Tex".

Tex, thought Tricia.

"I'm well aware you met Tex hon, you kept me up half the night with your grunting and grinding".

Paul, as ever, looked away.

"No harm done Paul?" Said Tina

"No harm done", and a trace of a smile appeared around Paul's lips. It's as much as you get.

The girls later went onto Naps, where Tina did indeed meet up with Tex and brought him home. Another sleepless night for Tricia.

Tex left early in the morning. Tina woke up, bright and breezy.

"Trish, we're going to look at wardrobes today".

"Wardrobes? You what?".

"Look at your dresses. They're spilling everywhere. We need to get you a wardrobe and put the coffin back in the living room where it belongs".

"How can a coffin be in a living room? Give me another hour in bed hon, you and Tex kept me awake all night and it will give you time to get ready".

One hour later Tricia was again woken by a dressed, but not made up Tina.

"Georgina is meeting us here in an hour, the water is on so get moving".

Tricia likes challenges like that and miraculously both girls were ready to meet Georgina at the agreed time. Georgina, who had spent the night with Dave, was scornful. It only took her half an hour to get ready.

Somehow Tina needed the bank again as did Tricia and Georgina needed some cigarettes so they stopped off at Sainsbury's before the furniture shop. Outside the ATM Tina and Tricia were immediately spotted by a family; well they were wearing extremely short skirts as the sun was shining. There were comments, giggles and wolf whistles. Tricia smiled and enjoyed the attention. Tina cringed. The family turned round to go into the shop only to bump into a six foot two inch fifteen stone schoolgirl.

"Life is fun" said Georgina.

"Enjoy it".

The girls hope the family have now recovered from the shock.

The furniture shop was closed. It didn't open on Saturdays. Tricia was relieved because she was running out of money. Georgina was relieved because it meant they could get to Paddys Goose at a reasonable hour. Tina was thinking about Tex. At the pub and all was smiles. Dave arrived, but later than Georgina would have liked and Tricia met Andy. A lovely gay guy with children of his own (a rarity in the village) so they had plenty to discuss. Tricia was a brave and sensible girl and left the pub before she got drunk. She had a walk round town, hardly creating a stir and watched a bit of the cricket.

When she returned Georgina and Dave had gone home for a cuddle and Tricia met Colin. Colin had just beaten Tina at pool in New York, New York and was, in his youth, a very good cricketer. We may even have played against each other. So Tricia again had plenty to talk about. Later Denise came in and started chatting to Tina and things gradually went downhill. They started playing games in the pub. Tina and Denise tried arm wrestling although there was a furious row about the positioning of the elbows so they gave up. Tricia stated how proud she was at being called elegant so they all tried to walk up and down the pub with a beer mat balanced on their wigs. All very silly. A drunk Tricia left for home with a similarly drunk Tina; but what had happened to Tex?

Far too quickly it was Sunday, although Tricia likes Sunday better than any other day of the week. There is less pressure somehow and there are more friends out. The girls decided to walk in through the canal and, for once, got no grief whatsoever. In Paddy's, Georgina, Tina, Tom and Tricia were having a conversation at the bar when Tex entered.

Tex immediately walked up to Tina who was sitting on a barstool; ignoring Georgina, Tom and Tricia who he all knew.

"Darling, I've got something for you".

"Not in here I hope" commented Georgina.

Tex bent down towards Tina's hand. An audible crack was heard in the pub as his back lowered. He felt in his pocket. Amidst the stale tobacco, till receipts, uneaten mints and fluff he managed to locate two leather bands which looked like they had come out of a Christmas cracker about twenty years ago.

"Tina, I want to commit myself to you so am placing this token of my affection on your finger".

Tina was totally phased so didn't reply. She merely placed the second band on Tex's digit.

Tom's eyes doubled in size.

Georgina and Tricia nearly fell off their barstools they were giggling so much.

For now though, Tex and Tina were engaged to be married.

The two love-birds stayed together for the rest of the day. Tricia went to watch the cricket, England were eventually to win this particular Test Match and returned to the pub to meet Julia and Tim.

"Trish", said Julia we've got this idea. What do you think?"

"Interesting and I will think about it" said Tricia "but I'm not sure that the flat is the best place for it".

Chapter 80

The Broken Engagement

Well, it lasted about six days, but that was about six days too long. Yes, Tina's engagement is officially off. So sad and by the way, this one took some digging out! But it's a Country and Western song just for Tex. Somehow I doubt we've seen the last of him.

> God in Heaven sent an Angel
> To relieve her ache and pain
> She went drifing off to Heaven
> On an Angel's snow white wing

Tina learns what SWOT means.

"I'm not sure about Tex, Trish"

"How do you mean hon? You're still engaged aren't you? You're still wearing his ring".

"I don't think its right"

Tricia had returned the following week anxious to find out how the loving couple were getting on.

"At work, when we wish to invest in something long term, we swot it".

"Swat it Trish?".

"Yes, I'll take you through it. 'S' is for strengths so what are Tex's strengths"

Tina thought for a while.

"He's good in bed and he's got a big thingy"

"That's just one, he's good in bed. Has he got any other strengths? Is he reliable for example?

Tina thought longer.

"Not really. He let me down last Saturday. I can't think of any more strengths".

"Oh well. 'W' is for weaknesses. What are his weaknesses?".

"He's got no money. He hasn't even got a job. He lives in a dingy council flat in the roughest area of Manchester. He isn't reliable and he can't even read or write so I can't text him".

"What, you can't text Tex?"

"No, how can you live without being able to read?"

"So, he's got everything against him except that he's good in bed". Tricia shrugged.

"'O' is for opportunities, though if he can't read or write I don't see many of those on the horizon".

"Can't think of any Trish".

"'T' is for threats, can you think of any of them"

"If I'm with Tex it may threaten my relationship with you and my other friends. He may beat me up, I've not yet seen him really drunk but I know he can be. He's not allowed to drink alcohol in Paddy's. He may even be an alcoholic, I don't know".

"Tina, I think you do know".

"Yes I do Trish, I need to break it off".

"That's a bit extreme isn't it Tina, the poor chap hasn't done you any harm".

"No silly. I'm meeting him tomorrow. I'll just give him his ring back".

"His band you mean".

With that the girls left the flat to go out on the raz.

"But if I haven't got Tex, what am I going to do for sex?".

"That's never bothered you before hon. And what's happened to Graham?"

"Oh yes, forgot about him".

The girls were waiting for a taxi on the pavement before the roundabout when they got beeped enthusiastically at by a white car. A taxi arrived and the girls climbed on board. No they didn't, they gracefully entered careful not to expose their panties. Tina looked behind. The white car was in the side road five yards from the taxi. Two guys were motioning to the girls to get in the car with them.

"Lets go" Tricia said to the cab driver. "Mancunian way then into the gay village". The cab sped off.

"They must have wanted sex" said Tina.

"I don't think we could take that chance. The danger song came into my head. It may have been fun who knows, but definitely too risky to find out".

A lucky escape, who knows?

The girls were discussing what might have been in the pub when they were joined by a man with the thickest beard you've ever seen.

"Hi, I'm Andrew and I've decided I want to dress and go out dressed just like you two".

"With that?" Tricia was aghast.

"I'll shave that off, but do you think you can help me?".

"Of course, what's your girl name?". Tricia was well aware of a certain tactic used by many admirers who wanted to get into her knickers, metaphorically speaking.

"Suzanne". Tricia started humming Leonard Cohen.

"And your surname?"

"Andrews, Suzanne Andrews because my first name is Andrew". Tricia was impressed. She knew many girls who didn't have a forename, never mind a surname. He was obviously serious. The girls agreed to help.

While all this was going on I was trying to avert a crisis going on at work. We had a major system down and one of my team had stayed behind in the office to test should the system get recovered. It came to a head at around eleven thirty when I had to make a decision as to whether to pull him out or leave him to find a hotel since his last train was due. I decided there was no guarantee that the system would be back that night so let him go home (indeed the system didn't come back until the following morning). I had a long chat with Kim who was looking after the incident and trying as ever to be all things to all men and one girl. Kim knows about Tricia so I sent her a text in the early hours of Saturday morning.

"I'm not sure I'm the right person to make important business decisions. But I'm good at frocks! Hugs Trish xx".

It gave Kim a laugh which is good. She has far too much on her plate which is unfair; but then Tricia knows all about life being unfair.

The girls, still sober, made Naps where Tricia met up with Knicki, a Ts and Tony, who thoroughly enjoys the company of TS's. Josh was around too and they had an interesting chat about Knicki's business. Maybe Tricia could help. As Tricia's life develops though she feels Knicki could definitely help her.

So the fateful Saturday arrived and Tina was still determined to give back the engagement band (well, ring is taking it a fair bit too far). The girls walked in through the canals and had a bit of a debate en route. Tina wanted some money and was going to go to Clone Zone to get it. Tricia couldn't understand. How could you spend money to get money? It cost money to withdraw money at Clone Zone. There was an ATM just off the main route although outside of the village where it would be free. Tricia often used it. She finally convinced Tina and they walked under Tricia's gobble and up the canal path to street level. They turned left and walked towards the ATM.

"No Trish, turn back, look!"

Tricia looked up. Outside O'Shea's, the Irish pub on the corner of the road were at least fifty drunken football supporters dressed in green and white. Celtic were playing Manchester City in a friendly.

"I think I'm with you on this one Tina". The girls rapidly retraced their steps.

Tina went to Clone Zone, Tricia went to get the drinks in; but no Tex so she had a chat with Tom instead. Tina returned and a few minutes later Tex arrived. Tina took Tex outside and they were out for a while. Tom told Tricia that he had heard through the grapevine that this wasn't the first time Tex had pulled such a trick.

Tina returned with a smile. She'd done it, but not completely.

"I told him Trish that he could always get in touch with me if he wanted a shag". Tricia wasn't sure. Surely you either break up completely or you don't. It wasn't her problem though. She shrugged.

Becky arrived and joined in the debate. Megan was working so they had to walk across town to meet her in a pub which turned out to be friendly, delightful and served good beer. Tricia was surprised when she met Megan. The wives' plan had been to save money to move to Australia but this had now changed, as Megan was about to. Yes, Megan was determined to change sex. It may have been something to do with her now short but dead good hairstyle. Tricia suspected it was and wondered whether she had anything to offer, but shrugged it off. Becky approves and supports Megan so all is well. Important and difficult times ahead though.

Becky and Tricia returned to Paddy's and carried on as if they hadn't left, leaving Megan to get on with organising her kitchen. They drunk and they drunk; goodness knows how Becky in particular managed it since she hadn't had a drink the previous month. They both survived though, and somehow got home in one piece.

A bleary eyed Tricia finally awoke on Sunday lunchtime. Actually see was woken by Tina.

"Wake up you dozy cow. I'm off to Graham's for a shag, see you next week".

The broken off engagement had clearly not affected Tina's sexual appetite. Tricia slowly got ready and walked into town. On the way she passed some Caribbean guys.

"A pretty girl like you must have plenty money in her purse".

"I wish hon, and thanks". They smiled.

It was to turn into a lovely day. There was a bike ride going on in Manchester called Skyride and may of the roads were shut to cars. The ride actually went directly outside the front of Paddy's so Tricia watched quite a lot of it while smoking far too much. She was also to cause quite a stir among the bike riders.

"Told you, you owe me a fiver!".

Tricia doesn't mind. She knows you can't fool all of the people all of the time and it was wonderful to watch families cycling together and the big grins on the faces of the children. To save herself from getting too drunk, Tricia went into town and bought a beautiful yellow and green dress. What was once running the gauntlet has now become a cake-walk. Tricia loves it to death, loves being herself and showing herself off and isn't at all concerned about the few comments she gets. She is still growing.

Back at the pub and Tim and Julia are there again. They like to come out on a Sunday evening. Tim was dressed so wasn't Tim at all, she was Katrina and she looked great. They were still discussing the idea.

"I'm happy to model anything Julia, you know me, but let's make sure we've got our target audience right and available".

Chapter 81

Careless Whisper

There is a joke about a wide-mouthed frog but fortunately for you I can't remember it. It was Pride weekend again and it was what I was concentrating on. I don't wish to look Gianfranco Zola even though he looks a happy enough chap. I must purse my lips and pout more, think Victoria Beckham.

But Pride was really only about one thing, selfish girl that I am. It was about my new wig which I simply adore. I am no longer just jingly-jangly Tricia, I am a thoroughly modern jingly-jangly Miss. Again I'll have to admit that I didn't really enjoy the commercialism of Pride but, by the way, I did get to see Frisky and Mannish; who were on the large stage at last. They played a very amusing version of the song.

> I'm never gonna dance again
> Guilty feet have got no rhythm
> Though it's easy to pretend
> I know you're not a fool

More and More Pride

A day late arriving (or a day early depending on your point of view) Tricia marched into Manchester at dusk. She can now pretty much pass at dusk; its just daylight she struggles with. She seemed to be walking well. She was walking taller than tall, I'm sure she'll tell you about that later, and she could see her hips swaying in the shadows. She thought back a long time. She thought back to her dance teacher Tara.

"Sit on your hips" Tara used to say and that was roughly what Tricia was doing. She smiled to herself. She felt good.

In the pub she met Dlara. A funny name but seemingly a nice girl who, like Tricia, was all over Manchester like a rash. Tricia felt she wasn't convincing enough though and gave her a host of hints and tips and shops to visit. Dlara took an interest in Tricia's Estrevon tablets and was going to buy some herself. They had a good time together when they weren't writing things down and comparing notes.

The following day was to a big one for Tricia as she was getting a new wig. No, not a cheap one, she has learned. She was going to a proper outfitters to take advice and spend some money. She also needed her eyebrows threading again. After umpteen pints at Paddy's where she met a totally drunk, out of control, Mancunian and a lovely Geordie who was desperate to be out just like her, Tricia waltzed off to Hudsons.

There she had a wonderful time but it was tricky to decide on both style and colour of the hair. For about an hour she tried on various wigs, some which would need to be ordered if they didn't come in the colour of her choice. For some reason Tricia couldn't forget about the third wig she tried on. It was called, ironically, Jordan so was easy to remember. Tricia was nearing the end of her allotted time and asked to try on Jordan again. It was shorter and slightly darker than her other wig which was now safely packed away so she could keep it as a memento. She walked out of the store wearing it and felt like a new woman, like a modern woman. She was delighted and got heaps of compliments when she got back to the pub. So Tricia has Jordan's hair. What other parts of Jordan would she also like I wonder.

Now, the trouble with Tricia's new wig is that it makes Tricia look much more like a woman and much less like a drag queen. So when she walks around town, which she frequently did during that weekend, she gets much fewer comments. In fact she hardly gets any comments at all. She is not altogether sure whether that is a good or a bad thing. But then when has she been altogether?

The following day was Saturday and Saturday at Manchester Pride is something else. It was far too much for Tricia who wished to ram all the whistles precisely where she used to be rammed herself. She couldn't move, she couldn't get served and she like me absolutely hates congestion. She had enough early on so went home for an early night. She did however meet a lovely non-couple called Claire and Jaime. They were ex classmates who met up years later. Claire was straight and with a partner. Jaime was bent and not, but was looking hard. Lovely people and they even complimented Tricia on her a wig. "Not a t-girls wig at all. A real woman's wig". Tricia was so proud. It was pride weekend after all.

But and there is always a but; no not Tricia's butt which she would like to be fuller and rounder nor the butt of many jokes, which Tricia has been in the past but less so now. What does pride come before? Tricia decided to get away from all the noise and mayhem and have a walk around town. She was just entering Piccadilly Gardens through the arch when a huge gust of wind came from nowhere. Somebody up there was laughing at her. It was perfectly timed for Tricia's entrance. Off came her wig which skipped elegantly along the pavement, closely followed somewhat less elegantly by an embarrassed Tricia who found it hard to keep up in her heels. Eventually though she managed to catch the wig up and somewhat more elegantly replace it where it should have been all the time; trying to ignore the sniggers of passers-by.

So Sunday arrived and the newly bewigged Tricia, who remembered her wig cap this time walked into town for the Proms in the Park, which started at two, with Tina. They gave themselves plenty of time to prepare in Paddy's; they got there before twelve! Lee behind the bar was looking forward to a fourteen hour shift. Fortunately Tricia was determined to show off her wig round town so couldn't remain in the pub for the full fourteen hours.

The girls had a few beers, saw a bit of Proms in the Park (naff thought Tricia) then some football. Tricia did go into town, saw a lovely dress but it didn't quite look right on her and bought a Mexican meal. She was taken for a woman at all times. She thought it was wonderful. Then back to Paddy's to be re-united with Tina and the few old friends who were actually attending Pride. There were so many of Tricia's friends missing which she thought a shame.

There was however a plan for the early evening. Tricia and Tina had promised Tracy (who owns New York New York) that they would be around for the parade of the drag queens. They must have been mad. Tina doesn't like drag queens because she thinks they distract from what we are trying to do. Tricia doesn't mind them but one thing she is not, particularly now, is a drag queen; she is a t-girl and proud of it. The girls however dutifully if not beautifully did turn up and got their pictures taken with the drag queens. Tricia returned to Paddy's as quickly as she could. The drag queens had clearly spent all afternoon getting prepared. They looked great but then they looked like drag queens. Tricia doesn't want that so shrugged and got on with her life. Tina almost throttled one of them.

Tricia had a few more beers before another early night. Well, we know all about how early Tricia's night's are. She was walking back through Deansgate with a spring in her heels and a pout on her lips (she was practising that all weekend) when she got beeped by a taxi driver. She walked around the corner by the station and up Bridgewater Road North. The taxi driver knew precisely where she was heading and parked in a side street off Bridgewater Road North. As Tricia passed he flashed his lights at her. Tricia smiled and walked on; sorry all. Was she safe? It was now pitch black (I told you Tricia left early) and she wasn't sure whether she was being taken for a single woman, a prostitute or a transvestite; although the latter is probably correct. Tricia had the danger song in her head. She knew what she was doing was right. She also had a good nights sleep.

In fact she had such a good night that she woke up eight in the morning and was desperate to get herself out early. Firstly though she was determined to sort out her wardrobe; well coffin really. The trouble with Tricia's wardrobe is that there is just too much of it. It has spilled onto tables, chairs, anything it could find. Tricia is reluctant to throw anything away though as all her clothes bring back such happy memories. She did however find a large bag which Monica had left behind so stashed all her worn-out or broken clothes in that to create some space. It looked very marginally more organised.

That done it was on to the serious stuff. What to wear today. She plumped for her green dress which zips and unzips up the front so is easy to get on and off. It was a statement of intent. She was going shopping today so would likely be trying things on. Shopping again Tricia? She so loves shopping for girly things. She walks into town proudly. Her first problem was to find a cash machine which actually worked since it was a Bank Holiday weekend and Pride was on. She finally found one outside Halifax and joined a long queue of girls.

She queued for about five minutes before her turn came. She got her money then turned around to an amazing sight. They are digging up the tramlines in Manchester which is a real pain and seems to be taking forever. But there, in front of her eyes, on a Bank Holiday of all times was a gaggle of workers working on the line. Tricia suspected they were on double time and if the year was full of Bank Holidays the tram line overhaul would be completed much more quickly.

So what was amazing about that I can hear you asking. Well, the gang of workmen were working only five yards away from the bank. In the past, before her new hair-do, she would have suffered a whole load of abuse from them. Now nothing; not a dickey-bird. Tricia was a bit miffed. Someone could at least have given her a wolf-whistle. Never mind, into Debenhams to look for a new white handbag. Shopping is fun. So Tricia shopped until she dropped; got back to see Frisky and Mannish who were superb and then met a shagless Tina in the pub. Tina was bemoaning the lack of action again during Pride but had an idea.

"What they should do Trish is have a shagging room".

"A shagging room"?

"Yes, a room; it could be a tent in the gardens, where everyone who wanted a shag could go".

"Then what hon"?

"You sit down and wait. Remember everyone that's there want a shag".

"You wait".

"Yes, you wait until you get picked up".

"I think I can see where you are coming from hon, metaphorically speaking. A bit like a sex chat room. Maybe you could partition the tent and put a couple of beds the other side so you could get an immediate shag".

"Yes, that would be good, but you'd need to know when they are free so you probably need some lights like a doctor's waiting room. It could be called the shagging zone".

"But you'd be waiting all day".

"Bitch. I don't do badly you know"

"Only joking, I know. I suggest you suggest it to the organisers; but don't hold your breath".

"I know Trish. I'm not sure even Pride is ready for a shagging zone yet".

And with that thought the sun disappeared over the horizon and Pride was over for another year. Tricia had survived because of some early nights. She wondered. Six days as Tricia is enough for anyone. She wondered again. Is it?

Chapter 82

Mad Dogs and Englishmen

With my new wig I think I pretty much pass and that's brill. Also brill is the fact that I can swan around Manchester doing what I want; but there is a bit of edge missing. By the way Tina is struggling to pass at the moment. Even dogs take a dislike to her.

Now, you know I'm mostly a very modest girl but this chapter is all about me. The thoroughly modern Miss. Though I'm so so much more confident now. Megan said to me the other day.

"Wow, look at you standing so tall and proud".

Comments like that only help, thanks Megan.

> At twelve noon the natives swoon, and
> no further work is done -
> But Mad Dogs and Englishmen go out in the midday sun.

The thoroughly modern Miss ponders a lot and sorts out her A/W9-10 wardrobe.

The thoroughly modern Miss who is Tricia Dale walked through Manchester with even more confidence than usual. Despite the fact that her earrings were ringing in the breeze, jingly-jangly Tricia can now be dismissed as history. She has one thing on her mind though. What should she do with all her flowers? Her new hair-do doesn't really suit them. Miss Tricia Dale would have to ponder a while.

Tricia was so confident she actually turned back on her walk into Manchester. She wanted as much exposure as possible, she wanted to test her new look as far as she could. She therefore walked in through Deansgate then crossed the road and walked back to pick up the canal so she could pass all the bars. It was Friday night, it was sunny, and the bars were packed. Not a comment, not a murmur. For the first time in her life she honestly felt she had passed. The thoroughly modern Miss had a broad smile on her face as she entered the pub.

She was in no rush since she was to meet Megan and Becky later. Tina was to join them as was Dlara. Sadly Dlara turned into bad news by spouting off about religion to Megan. Tricia had earlier made a rash promise to meet Dlara the following lunchtime at Boots. To show her where she could buy Estroven. As luck would have it though Dlara didn't turn up, leaving Tricia free to buy a beautiful black and white check dress. Bang in fashion. Walking around town was a joy and if there were any sniggers, well she couldn't hear them. There was however a downside. She often liked the attention she got. How could she get people looking at her again? This could become boring. More for Miss Dale to ponder about. For the meantime though going into shops and trying things on without comment or insult was great fun. It was to take only a week for Tricia to come up with a solution to her problem. Or had she?

While Tricia was shopping and unbeknown to her because her phone was in her handbag surrounded by the kitchen sink, she received a text from Tina.

"Trish, hurry up, Kimberley is getting a new wig. You may be able to help. We are in the pub".

Tricia would willingly have rushed back had she received the message but was so busy and happy shopping she carried on ... and on ... and on. When she finally got back to Paddy's, Kimberley was already there proudly wearing her new rug. Tricia put her head in her hands. It was exactly the same as her old wig only slightly shorter, so marginally better. What was even worse was that it cost her £99. About the same price Tricia paid for hers. Tricia shrugged. There are some times in your life when you can only say 'if only'.

"Next time Kim arrange with me first, please".

Tricia said 'if only' the following day too because the Birchplace girls were in town. She was having such an entertaining and drunken afternoon that she decided to break her rules and take a wakey-wakey pill. For once the wakey-wakey pill appeared to work and she was to last all night, though can remember little or nothing about it. She staggered back to the flat as the birds were starting their morning chorus. She managed to unlock the door so Tina had not returned. She had clearly pulled but with whom? Tricia cast her alcohol addled brain back to Naps. She hadn't seen Tina with a bloke all night she thought to herself. For once Tricia's alcohol addled brain had remembered correctly. Tina had gone back to Peta's hotel. So Tina's last two romantic(?) liaisons, since Tex, had been with transvestites. Had the worm turned? Tricia was spending the whole weekend pondering.

On the Sunday, despite thumping heads, the girls spent a wonderful afternoon with Georgina and Lesley. Georgina had a bit of a predicament and was pondering herself. Could she trust Dave? That was an important question which for now was left unresolved leaving a lot of friction between her and Dave. But no, not that sort of friction.

The thoroughly modern Miss encouraged by a whistle and a "pretty girl" from a passing cyclist repeated her round-about walk through all the bars the following Friday with equal success. She met up with Georgina and Rita who was in town for the weekend but had, for Tricia, a quiet night. She wanted to be out and about early the next day. A skint Tina went back to her Friday night fun with Graham so clearly hadn't completely turned.

Tricia was indeed up and out early on Saturday and walked all the way into town along Deansgate. The first time she had done that and it displayed her greater confidence. She spent three hours shopping but didn't buy a thing. She was prepping her Autumn/Winter 2009-2010 wardrobe and tried on many coats and dresses. She saw a cerise coat which she really liked but didn't buy. It was so bright you needed to wear sunglasses. It screamed out look at me. She also found two lovely dresses she just adored and a purple coat. She was looking for a coat with a belt and a hood but couldn't find one.

Back at Paddy's and Tom got his marching orders.

"Do you want it now or later" he said to Tina in a voice so loud the whole pub could hear it.

"Drink up and leave please" said Steve behind the bar.

It was an afternoon like that. Dave and Georgina had a blazing row. Georgina stormed off to New York New York. Tina and Tricia hatched a plan. Tina went to appease Georgina leaving Tricia to discuss things with Dave. We will know in due course whether the plan worked but at least Dave and Georgina were talking later in the evening. In the meantime Tricia met Carolyn who is the butch part of a lesbian relationship but helps Tricia become more girly when they meet. Tricia's shoes were killing her because one of the heel taps had come off so one shoe was a quarter of an inch higher than the other.

"Rip the other off hon, I always throw them away anyway".

She also told Tricia to:

"Dress and wear whatever you want to. Its your life and you should do what you want. Its short enough anyway. And anyway, you of all people should know that".

Tricia nodded; Carolyn was right. She was to remember one piece of advice but not the other.

The following day even Tina was up and dressed relatively early giving the girls a chance to re-run the Grand national course. It was a lovely summers day. It was also September so could be the last summer day of the year. The target was to get to Paddy's for opening time which was, as it is every day except Christmas Day twelve o'clock. The race was going well until they passed some fishermen just before the water jump.

"Bloody hell, they're blokes"

Tricia, glad to be recognised for once (I wonder why) smiled and waved at them. Tina muttered under her breath (for once).

They crossed the water jump, with elegance of course and proceeded down the tow-path. Tricia was hobbling a little in her shoes (what had she forgotten to do?) but Tina was striding along confidently when .....

"Woof, woof, woof, woof, woof!"

A dog on a bank on the other side of the canal rushed towards her. Both girls thought it was going to swim across but it stopped just before the edge and started barking at Tina again with even greater determination.

"I don't think he likes me very much Trish".

"Or of course, it may be the rutting season hon".

Sadly, we will never know.

After a couple of pints at the pub, and the removal of a heel-tap, Tricia was to be found in town doing what she does best, shopping. There was a particular bright cerise coat she was determined to buy. It was Tricia. It made her stand out and it may even solve the problem of people not taking notice of her. Who knows?

She returned to the pub in ebullient mood and warned people to put on their sunglasses before modelling her new purchase. At the pub she met Josie again. Josie and Tricia get on like a house on fire and are quite happy taking the mickey out of each other. Josie constantly criticises Tricia about the length of her dresses and skirts but I need to explain. Josie is transsexual and one of the first people ever to go through the operation. She was seventeen at the time. Now, I hope she doesn't mind me saying she's around sixty, she looks fantastic. Dressed twenties style with dark glasses and cigarette holder she is definitely her own woman, and fantastic fun too. She teaches Tricia a lot and is very patient with her. She loved Tricia's coat though.

"I don't care what you look like as long as you are yourself" she said.

"Does that mean you like it?" whispered Tricia.

"Actually, you look lovely".

Tricia later met three straight girls Marie, Nicky and Jo who said the same thing. The thoroughly modern Miss was so happy.

Chapter 83

Happiness

I'm now in a place I never want to leave, but know I will. I'm very, very happy. I am myself. I truly am Tricia. I look like her, I feel like her and I live like her. It's wonderful. Further down the line I know things will change but for now I must just enjoy being myself. There are trips around the corner too. By the way, I never thought I would ever use Ken Dodd. Iain's Dad would have had a right go. You can't use never and ever in the same sentence. It's clearly never or not – so I'm sorry; but then he was never tickled by Ken Dodd either.

How tattefelarious!

> To me this world is a wonderful place
> And I'm the luckiest human in the whole human race
> I've got no silver and I've got no gold
> But I've got happiness in my soul

At last Tricia learns to live by some rules and escapes a couple of dead tricky encounters.

I arrived in Manchester late, and tired. The rain was pouring down, the sky was dark as far as you could see. Going up on the lift I realised that tonight I was not going to be Tricia, tonight I would be Iain. I had four days of Tricia to look forward to but simply didn't have the energy to light all the candles and get myself ready. Tricia would have to wait. So I just dumped my bag and walked back out of the flat to watch the football. It was a good decision. After all, you can't be a girly girl all the time...... or can you?

Tricia (or Tamsin) had had a number of chats with Alex who was interested in her story. On Thursday morning it came to a head. If Tricia wants to write as a journalist, which she does, she would have to come out completely. Pictures of her and me; my name in the papers. This is not a problem for Tricia personally, but how would the family react? Tamsin told Alex she would make her decision by the end of the weekend. Scary but fun too, and Tricia likes that combination.

Tricia was up and out bright and early the following day. She went straight into town and spent some time shopping in her new Autumn coat; the perfectly modern young lady. No reaction whatsoever. Back at Paddy's and Tricia met Georgina. Dave had not listened to her so had lost Georgina's trust. Georgina and Dave were an item no more. Georgina was also miffed that the TG sauna had been called off.

Now, Tricia doesn't get the idea of a TG sauna. She would be baking hot even in her short wig and her make-up would surely run everywhere.

"I agree" said Georgina. "Actually it's just an excuse for a knocking shop. I probably wouldn't have enjoyed it anyway".

Tricia had a cunning plan. She left Georgina and went to the Chinese buffet where she enjoyed a four course meal. She ate and she ate and she ate. That will keep me going all weekend she thought. After about twenty minutes sitting down eating, the guys opposite finally twigged who she was.

"Bloody hell, you look fantastic".

Tricia smiled, then her phone beeped. It was Becky.

"Fancy the cinema tonight, I've got some free tickets"

Of course she did.

You'll have to bare with me here because it's dead confusing. Becky and Tricia drove to a cinema in Didsbury where they watched a play. The play, Shakespeare's 'All's well that end well' was being filmed from the Gielgud theatre in London. It was a live performance and was extremely well done. It was being simultaneously screened in many cities throughout the UK and would later be screened across the world. It was sponsored by Classic FM. What a jolly good idea, and you just had to apply for the tickets. They were free.

They got back into town and picked up a pretty dishevelled looking Megan who was opening her new venture, 'The Black Lion' and took rather too much advantage of the complimentary beers. Apparently the pub had eight hand pumps! Tricia must try it.

The wives left just before closing, while Megan could still stand leaving Tricia with half an hour to kill. She desperately needed some cigarettes so walked around the village looking for anywhere which would sell them. A pissed up young guy shouted "Stacey" at her. Where that came from goodness only knows. Gavin and Stacey? Stacey off Eastenders? Tricia has no idea but doesn't particularly care. She had been called worse. She couldn't find any fags though, for once.

"Trish you silly girl" said Paul behind the bar. "There's a fag machine here. It lights up when you put money it. So Tricia was sorted and immediately went out to the back for a puff, the first for a very long time. A black guy was out there smoking away. Did he come onto her? Hands on her boobs, fingers on her backside, he was all over her. When he took her hand and placed it where no hand should ever go, particularly in the smoking area of the Irish pub, Tricia felt she ought to get hold of the situation rather than what she currently had hold of.

The thoroughly Modern Miss, who is Tricia Dale does not differ from jingly-jangly Tricia in this respect. The man was quite dishy as well as very large. It may well be true what they say about black men. She wasn't therefore against the idea of a liaison, but where? Equally her rules state that she must at least have a chat with the guy so she could check him out. Yes, even Tricia now has some rules.

"Firstly hon not here. Its my pub and I don't wish to be thrown out. Secondly, we need to think about where. There are cameras everywhere in the village to protect unsuspecting young ladies like me. And finally, we need to have a chat first. I'm getting myself a last drink, you get yourself one and we'll talk it through".

Tricia removed her hand from where it should never have been and ordered another pint. He walked out of the pub in a strop. He only needed a twenty minute chat and he probably would have got what he wanted. But Tricia was aware that most men in the village were like that. If they want fun, they want it now. Twenty minutes later is not good enough. At least she hadn't been knifed or robbed; how could she be sure without talking to him? She marched back to the flat and got loads of beeps from passing cars. She was looking good, she knew.

On the Saturday morning Tricia was a very clever girl. She managed to put up a canvas wardrobe all by herself. Tina had already erected anther one so now at last she had some room for her growing collection of skirts and dresses. The coffin would have to stay for now though to house her long dresses. And anyway, mused Tricia, how can you have a coffin in the living room?

Tina and Tricia, tired after all the hard work, went to the pub where Tricia met mad Steve/Steff (not much evidence of Steff though) who had plenty to think about. He now had a boyfriend and they were supposed to be going shopping in the morning. The boyfriend didn't turn up and Steve had to phone him. Apparently he had no money; not a good way to start a relationship. Tricia advised Steve of the three strike rule she uses. Anyway they were back together the following day.

Now, what do you do when someone tells you that he's just been cleared of attempted murder and was lucky to get off. Well, that happened to Tricia after Tina had gracefully taken the easy way out and done a runner to New York, New York to play pool. Tricia had a long chat with Darren who was very frightening. She hoped she had managed to calm him down a bit, but suspects not. At least they parted on good terms so she could watch the football in the Waldorf. Lucky girl? Lucky United who scored the equaliser against Sunderland in injury time, but didn't deserve to.

Looking dead glam in sparkly gold dress number two with gold leggings and very, very gold new handbag; Tricia hit Naps with Tina and danced the night away. She hadn't done that for a while and thoroughly enjoyed it. She looked in the mirrored dance floor and guess what; she saw Tricia looking back at her. She was happy. Tina picked up another, yes another t-girl, and managed to do things to her Tricia certainly couldn't. What is happening to Tina, she thought.

So to the Sunday and most likely Tricia's best day ever. She learnt what it felt like to be a girl. Her make-up, even her eye-liner went on perfectly. Maybe Tricia is improving. They say that practice makes perfect and Tricia is certainly practising a lot. When you feel great inside you look special outside and Tricia walked around Manchester like she owned it. She got many compliments in the pub and guess what? She was wearing her black jeans so wasn't being girly-girl at all. Cerise coat and pink top did help though.

"You look fantastic", said Ray.

"I know", Tricia smiled. It was wonderful to feel like a woman as well as look like one.

Chapter 84

New York New York

Ha-ha. Funny to choose this song now as, by the way, New York New York's football bar is shut for redecoration. I did have a great time discussing New York with Steve though. I think I'd like to go; all those fantastic shops. I'm not sure Iain would approve but I could try to use baseball to convince him. I know he's always wanted to go to a baseball match.

> Start spreading the news,
> I'm leaving today.
> I want to be a part of it -
> New York, New York.

In which our girls are in peril, there is bad news and good news and travel seems to be on their minds.

The weekend started with a bit of a scare. Tina fancied a Friday night out again and so Tricia waited as patiently as a Saint for her to get ready. For once they were sensible girls and used the traffic lights rather than trying to hobble across the dual-carriageway outside the flat in their high heels. Or were they? The traffic lights changed rather earlier than anticipated. Tricia heard the beeps and sprinted (I'm not sure that's entirely true) to the other side. Tina didn't hear the beeps and nearly got run over by a car which seemed to accelerate. The car got stopped by the lights at the roundabout. Tina chased after it cursing and swearing.

"Wait Tina, what if he gets out"?

Fortunately he didn't and he moved into the middle lane where he could watch Tina glaring and waving a fist at him. Not very ladylike. Tina returned.

"The funny thing is Trish, I didn't know what to do".

"Thank goodness nothing happened hon. He might have had a knife or anything. Anyway, it might have been an accident".

"Accident? He deliberately tried to run me over. You think too well of people".

Tricia thought that maybe she did.

At the pub there was some good news and some bad news. Tricia always likes the bad news first in such circumstances. Georgina and Dave had officially and unreservedly split. There was to be no reunion. They have however agreed to drink together so not all bad.

The good news was in fact Tricia's. She had accepted her agent's proposal to reveal all. Yes, it was agreed following discussions with friends and family. Her Agent is very interested in the story at wishes to meet Tricia in mid-November. Whatever happens, it will be an interesting encounter for Tamsin. Will she remember not to be Tricia though?

The girls are keen to get out of Manchester. Tina wants a weekend away in Blackpool. Georgina wants to visit Hadrian's Wall. Every weekend in Manchester can get predictable and, as we know, Tricia is very keen to expand her horizons. Interesting times ahead if the girls can fit it in and Tricia can afford it. She has strict instructions to cut down her clothing allowance if she wished to go on these two trips. The pub have already decided their travel itinerary. About a dozen of them are going to Benidorm next week. Blackpool or Benidorm? Tricia isn't sure about either.

A lovely Friday night followed by a lovely Saturday. Tricia met Mark's boyfriend, Tony for the first time (a different Mark from Mark/Morticia). He was so happy and it was wonderful to see them kissing and cuddling. It was clear they were so happy together. Tricia loves a bit of romance. It makes the world go round.

She also met a real girl, Jen but struggled with her a bit.

"Jen, what is the one thing that will really make you happy? What do you want from life above all else"?

Jen didn't know. Tricia tried and tried to find some direction for Jen but in the end had to give up. She did ask Jen to keep thinking about it though.

Tricia then met Steve and had a long chat with him.

"I'm like you Trish; I long to dress but my hands are too big. And I could never be as brave as you".

"Never say never hon".

Steve told Tricia about the time he spent in New York. About how important it was to integrate with the community but if you did so the rewards were tremendous. About what a marvellous place it was. Tricia was intrigued and got more interested as the conversation went on. She thinks she would really like New York and wouldn't mind giving it a try. Maybe that's her first trip abroad sorted.

Then the night went sour. Tricia decided to go to Napoleons but it was pretty empty. She went upstairs to an empty dance floor and did what she enjoys most. She danced to a few records to warm herself up then returned to have a few sips of her pint. But where was it? She had put a beer mat over it so it should not have been taken. The only guy upstairs confirmed that the bar staff had taken it. Tricia had a sissy fit (she was good at that) and searched out Jaye. There was three quarters left; but then as we know, Tricia's glass is always half full.

"Jaye, I know its vile beer, I know it's overpriced but when you are dancing you need some liquid inside you. And I didn't take it onto the dance floor with me because you told me not to".

Jaye said he would have a word. Tricia marched out of the club in a huff. I suspect she will be back though.

Back at T-Girl Towers she fell into a deep sleep. So deep in fact that she was unaware of the shenanigans going on next door where Tina's Asian guy managed to get through five condoms. But only four lubes?

Another day another dollar, as Tricia assumes they say in New York as well. She met up with Megan and Becky again. Megan re-iterated her good news. Her restaurant had been given an excellent write up in the local paper. Her burgers were apparently to die for. Tricia knew about that but what about her baps? Are they to remain? This has meant Megan has become extremely busy and is finding it difficult to find any free time. No peace for the wicked; but then Megan could hardly be described as wicked.

Tricia went for her normal Sunday afternoon shop. She doesn't buy anything, good girl that she is, as she is saving up for trips away from Manchester. She does however stop to have a cappuccino. It makes a change from the beer and is good for her. The comments she now gets are far less derogatory than they used to be.

"I'm sure that's a man" was said a couple of times. You see, now they are not so sure. One she liked though was "Pretty Adam's apple". Tricia doesn't try to hide it. It is part of her after all. She was walking back to Paddy's when she bumped into two guys coming out (though they already had).

"I wouldn't go in there love you'll get molested. The place is full of fellas".

"Goodee" said Tricia and rushed in.

Inside the pub she was own her own for a while, which she enjoyed, before Kimberley joined her. Then Marion and Elsie joined the table and they had a lovely evening talking about girly things. About make-up, dresses and hair-styles. Tricia learnt a great deal from these two elderly ladies as did Kimberley.

Who needs fellas anyway? Tricia thought to herself.

Chapter 85

Outside the Wall

Another first for me, YAY, my first time on a bus; although it was a bit of a rickety bus. The AD122 runs from Carlisle station. Now what was I doing that far North? I made sure I wore my thick woolly tights on under my jeans. So I have now done trains, tubes, trams and buses. That just leaves boats and planes. Megan, Becky and I are trying to organise a canal trip next year so it looks like boats next. I have also been out of England for the first time. Well, only about two paces into Scotland but surely that counts? By the way, I loved the album but was never convinced by the film. I think the wall may be down though. Well, it is for me anyway. How about you?

> All alone, or in two's,
> The ones who really love you
> Walk up and down outside the wall.

Hadrian's Wall

Tricia had another experience that all real girls learn when she went to Hadrian's Wall. She had arranged to meet Georgina at Piccadilly Station at eight. It was a half hour walk to the station so Tricia really should have been up at six. She stupidly set her alarm for half six thinking she would have plenty of time, and duly awoke on the dot of half six. As is usually the case in Manchester, Sindiy was already awake and needed attention. Tricia was travelling on trains and buses and didn't want the journey spoiled by Sindiys interruptions so she did what she needed to.

Normally in Manchester, Tricia has all the time in the world. It doesn't really matter if she gets to the pub at twelve or half past; but now she had a deadline. By the time she had seen to Sindiy and made her bed it was ten to seven. Quick girl quick. She put the kettle on and tried to get dressed while it was boiling. Big problem. She wanted to wear her check blouse but it was pitch black and she couldn't see to do the buttons. She struggles with the buttons on that blouse in the light. Eventually, frustrated she gave up and opted for her "Those shoes look fab .... I just have to have a pair" pink t-shirt with her black jeans and cerise coat which people can see a mile away. She put on her walking shoes, thanks Monica, and at least she was dressed.

The kettle, well saucepan of water really, had nearly boiled dry so she had to top it up with more cold water. Time was running out. After carefully shaving there was only ten minutes left, things were getting frantic. Tricia rushed around finding her bling and putting it on. New black earrings will work with the outfit, she thought; then perfume. Wig, that's quite important too. By the time she had straightened it, she hoped, she couldn't really see enough to be sure, there were only three minutes to go. She couldn't go to the station naked. She quickly powdered her nose then painted her lips before packing her handbag. Fortunately she remembered to take her nail-varnish and foundation so her make-up bag was bulging. She felt under dressed as she strolled through Manchester to meet Georgina. Surprisingly though she didn't get any comments. She was five minutes late but there was still plenty of time to get the train to Leeds. Georgina looked resplendent in her tiny kilt. Very apt for Scotland, Tricia thought.

It was to be an extremely long but disappointingly uneventful journey. Manchester to Leeds, then change trains. The reason for going to Leeds was that the journey from Leeds to Carlisle (their ultimate train destination) beyond Settle is supposedly the most picturesque in the country. It certainly was spectacular. It made Tricia proud she was an English girl?

It was rush hour in Manchester so Tricia didn't have a good enough seat to properly do her make-up but at Leeds they found a table they could share and made themselves up with some relish while waiting for the train to start. No eye-liner for Tricia though. She still struggles with that.

Eye-liner is Tricia's make-up bête noir and very very noir it is too. She can spend fifteen minutes putting it on and taking it off and putting it on again

again. The trouble is, even when she puts it on perfectly, her eyes water which smudges it and makes it go all blobby. She gets really frustrated which doesn't help matters. It has moved up to second in her make-up regime which now goes foundation, eye-liner, concealer, powder .... If she puts the concealer on before the eye-liner, she had to reapply following the six or seven botched attempts to get a line around her eye lids. Today, on the train, with her little make-up mirror. No way! She would have to do without.

The girls arrived in Carlisle at the appointed time; Tricia pointless thank goodness. Now, Carlisle is apparently the most gay-phobic city in the UK so how on earth will it take to two t-girls strutting their stuff around it? Actually surprisingly well. The girls eventually found the bus stop to take them to Hadrian's Wall but the bus wasn't due for over an hour so they decided to have a pub lunch. As on all occasions in new areas, could they find a pub? They walked round Carlisle for about five minutes before finding one, in the other direction from the bus stop, about one minute away. But the walk was fun. The looks on people's faces had to be seen to be believed. It was clear that not many t-girls had ventured this far north in the past.

The pub was friendly and welcoming. Tricia was a bit miffed that none of the four hand pumps served real ale so she settled for a pint of Theakstons. They were served lunch by a lovely old lady who insisted on calling them 'sweety's' .

The AD122 turned up on time and the girls spent just over an hour being thrown up and down on not very well upholstered seats. It is on occasions like this that Tricia sometimes wishes her own seat was a bit better upholstered; but, she supposes, that is one of the prices you have to pay for having the body of a super-model. The bumping up and down did little for Tricia's bladder, which was now full of beer, and she couldn't wait to get to Birdoswald Roman Fort where she hoped she could find a 'Ladies'.

The bus eventually reached the Roman Fort and Tricia rushed off as quickly as she could. She found that there was a Ladies, but it was in the Heritage Centre and that would cost £4.50. Now, Tricia doesn't mind spending a penny but £4.50 was a bit steep. There was only one thing for it.

In such unfortunate circumstances there is one major advantage of being

a girl like Tricia. If you see a quiet place surrounded by trees and bushes
....

Tricia remembered to place her handbag upstream (so to speak) before a large torrent erupted from between her thighs. As is usual when this happens it took quite a while to turn off the water works.

Fortunately for Tricia, Georgina was on guard and they don't think anybody noticed. A pretty girl standing up to do her business. What would the history lovers say?

Hadrian's Wall was exactly what you would expect; a wall. Tricia and Georgina were under-whelmed. They walked about seven paces of the seventy odd miles on it before giving up. It was dangerous in such high heels and Tricia didn't want to fall over again. They took a few pictures then waited for the bus to take them back. A passing walker commented that Georgina, in her kilt, was on the wrong side of the wall. But what is the right side?

Waiting for the bus though was quite entertaining. Many of the walkers appeared more interested in Georgina and Tricia than in Hadrian's Wall; cars kept turning round and coming back for a second look. Georgina suggested that if the Heritage Centre could charge £4.50 for a pee, we should be able to charge at least £3.00 for a gawp.

The bus journey back to Carlisle was enlivened by the cheery driver giving us a running commentary on the history of the Wall and the surrounding area. He also suggested, cheekily Tricia thought, that Hadrian may have been the first ever transvestite judging by his statue at Brampton. "I am a t-girl not a transvestite", muttered Tricia under her breath.

The bus got them back in perfect time for the train to Leeds. The girls fixed their make-up before trying to have a snooze. It was getting dark by now but even so Tricia could only manage twenty winks. She struggles to sleep on the move. At Leeds they just had time for a couple of puffs before the Manchester train was due. They couldn't find any on the station so had to make do with two cigarettes instead. Dragging in drag again? I don't know Tricia, isn't it about time you gave up? Think of all the lovely dresses you could afford.

The girls rushed across to the platform for the Manchester train; Tricia, in her heels slightly behind Georgina. A girl was coming up the escalator in the opposite direction, turned right at the top and bumped into Georgina. Tricia could see everything. The instant look of complete shock on her face, quickly followed by the broadest grin you have ever seen. Life is such fun being a t-girl, or a schoolgirl come to that; and not only for them.

Back at the pub and our intrepid travellers are so tired they are about to drop off. Just then the pub doors opened.

"Hiya girls, how was your trip". It was Megan and Becky. Yay thought Tricia, they'll liven me up, and indeed they did and Megan had some very good news....

Chapter 86

Pennies From Heaven

Despite the rain, although we were to have lovely Saturday afternoon for once, this was a lovely melancholy weekend. I think the amount I had achieved finally hit me. As luck would have it I had plenty of time on my own; but that is what I wanted and needed. It was Katrina's birthday and so was good to see her rather than Tim in the pub. As for the song by the way, it really felt like it was raining pennies from heaven; and its not a bad philosophy for Manchester.

> Every time it rains it rains
> Pennies from heaven.
> Don't you know each cloud contains
> Pennies from heaven.

Peace, Happiness and Contentment.

Tricia is sitting in her pub. Friends have come, friends have gone, friends will come. She knows that because it's Katrina's birthday today. She bought Katrina a card. Its good to have sisters. Outside it was a typical Manchester day. The rain was pouring down from a sullen, soggy sky. To make matters worse there was a gale about to start howling. Tricia was lucky; she had walked in earlier when all was calm, albeit cold.

As we know Tricia enjoys sitting on her own. She enjoys getting into a space I can't reach. She shuts her eyes and waves of emotion flood over her. She is happier now than she has ever been in her life; than I have been in my life. She is at last herself; she is at last displaying her true feelings, wearing her heart on her sleeve. She is content and she is proud of herself. She shakes internally. Life's worth living when that happens.

It is now 16:30 on Saturday 31st October and Tricia is sitting on her own in the pub. It is Halloween. Tricia shuts her eyes and the waves of contentment return. She has just spent two hours walking around town looking for a new dress. She thought she had found one but, when she tried it on she could see it wasn't quite her. In any case she was eager to stick to her budget so she could afford Blackpool with Tina next week. The weather was, for once, spring-like although Tricia noticed the rain clouds starting to gather menacingly. There had been a buzz around Manchester which Tricia had enjoyed. How things perk up when the sun shines. The girl in the café who knows Tricia had picked up on it to. She couldn't wait to emigrate however, to get more of it.

Tricia woke up in the morning with just one thought on her mind. 'I was born to be a girl'. She was so looking forward to getting dressed, putting on her make-up, getting out and being Tricia; a proud girl, a brave girl, a girl with attitude. Tricia doesn't now care about any comments; maybe that's why now she doesn't get any.

It is now 15:35 on a Sunday evening and the rain, once again, is lashing down. Guess where Tricia is? She had enjoyed a lovely chat with some Scottish guys about English food in the dripping cigarette shelter. She recommended lamb's hearts. She knows more about food than she lets on, but don't tell Megan. She also had a lovely chat with some Irish guys about football and the theatre of dreams. They were up for the match which Tricia saw in the straight pub down the road. They were all young lads but they totally accepted her for what she was. They also all agreed what a chilled city Manchester was. She knows more about football than she lets on, but don't tell Tina,

Tricia was sitting in her pub on her own. It was 16:45 on Sunday and the rain was still lashing down. She shut her eyes and the waves of contentment came back to her. She has respect for herself and, in general, other people have respect for her. She was confident, she was brave, she was happy. She is living her life as the girl she wishes to be and is so proud of herself. She is about to go back to the straight pub to watch Manchester City. Actually, and whisper it, she quite likes Manchester City. For years and years they have been the underdogs but now they are fighting back. Tricia likes that;

it is a bit of a mirror of her life. She knows she will again be treated with respect at the pub, although all including her will share a joke about the situation. Then she'll go for a meal (she's not sure yet, she may try the curry buffet) then sleep. The next day back home, to Sheffield and Chesterfield and to climb back on the wheel.

Tamsin, please get me into a place I will love permanently. You can do it! November 17th?

Somehow, Someday, Somewhere.

Chapter 87

I do like to be Beside the Seaside

By the way, I don't. Even I thought Blackpool was tacky, Iain was positively dismayed. They kept saying that they were the gay capital of England but I know better than that. Brighton may have a shout but Manchester is far better. It's got more than six clubs and pubs for one thing. Still, Tina and I had a good time and we did meet some lovely people. But the weather; it was just too wet and windy. Worse even than Manchester!

"When I grow up I wanna be famous"

Actually I don't. But I surely need to leave something behind don't I?

> You save up all the money you can till summer comes around
> Then away you go
> To a spot you know
> Where the cockle shells are found.

Lock up your sons, the girls are visiting Blackpool!

Tricia had it all prepared; Tina, prepared, what? The plan was to go to Blackpool on Friday afternoon but traffic is notoriously bad on Friday afternoon so we aimed to leave at two thirty, three at the latest. The weather was filthy. Cold, windy and it was pouring down. Tricia was ready on time as always, looking delectable in her blue wool dress. I'm sure it won't surprise you to know though, that Tina was not. It was to take Tina a further hour to get ready so the girls left far later than anticipated and just before the biggest downpour of the day.

"Turn left" the charming voice of the sat-nav said.

"Why turn left Trish we should turn right".

Tricia said nothing. She quite liked being dominated by women. And a woman with such a lovely, English, Radio Four voice at that. Tricia would have followed her to the ends of the earth. But Tina? No, Tina knew best. Tricia couldn't believe the patience of the sat-nav lady who would pick up the route and redirect them in the right direction after Tina disobeyed her earlier instruction without a cross word. Tricia thought she probably wasn't much fun, but in the end and thanks to the lady the girls arrived at their destination. The omens weren't good though. It was still pouring with rain.

Tina went to park the car leaving Tricia with the hardest task of the day. Lugging the suitcases up the stairs to the room. Tricia only had one suitcase but it has to be said that it was extremely large and heavy. Tina had five. I ought to explain at this point that the girls were only staying for two nights. They clearly brought their capsule wardrobes with them. Fortunately the car that they travelled down in was an old Volvo so they could fit everything, including themselves in. Tricia was hot and sweaty when she had finished so needed to re-apply her make-up. She though aloud while doing so.

"If we are only staying for two nights how come I have packed three skirts, three dresses, three handbags, one pair of jeans, three pairs of shoes, three coats, umpteen t-shirts and blouses and my entire underwear, jewellery and make-up collection". Sometimes, she mused, it was so hard being a girl. But both girls agreed that it was good to have options.

They started to unpack and fortunately had a large wardrobe to store all their gear.

"Trish, I've sorted it, we're not going to go hungry this weekend"

"What the ...." Tricia was to say the least slightly alarmed. No wonder Tina's bags had been so heavy.

Tina had produced two cans of hot dogs.

"What on earth are we going to cook them in hon"?

Tina produced a pewter mug.

"It's easy Trish. We just boil the kettle, put the hot dogs and the boiling water in the mug and let them heat through".

"Have we got any rolls"?

"I will be rolling more than enough for both of us tonight".

"Have we got a tin opener"?

With aplomb Tina revealed .... No she didn't, she shook her head.

"I knew I'd forget something Trish. We'll have to buy one in Blackpool".

Tricia shook her head in despair.

The girls changed, touched up their make-up and went out to boogie. Tina knew most of the pubs and clubs as she had been before, so it was a breeze. Actually it was far more than a breeze as the girls literally got blown to their first port of call; The Flying Handbag. Tina, as we know, loves breezes as they lift the hem of her shorter than short skirts to reveal her knickers in all their glory. Tricia was a little more conservatively attired. Blue dress with zips and her skin-tight black leather look leggings. Dead sexy nevertheless. At the Flying Handbag they met Steve and had their first taste of a drag queen; although taste doesn't come into it. Steve was helpful and informative; telling them the route they should follow and when to get to certain places.

"It will be quiet tonight though girls with the wind and rain playing up like it is".

Tina looked up at the video playing above the bar.

"Look Trish, she's wearing the same dress as me. Who is she, she's quite tasty"?

Tricia looked up at the video playing above the bar.

"There is a slight resemblance but her dress ends at her knees and not her backside and is rather better cut. Oh, and by the way, she's Kylie Minogue".

"The name rings a bell Trish but its not my kind of music".

Tricia shook her head again. Tina's mind and experiences were clearly single tracked; and they hit the buffers at about 1980.

The next stop was Pepes. An underground bar which appeared to be frequented by elderly gays into leather. Tricia felt she should be ok in here because she was wearing her leather leggings but the guys didn't notice her. After all she wasn't an elderly guy was she?? Pepes was quiet however so after a swift drink the girls crossed the road to Taboo.

Now if there is a definition of tacky, Taboo could certainly be it. It had bright glitzy lights outside but inside the paintwork was peeling about as much as the upholstery on the chairs. The girls were greeted with a barrage of noise from the resident drag queen. The noise however was not directed at them for once which surprised Tricia. They were such an easy target after all. They saw some other t-girls so went to sit next to them; but they were involved in their own conversation and carried on with their knitting.

The girls went up to the ladies to powder their nose and Tina got into a confrontation with a drunk who apparently didn't know what he was talking about. Tricia knew he didn't know what he was talking about and did what she normally does in such situations. She kept smiling, that way there will be no problems. He was a red rag to Tina though who started shouting back. Tricia muttered under her breath "what is the point"? Eventually a young girl came in and took the drunk downstairs. Thank goodness for Superwoman, thought Tricia, they almost came to blows.

After a lecture from Tricia, which was not heeded, the girls set off for Mardi-Gras. They had been warned not to be fleeced by the lesbians on the door so Tricia smiled her brightest smile. They wandered down to ..... a drag queen in full flow. Tricia deliberately walked in her eye line but received no comment whatsoever, she was well miffed. What, she thought, do I have to do. At last the girls met up with another girl like them, Zandra, and had a good chin-wag in the smoking fire escape. They decided they wanted a dance and noticed a dance-floor tucked behind the stage. Yay! Tricia could strut her stuff. Actually though she couldn't; and that is the problem in the drag queen capital of the UK. Whenever the music got going (as did Tricia) the drag queen would turn the volume down, make some inane joke, then turn it up again. An example:

'You can dance, you can dance, having .....' [music down]

"You couldn't dance at all in those dear could you. They must be at least eight inches. First time you've had eight inches? I don't think so" [music up]

"..... dig in the dancing queen".

The only thing Tricia could think of when the drag queen interrupted was to dance in slow motion. Then it took time to get the rhythm back. Then, as soon as she had, the drag queen would interrupt again. Tricia gave up and went back to the Flying Handbag; not before advising one of the knitting circle how to dance.

"Honey, you've waited all this time to get some tits; so stick them out and show them off!"

Tina joined her and the girls made a surprisingly good decision at closing time.

"Lets not go to the nightclub tonight Trish, lets be fresh for tomorrow, after all we've only got another day". Tricia, for once, agreed. I'm not sure how fresh they were in the morning though!

Chapter 88

My Little Stick of Blackpool Rock

If you ever go to Blackpool, whatever you do don't go in November when the weather forecast is dodgy. I can't remember a worse day. The rain was lashing down horizontally because of the gale force wind. I wrapped up as warmly as I could; thick woolly tights under black jeans. I didn't warm up or dry out all day (although, as you know, the latter is normal). All in all it made Manchester feel like the Costa Del Sol. Tina and I didn't pull either, not that I was bothered, even so we had a good time. Oh, and by the way, this got banned by the BBC. How times have changed. Sindiy didn't even twitch!

A fellow took my photograph it cost one and three.
I said when it was done, "Is that supposed to be me?"
"You've properly mucked it up the only thing I can see is
My little stick of Blackpool Rock."

Here Come the Girls

The girls woke up to a furious thunderstorm with the wind knocking tiles off the roof. Tricia opened her eyes and after a while realised she was in Blackpool, not Manchester.

"Oh well Tina, at least we can have some breakfast. It may calm down during that".

"Oh good Trish. Bacon, egg, sausage, mushroom. Just right to get inside us before a brisk walk on the prom".

"What, in this? And its a continental breakfast".

"What's a continental breakfast?"

After their coffee and croissant (Tricia) and tea and toast (Tina), the girls went back to their room to prepare for their brisk walk. There was no sign of the weather breaking up.

"Are you sure hon, its horrendous out there"

"Perfectly sure Trish. It'll blow away the cobwebs. And anyway the pubs don't open for another hour".

"Blow away the cobwebs? They'll be banished to the four corners of the earth".

There then followed what could quite possibly be described as the most unpleasant walk in Tricia's young life. Pouring with rain the whole time, her umbrella useless because of the hurricane, Tricia thanked goodness she had packed her jeans. Walking to the beach was a case of two steps forward and one back. The girls hit the promenade and turned left. Then the wind, which was now behind them, really got up. Tricia, holding onto her wig with all her might, couldn't control her legs in high black heels and was forced to run along the prom totally out of control taking tiny little steps. Fortunately nobody could see the ridiculous sight she made. Other people weren't stupid enough to go out in such weather.

"This is no fun Tina, lets go back to the gay village"

Tina agreed and they waited outside a pub for a bit for the rain to die down which it sort of did before moving on towards Taboo.

"This is the best street in Blackpool, look at the shops Trish".

Tricia looked around and her heart sunk. There were charity shops everywhere. It was Tricia's worst nightmare and Tina's dream come true. Tricia had to think fast. She didn't want to be hanging out outside umpteen charity shops in the wind and rain.

"Right hon, I shall go to Taboo's, you can do what you want and meet up with me later. Send me a text". Tricia couldn't stand charity shops but an afternoon in the bar?

At Taboos Tricia met Neal and spent a long time talking with him about the pleasures Blackpool had to offer for the gay scene. Neal was clearly proud of the place and got it across well. Sadly it didn't make Tricia any more enamoured. The girls agreed to meet up at the Flying Handbag and shoot some pool. Neal came along with Tricia but was somewhat reluctant to go in and be seen with a couple of t-girls. How strange, thought Tricia who by now had drunk the pre-requisite number of pints for her pool purple patch to begin. For five games she was unbeatable. A young flashy upstart, brimming with confidence challenged her to a game. He shouldn't have done, she won.

"I'm so glad you beat him" said his girlfriend. "I've a weapon now he can never live down".

"So have I". Tricia left it at that.

Outside having a cigarette, it was at least covered but still freezing cold, they join an argument between a young boy and a couple of older girls.

"I'm not sure if I am gay though". Tricia later established that the boy was only sixteen.

"Oh you are, you definitely are" said the girls.

"Whatever you do hon, take your time before you decide to do anything. You're very young" said the voice of reason who was Tricia.

Back to the pool table and Tricia's purple patch was over. She promptly lost to Tina.

What was brilliant though, and gave both girls a great deal of confidence, was how everybody insisted on telling them how good they looked. Gays, straights, lesbians alike; it was wonderful. Tricia sent a text to Megan and Becky:

"The Manchester girls have given Blackpool the wow factor"

Back to the hotel for a change for a change. The girls were off to see the world famous review, 'Funny Girls'.

Now those of you that can still remember the story will know that Tricia has seen La Cages Aux Folles in London. This means that Tricia's criticism should be taken with a pinch of salt. After all it cost £40 to see La Cages Aux Folles and only £8 to get into Funny Girls. The difference in quality, Tricia felt, justified the difference in cost. The problem was that everybody had told her how good Funny Girls was so she went in through the door anticipating great things. The girls were treated with canned music whilst waiting for the show to start. Fair enough, thought Tricia, who as we know is fair enough. When the show started guess what they were greeted with? Well, what would you expect from the drag queen (and charity shop) capital of the UK. Yes indeed, possibly the foremost drag queen on the circuit opened the show. The drag queen who has climbed the greasy pole the highest (bet its fun sliding down). She was good, thought Tricia, but not that good. There then followed a song performed by other drag queens which was good, thought Tricia, but not that good. That was followed by canned music for another half an hour before the whole sequence was repeated. At least it was different song this time.

"Trish, I don't fancy hanging around for another half an hour, can we go?".

"You said it Tina, Flying Handbag?"

The verdict on 'Funny Girls'; disappointing.

So the Flying Handbag turned out to be the end of the Blackpool trip. Nice and symmetrical because it was also the start. It did though end in some style despite the drag queen half way up, or was it down, the slippery pole. Tina, who by now had far to much to drink, went into full socialist mode with a wind-up merchant. Tricia fuelled the flames and he was extremely good. The argument lasted for ages until finally:

"I don't suppose you know who you are talking to?"

"No" said Tina, eyes firmly shut.

"I'm the socialist MP for Blackpool North".

Tina stormed out of the pub in a hissy fit.

"Well Trish, she doesn't know I'm not". He said after Tina had gone.

She does now; ha-ha.

The following day the clouds had lifted but it was still windy. The girls packed up and left. Tricia was relieved to return to the home comforts(?) of Manchester. She didn't really like Blackpool; it was too cheap and tacky. She will likely return though; maybe next summer. It will be better in the warm so maybe she isn't being particularly fair. As for Tina, and as they discussed in the car:

"I don't know Trish. We go all the way to Blackpool; there are blokes all over the place; everyone says how good we look; and I never get a shag".

"Never mind hon, I suppose the hot dogs made up for it. All that meat"?

"Hot dogs, no Trish, I forgot to buy the can-opener.

And we forgot to buy any Blackpool rock.

Chapter 89

One Life

I'm cheesed off because there is no way I am going to Manchester and living in the flat this week. It's far too cold. I'll catch my death as my Mum would say. The barnacle said I could stay at his house but no chance. I know that Georgina, Megan and Becky would let me stay at theirs, but that means lugging all my clothes and make-up around in the freezing weather so that isn't much fun either. I've made my bed and I have to lie in it. The pity is that it is in Chesterfield and not Manchester so I will not be wearing my baby doll. Actually though I suspect it's probably good for me as it will give me time to think. And, by the way, I am only just beginning to realise that this is our life.

> Crying over my mistakes, forgetting
> all the breaks I've had
> In my life
> I was put on earth to be, a part
> of this great world is me
> And my life
> Guess I'll just add up the score, and
> count the things I'm grateful for
> In my life
> This Is my life

Happy, though early New Year Thoughts?

I will not say anything about global warming because I know it is happening but England is so cold it's unbearable. I am worried about many things; money, my life, my family, my future but none of that seems to matter. I just want the bloody snow to go away and for it to warm up. It was -12 in Manchester and with no heating am I going to risk going up? Dream on.

However there is no point in moping. We all know Tricia's glass is always half full. This story, my legacy, is being written. And I know is sellable – but where? The plan is still to give up work to write and move to Manchester to be with my friends. I really do wish to be Tricia all the time, even at -12 if I had electricity, and not just play at it. Although I suspect you could hardly call what I do playing at it.

My original goals still stand. When I first started this I was determined to get myself out. I think that is a definite tick. Secondly I wanted to help others like me. I try so hard at this but it is difficult because guys like me are so scared of revealing their deepest feelings and fears. I am though currently in contact with two new girls who wish to come out with me in Manchester. We'll see. From what they tell me I can see how petrified they are but I will try to help them as much as I can. The final goal was to document what I am doing and that is happening. It gets harder to write because I have now done most things I can. That though is another reason to move to Manchester and live as Tricia 24/7. There will be more opportunities and I would definitely mix more with straight and genuine girls rather than just at the village. Going up for a couple of days only is limiting and, if I wish to see my friends, I can still to go to the village.

As for the dreaded chop. It's still in mind but until I live as Tricia full time I won't know whether it would be right. My hormones at last seem to be taking affect, albeit very slowly. I would so love some boobies, even now. I would be so proud of them and my walk would develop even further if they were present. One day...

I must keep trying. I must keep pushing Tricia. She loves having a good time but needs to help me more; after all it is the only way she will get what she wants. I think she understands.

I think what I am doing here is writing my New Year's resolutions, something I gave up many many years ago. They seem relevant now, they seem important, they could be a way to chart out my life. Work is dire and is actually getting worse. I didn't believe it could get any worse but it is. I need out but more important, I need Tricia out. Who knows where the road will lead but I know one thing. It will be fun finding out!

The bloody snow has started again so it will certainly be a while before I return to Manchester. I must keep thinking and working on things here in the meantime. I really want to be free but for now I'm in limbo and it's extremely hard to motivate myself in the short term. I have to be strong and I have to be stoic. I am an English girl after all. The snow, the work, the family, the finance and the cold must lose out to the brain and the heart and the mind. They, after all, define my soul and define who I am.

Chapter 90

Greasy Chip Butty

Well I had my interview and I enjoyed it, but Tamsin's first chance to get herself out has gone. The girl who interviewed me was very nice but her company wished the impact I had on my family to be foremost and not my own life. If I am going to come out there must be no strings attached so the magazine article is not going to happen. But the following weekend; poor Iain. Oh and by the way this is Sheffield United's football club song. Sheffield is where Iain works.

> You Fill Up My Senses,
> Like A Gallon Of Magnet,
> Like A Packet Of Woodbines,
> Like A Good Pinch Of Snuff,
> Like A Night Out In Sheffield,
> Like A Greasy Chip Butty,
> Like Sheffield United,
> Come Fill Me Again,
> Na Na Na Na Na...OOOOHH!

Poor Iain; brave but stupid Tricia

This is amazing. After three weeks away I go back to go Manchester. It is still cold and dark but at least the snow had gone. I decided to go up on the Saturday morning without realising which football games were on. I was pleased enough to get a seat on the train but then, at Sheffield, the carriage was invaded by a hundred or so Sheffield United supporters singing and dancing. They were playing Bolton in the cup in the afternoon. Having a bald head was not a good idea on that train carriage. I took a tremendous amount of stick, more than anything Tricia had to put up with. One comment made me smile though:

"What are you going to Manchester for; a wig?"

They obviously quite liked me despite taking the piss on the whole journey to Manchester. They all shook my hand when they got off

If only they knew that my holdall contained my newly washed bras, tights, leggings and tops. If they had opened that up? Then, with them all gone, Tricia entered my thoughts for the first time.

What if Tricia did open up? What if Tricia showed them and told them all she knew? Dead risky and likely too scary too. Something deep inside her told her she could though. So Tricia, brave and foolish girl that she is, went to Manchester Piccadilly station after the match. She sat upstairs and ate a KFC so she could watch the crowds for the lads on my train earlier. There were police everywhere. There were Manchester United as well as Sheffield United supporters everywhere. If Tricia can put herself in this situation surely she can do pretty much anything at all. She never did find the lads on the train; but at all times she was in fact very safe at the station.

As for the rest of the weekend. Well nothing really mattered or could compete after that. She met Mad Steve, not Stephanie (who was still waiting for her make-up). Steve had allowed her boyfriend to move in with her, silly girl, think! She now wishes to get rid of him but can't. Tricia said she would try to help but wasn't entirely sure how she could. Anyway, Steve now has her phone number which probably wasn't very wise of Tricia.

If anything Tricia felt even more confident and proud of herself after her extended break. She walked around the village bars with Tina, admiring herself in every mirror he could see. Careful, she thought, you'll end up like the worst transsexuals. She was so happy though that it was indeed Tricia looking back at her from every mirror, and she was very pleased with her look. She was, after all, just a normal young woman enjoying herself in a few bars; wasn't she?

In the smoking area outside The Irish Pub (at the back) an interesting conversation developed. Three girls were discussing bras and cup sizes, comparing their measurements, bemoaning the fact that bras don't seem to fit properly any more, complaining that the straps slip without prior warning, swapping information about where to get the best bra fitting, sharing notes about where to buy the prettiest bras and where they each bought their bras, discussing the advantages of gel filled bras and padded bras, agreeing about how lovely it is when a bra fits perfectly. The interesting part was that one of the girls was Tricia whose own yellow bra straps were proudly on show on her shoulders. She was extremely knowledgeable and contributed as much to the conversation as the other two real girls. She is learning well in many parts of her life.

She went to Napoleons and stayed for the first time in months and thoroughly enjoyed herself. She is still the dancing queen. She chatted with loads of people, including a long chat with Jaye. It was clear there were no scars remaining and Tricia would be welcomed back whenever she was sober. She walked back confidently through Manchester in the early hours, happy and content. Two hours later Tina arrived back at the flat, an Asian guy in tow. Tina was a star though. The Asian guy was apparently only after kinky sex and was desperate to get into Tricia's room so they could have a threesome. Tina kept him out though. Eventually he left to scour the streets for any woman, male or female, he could find so he could get the threesome he desired. Did he find one? I think we all know the answer to that. It was, after all, about half five in the morning.

Sadly to the downside of the weekend; well it was only a day really as I came back on the Sunday on a much quieter train to be with my daughter and prepare for a busy week at work. Julia and Katrina are giving Tina the cold shoulder. Georgina is ignoring Tina. This is not good at all. Tricia is loyal and will stand by Tina but she doesn't like the way it affects her friendships with others. Next week, when Tricia has an extended stay, she must try to do something about it. Precisely what she isn't sure. She is going to have to be a determined and diplomatic young lady. But then we know that she is precisely that.

Sheffield United lost two-nil at Bolton and were left to concentrate on promotion to the Premiership.

Tricia Dale left Manchester early to concentrate on a presentation she needed to write for Wednesday.

Tricia Dale

Woodbines were non-filtered cigarettes

Magnet is bitter beer

A butty is a roll (but not that type)

Chapter 91

The Meaning of Life

I'll have to leave Trish to write this one. Despite the fact that I've spent my entire life thinking about it only Tricia has got close to understanding; I still don't think she fully has though. I think in my life I have only seen about half a dozen transgendered people. There was one in particular who almost made me cry. He was in the middle of my market town on a Sunday before the shops had opened. The town was almost empty. He was walking through the narrow passageways where he would be seen by the fewest people. His head was down, his shoulders slumped. It was clearly the bravest thing he had ever done in his life. I didn't know whether to approach him or not so I didn't. I willed that he was happy though. By the way,

> And just what-- what-- what-- what do we fear?
> Well, ce soir, for a change, it will all be made clear,
> For this is 'The Meaning of Life'. C'est le sens de la vie.
> This is 'The Meaning of Life'.

In which Tricia tries to explain

Oh dear, Iain has given me a task and I'm not very good at them. I just want to be who I am and not think too much or worry about it. He says I am in a better position than him; whatever could he mean? I will do my best though and I do know as much about it as anyone else I suppose. I'm sorry about my English; I missed a lifetime of education!

Iain has told me that when writing it's easier to start with questions. You can then put the answers into paragraphs and end up with a conclusion.

It will make it flow better. But there are so many questions I can't answer; and I can't get anywhere close to a conclusion.

So questions. What drives me and people like me to do what we do? Why, when all the when all the world around us is staying 'stop, stop' do we carry on and go even further? Why are we so desperate to hide it all in early (and for most) later life? Why do we put up with the ridicule and the humiliation? Why do the feelings get stronger as we get older? Why do we risk alienation from our families and live in constant danger of losing our friends? The only answer I can think of is straightforward. It's because we have to.

I have met many, many girls of my own persuasion and so it's certainly fair to say I have a decent sample. The thing is that, although we are similar in that we like to crossdress, our motivations for doing so are completely different. There are as many shades of transgendered people as there are straight people. All I can do is point out the trends. I don't like labels or categorisation of people but I do understand that it happens and I can't stop it. So here are my broad categories but I will stress, not every transgendered person will fit into these.

So dive in girl! The first type of crossdresser I know are those who don't really care what they look like. They are quite happy just putting on a frock. They won't use make-up or spend hours getting ready. They may even have facial hair. We are all follically challenged but they will not spend an age removing all their body hair like I do. They normally start after puberty; often very late in life. Putting on a dress releases their stress and makes them happy inside. They don't need to prove anything to anybody so won't go out in public in general but they can be seen around the village. They are just expressing a facet of themselves for the time being. Good luck to them.

At the other end of the scale are the transsexuals. They will spend hour after hour carefully removing every single body hair follicle. They care about their appearance to the n'th degree and are desperate to pass as the woman they desire to be. They generally start to crossdress before puberty often as early as at three or four. Eventually they will go through the operation, have it cut off and become post-op. Interestingly where I have seen many very happy crossdressers, I haven't seen many happy transsexuals. They always seem to want more. They are searching for perfection so they are searching for something which doesn't exist. I get on well with them and although some are a complete pain to be with since they are more interested in their appearance than who they are talking to; others are great fun and a laugh to be with. Most are though, in short, obsessive.

I'll pick up drag queens here, no not literally although I do wonder what happened to Eric, but I don't think they are anything to do with people like us. They do it to make money, and that is all. If they did harbour a secret desire to crossdress then I suppose they have the perfect alibi but it just doesn't seem right. If they wished to be feminine they would not caricature the feminine form like they do. Having said that, I always get on really well with them and we have a laugh together. I have no doubt that most, if not all drag queens are gay and so are part of my community. They are simply not like me or girls like me. I absolutely don't miss Blackpool; though if truth be known, I wouldn't mind being Miss Blackpool.

The next category is transvestites. Do we know any transvestites? I think we do. Transvestites are primarily sexually motivated so they primarily dress to attract men. So very short skirts, fishnets, tight clothing and fetish gear are what they shop for. Make-up is shovelled on with a trowel. It is of course a look that gg's shy away from in general (although some do love it) so they fill a niche in the marketplace. I used to think I was a transvestite but am now aware of what a good girl I actually am. Classically transvestites start dressing during puberty hence the sexual attraction link. TV's are normally very nice people who can have a laugh at themselves. I think that's important.

So what is left is girls like me; t-girls. We want to be girls and want to be taken for girls but know deep down inside (actually not that deep at all) that we are not. We try our best to portray the most feminine image we can but know precisely who and what we are. We really do have the ability to laugh at ourselves. We don't necessarily want the chop or to develop boobies but we aren't altogether against it. We are not yet recognised by the medical profession but maybe that is correct. Maybe the truth is that we still don't know and are still working our way through it. We are somewhere between transvestite and transsexual but tend to be on transsexual side as we normally start dressing before puberty. I started dressing when I was five but I'm still not sure if I am transsexual. I know I am very, very close but very, very close is not close enough. I will only know if and hopefully when I can dress all the time.

So there we have it. Like anything else in life we are a diverse bunch but that's what makes us fun and makes life worth living. We also know we give fun to others. So if you see one of us walking about in town all you need to do is smile. I promise we will smile back. If we're out there with you, we are brave enough to do so. The pity is that so few of us will be out there with you.

Is that ok Iain? Its not very funny.

Chapter 92

Follow the Yellow Brick Road

It's a great laugh now I'm pretty much passing. I can keep my head down (though my shoulders back) and walk around town unnoticed. Or I can flirt outrageously and shock and surprise people.

"We love how it feels, putting on heels causing confusion". Indeed.

By the way, its about time we got back to where the story started.

> Follow the Yellow Brick Road.
> Follow the Yellow Brick Road.
> Follow, follow, follow, follow,
> Follow the Yellow Brick Road.

In which Tricia gets mugged, propositioned, drunk and enjoys herself.

Fed, watered and looking quite foxy; the non-reversible reversible fury jacket; the dead animal as Georgina calls it, entered the pub at six o'clock on Friday night. Inside it was Tricia. It was likely going to be a quiet weekend as Tina, now known as the wicked witch of the North, had to stay in to provide a tax return to Her Majesty's Government by Sunday at the latest. You see we do occasionally return to the Wizard of Oz - if only briefly.

Speaking of which, or witch or whatever; Tricia hadn't heard from Kimberley for a while. She tried to phone but she couldn't get through. She really hopes Kim is ok. Anyway it turned out to be a quiet night.

Tricia got extremely drunk and talked to loads of people, but somehow remained sober enough to walk home so didn't go to Naps. The latter however was probably good since Tricia had heard through the grapevine of scurrilous things going on in Naps the previous Wednesday night. Tina was apparently involved and Jaye apparently saw everything, but was not telling. Since I wasn't there either I can't add to the rumours so you will have to use your own imagination. I doubt you'll need to dig too deep!

Walking in the following morning; a beautiful cold and crisp winter's day, Tricia fell for the oldest trick in the book from someone from the oldest occupation in the world. She was in straight City when she was stopped.

"Wow, you look amazing". A not unattractive elderly woman stopped her.

"My name's Debbie, I'm a street girl and I love your look, especially your lippy".

"Hi, my name's Tricia".

"Where did you get your lippy?"

"It was given to me actually".

"Can I see? Your make-up is fantastic, you must have spent hours working it"

At this point Tricia should have walked off but with all the flattery she was being given would you? She stupidly opened her bag and fumbled around for her lippy which was of course at the very bottom of her make-up bag, which was of course at the very bottom of her handbag. She should have known. It always is.

"There!", a triumphant but naive Tricia produced her lippy. Her perfectly packed handbag was now in disarray.

"Mind if I try it, and I love the foundation too, it really suits you; can I borrow some of that?"

Tricia produced her tube of foundation now floating with umpteen other, more valuable things at the top of her handbag.

Debbie toyed with the make-up.

"Do you mind if I have it; I'm only a working girl?"

"Well you can have the lippy but not....."

Debbie was gone.

"Bugger off tart!"

Tricia could have chased and caused a kerfuffle; but in such high heels?

Anyway, she thought, I'll just have to get some more make-up. Good!

Anyway, she thought, I have just been mugged for lippy which was left behind the bar at Paddy's and foundation which cost £1.95. It could have been a lot, lot worse.

But then she really thought. Was it good being complemented on your make-up by a lady of the night? Even if it was morning; especially if it was morning. Tricia was very confused.

She had choices though. Should she go straight to replenish her make-up, or should she go to the pub first? I think we all know the answer. She was at the bar talking to Georgina, Waldorf and Statler when she got nudged.

"You are the dream of my life".

An elderly guy with a strong Glaswegian accent clearly had the hots for her.

"No I'm not. I am Tricia I am she". Said Tricia.

"You are an amazing person"

"I am who I want to be". Said Tricia.

For the next half hour while the Glaswegian wasn't drooling over his pint he was drooling over Tricia. Tricia didn't understand a word he was saying but then again she wasn't sure he did either. Eventually he left but not before falling over in the pub before he reached the door.

"Love you darling".

"Me too." Said Tricia waving frantically. She knew when she was out of a bad thing.

Why, thought Tricia, do all the drunks love me so much?

It was clearly time for her to disappear, to go shopping in the City with a heart and soul as big as hers; so off she trotted. Tricia is starting to recognise who almost recognises her and plays up to it. It is normally the young who have an inkling but she also likes to shock the old. She has started winking a lot, widening her eyes, blowing kisses. She loves flirting with people. Walking back to the pub from the centre of Manchester, and remember she had not topped up on lippy or foundation; that was the purpose of her visit; two guys were passing her. Tricia winked outrageously and listened.

"Bloody hell, that's a bloke and I wanted to shag it"!

Tricia merely smiled. She knew she was a good winker. She had been told often enough.

Back in the pub and she notices a girl looking remarkably like a younger version of herself chatting with a guy. The girl was wearing the sort of clothes Tricia likes so obviously looked dead gorge. Something was wrong however. She definitely looked like a very attractive young lady but her actions, her demeanour; her gestures gave her away immediately. And girls do not lean forward at the table if they are talking to a guy. They can lean any way they want but not forward. Just then Tricia heard a comment from the gays at the table opposite her:

"I like big nipples on a man, they're gorgeous".

She decided to go outside for a cigarette where the discussion was about getting your electricity put back on so Tricia listened intently. Apparently if she had a kid under ten with her, and the younger the better, they would turn it back on. Tricia pondered. She is though, we know, a very rounded girl and totally understands that some things in life are beyond even her. And pregnancy is certainly one of them.

The night then, like many other Saturday nights, fizzled out before Tricia's mild and bitter eyes. She must have walked home however because somehow she woke up in her own bed, albeit much the worse for wear. She struggled into town to meet Tina, tax return duly completed, in Coyotes for the football. They missed each other; goodness knows how in such a small bar, but met up again in Paddy's and decided to go round the village for a change. They wanted a dance in New York, New York but it was too quiet so they went to the New Union for a game of pool. There they got thrashed by couple of girls. Tina was quite annoyed but as Tricia explained;

"We played like a couple of tarts; but that shouldn't surprise anyone".

Tricia knew that if she chose to live her life as a woman there was absolutely no shame in being beaten by them; particularly since the girls were younger and their eyesight far sharper than her own.

Back in Paddy's, Julia and Tim still haven't relented over their split with Tina and neither had Georgina. Manchester City won so the barnacle was there, desperate as ever to get into Tricia's knickers; a rather fetching lacy green pair actually. Fortunately there were plenty of friends at the back of the pub so Tricia could safely escape. After goodness knows how many beers she can remember this time trudging home at about half ten. She collapsed on her bed and was not to re-appear until after midday on the Monday. Fortunately I had the day off work. It was Georgina's birthday but sadly Tricia was just not up to it. She changed back and went home as me.

It is however becoming clear that things have to change. Let's hope things happen soon so Tricia can continue to follow the yellow brick road, in Manchester. Maybe though there are a few more things beyond her that she ought to be aware of.

Chapter 93

She

What a great weekend! I didn't go up until the Saturday but the shorter time helped in a way. I met many, many friends; made some more and had a lovely Sunday afternoon in town. I did get rather drunk and wasn't a particularly good girl on Saturday night; but then I wasn't very bad either. I think I may be ready for a relationship. Not just sex but a proper relationship. I know I'm a dark horse but I am not a nag! Elsewhere there are problems everywhere as Iain will explain. Oh and by the way, sorry if you sing it all day.

> She may be the reason I survive,
> The why and wherefore I'm alive,
> The one I'll care for through the
> Rough and rainy years.

And when she is good she is very, very good. And when she is bad she is …. Not so bad really.

Having washed her grey jacket during the week, Tricia was early at Paddy's. She had arranged to meet Megan and Becky in the pub at four but was so eager to get out she actually got there at three. The wicked witch was stuck in the North but would be along later. The super bitch was in the pub, but more about that later.

Tricia hadn't seen Megan or Becky since before Christmas so it was wonderful to meet up again. Megan was keen and eager to discuss new work ventures; Becky's job was, like mine, precisely that. Tricia is glad. She wants them both to be happy because they are such lovely people.

After the girls left, Tricia went into the more salubrious part of the pub to have a chat with Peter, Les and Mary. The wicked witch (not fair so from now on it's Tina) turned up and they spent a good couple of hours talking. Now, what needs to be said here is that Tricia was totally innocent. It wasn't her fault that the Unicorn had run out and she had to drink the Bombardier which is much stronger. It was not her fault therefore that by half nine she was four sheets to the wind.

It also wasn't her fault that the Barnacle walked in and immediately made a bee line for her. The inevitable happened about half an hour later as the Barnacle's lips clamped around Tricia's. Tricia was a good girl though. She didn't open her mouth the whole time so no tongues. Her secrets remained secret. Well, that's what she thinks at least.

Goodness knows how she managed to prize herself away from the Barnacle but she must have done. She can vaguely remember talking to Tina in Napoleons at about three in the morning; just a flash of recollection. Then she woke up in her own bed with a slitting headache. It was eleven o'clock on Sunday morning. Tricia exhaled; saw the familiar plane of condensation leave her lips and promptly went back to sleep. Eventually she got the courage to wake up and decided to dress in her blue roll-neck top with tights and leather look leggings. Adam would not be giving her away today.

A walk into the village in the freezing conditions enlivened Tricia and she arrived in the pub at around half two. Georgina, Dave and Suzie were in their normal positions on the bar stools. Suzie was looking particularly resplendent in transparent top with no bra. There were nipples everywhere! One day, thought Tricia. Georgina was off on business in the evening but Dave and she were in sparkling form. Although not an item they still get on really well together which was more than can be said for Georgina and Tina. The feud was still not resolved.

"Did the wicked witch say anything to you yesterday Tricia".

"Well, she said she thought you were a bitch".

"Tell her I'm not a bitch, I'm a superbitch.

Tricia sometimes struggles with her girly friends.

It was time for Tricia's walk into town. She needed some black nail varnish and had collected coupons from a magazine for some free make-up. She struggled for half an hour on Saturday to get her black nail varnish to look right and was blaming the brush (not herself of course). Eventually she realised that the brush was innocent. The problem was that she hadn't closed the nail varnish properly the last time she used it so it was thicker than it should be.

Walking around town was a joy. Tricia felt so girly. She picked up her free make-up and looked around dozens of stores but couldn't find anything that stood out. But then neither did Tricia. There was a lovely moment when, after enjoying a coffee, she walked back into town and some fourteen year old girls crossed her path.

"Is that a girl or a guy?"

Tricia turned round and winked.

"Yay, it's a guy, brilliant!"

They didn't really know. If Tricia can fool fourteen year old girls she can fool anyone. And she can only get better.

Back at the pub she bumped into Josie; yippee! Tricia loves and thinks a great deal of Josie. They have a laugh together. They can happily slag each other off, slags that they are, without hurting each other. Josie also helps Tricia to become herself. They had a wander around the village but all was too manic. Even on a Sunday night. Tricia was happy though. She was being herself with somebody who respected her and whom she deeply respected herself. Facelift Josie? Go for it if you want to, make sure you do.

Tricia managed to stagger back to the flat and managed to get into work on Monday morning. Just. I was a bit of a dead loss at work though. Things have changed; I have changed.

"The meaning of my life is She".

Chapter 94

Spread a Little Happiness

I am aware now that I make people smile. I no longer cause derision as I am so much better than I was and, if anything I'm even happier than I was. I walk around everywhere with a smile on my face and that rubs off on others. So, and by the way.

> Even when the darkest clouds are in the sky
> You mustn't sigh and you mustn't cry
> Spread a little happiness as you go by

In which Tricia finally realises that she, herself is fun.

I know I moan about the weather but what can beat a crisp English late winter day. Very cold in the shade; merely warm in the sunshine but little or no wind so you feel invigorated. Tricia felt invigorated when she got to it but was to suffer frustrations beforehand.

The first frustration was my fault. Tricia had a chance of an extended stay and wanted to go out on t-girl Wednesday night for once. Work however had other ideas and work has to come first. What work doesn't understand is that any target it sets must be both achievable and realistic. After all, Tricia couldn't just drop everything and become Tricia in three days. It has taken her two years so far and she is still learning. Work however doesn't do reason.

"This has to happen tomorrow" said work

"It wont", I confidently say.

"The deadline was last Friday".

"Ha-ha-ha-ha-ha. We are at least three months away from getting this working, probably longer".

"But we promised"

"You might have done, but you didn't ask the people who are actually doing the work first, did you?"

So I had to go back into work on Thursday to try to ensure the project went in on time. It didn't of course but I managed to progress things to the next major stumbling block. Early June at the earliest I think. I did try my best but sometimes the best can never be good enough. Having tried to sort out what couldn't be sorted out I left work far later than I wanted to on Thursday lunchtime. Tricia was dead frustrated. On the way to Manchester I managed to pick up some gas canisters. This however was to be the cause of Tricia's next bout of frustration.

Tina hadn't told Tricia that the gas had completely gone which didn't help matters; so it was good that Tricia remembered to pick up some more. Tricia, running out of time and light, tried to change the gas. It just wouldn't play. At one stage her eyebrows got singed; which didn't bother her. After all it made her eyes even more attractive. For fifteen minutes she tried and she tried but the canisters kept hissing at her. She was used to being hissed at by guys, but gas canisters? Finally she gave up and had a dry shave. Far from ideal but it would have to do. Tina did eventually manage to get the gas back on but it required a huge feat of engineering that was way beyond Tricia.

Things were to get better from then on though. Coming down out of the flat the lift stopped on the fifth floor. A tall young gangling West Indian, looking menacing, entered. Calm Tricia, calm. Look your best. Be as girly as you can. The lift reached the ground floor and the door opened. The menacing Caribbean smiled and beckoned Tricia out. For the first time she understood the term 'ladies first'. He didn't guess and Tricia skipped out into the hall with a smile on her beautifully made-up face.

That night, and indeed all weekend she bumped into friends old and new. It was lovely to meet Val again who hadn't seen Tricia since her face-lift or wig-change, call it what you will. Val was well impressed and told Tricia she was getting better and better. Tricia also met a lovely Irish girl called Siobahn who she will keep in touch with. She learnt that Michael had testicular cancer but was going to get a plastic ball. Tricia was sure she wouldn't have worried about that but wished him luck in any case.

Tricia left the pub early, good girl that she is. She got back to the flat at around eight, just in time to bump into Tina who was going out. Except Tina of course wasn't quite ready so Tricia sat on the bed and chatted to her while she was doing her eyes. On her side Tina was halfway through a large glass of wine.

"The trouble is Trish; I always pull better when I'm drunk".

"The trouble is Tina; you always pull better when he's drunk".

Tricia was to be woken up at four in the morning by some extremely drunken foreplay. The guy apparently wasn't up for it the following morning though. Tricia suspected guilt to be the cause but then she may have been wrong.

Saturday started off badly. It was freezing so Tricia didn't get up as bright and early as she meant to. Then Tina had a go at her because they never walk into town together now. Actually they did the previous week which Tina had conveniently forgotten about. Anyway Tina was still in bed with no sign of moving so Tricia left. She went to the Vine, a straight pub next to the Town Hall, to see if the football was on.

It wasn't but it was fun anyway. Having bought herself a rather expensive pint Tricia settled down to read her paper. Shortly some City supporters came in and sat on the table next to her. Fifteen minutes later the table went silent. They had finally realised she wasn't really a girl at all. They didn't know what to say or what to do. After a minute or so they pulled themselves together and carried on with their conversation. Tricia slowly drunk up. When she left the silence re-appeared (can silence appear?). Tricia lit up outside the pub and listened to a gaggle of noise inside. She had made her mark.

Tricia was determined to be a good girl that afternoon. She met Georgina and they went to the Chinese buffet; sure to keep her sober, and then back to the pub. She was about to go shopping as she needs a large handbag; she will tell you why later. She had one sip of her last beer left when .....

in walked Megan and Becky. Oh well! She was drunk again by nine but at least she had the common sense to stagger home then.

Sunday arrived with Tricia really needing some time to herself so she made sure she got it. No talking to anyone, get out into town and be as girly as she can. She had £50 to spend but couldn't find a large handbag which she liked. She will have to go away and think about what she really wants. She enjoyed her shop immensely though.

The funny thing about Tricia at the moment is that she passes at first glance. Some people can spot her though. She was on the second floor of the Arndale, where all the girly shops are of course, when a young lad and his girlfriend doubled back to check her out. Shocked, they burst into laughter. But not nasty jeering laughter like she used to get. The laughter was more an astonished giggle. Tricia realises she now has to re-learn. To learn how to really be like a women. To develop nuances and impulses like any other woman. She is good, very good, she knows that; but there are still many miles to travel.

She went into a straight pub to watch the football with only smiles and admiration from the girls behind the bar. Girls know you know. Blokes now hardly have a clue. Is that why she wishes so much to be a girl? She doesn't know.

But Tricia does know what she wants and so do I. I had Monday off work but Tricia didn't get out. There are more important things for us to do. This could be the week when Tricia breaks free. I must be strong. I must do what Tricia wishes and needs. I must be brave even though there may be a huge well of tears. Sorry Mum. I need to come out. NOW!

Let's go to the show.

And the man in the mirror is no more.

Chapter 95

Tonight

My other half is having a quick beer before we change. It does take time to change, far longer than I think as I found out this week. I was really happy as I was going to meet a couple of work colleagues in the middle of Sheffield on Tuesday night. I was well looking forward to it. But there was the weekend first and Sunday would certainly be interesting as both major Manchester clubs were playing. You certainly need bollocks to walk around town when City and United are playing. But I have bollocks; well at least for now..... and by the way Tuesday night was one I will never forget.

> Today, the world was just an address.
> A place for me to live in. No better than all right

A time of conflict and high emotion.

The weekend was a bit of a side-show for Tricia as late on Friday night she had arranged to meet Lesley and Kim after work on Tuesday in Sheffield. The hotel room had been booked and she was raring to go. The trouble was how to get all her girly gear from Manchester. She recalled the time before she moved in with Tina when she had to strut her stuff in hotel rooms. She learned then that the secret was good planning and simplicity.

Work was still horrendous and time consuming so, despite the milder weather and lighter evenings Tricia couldn't get up to the flat until Saturday lunchtime. It would appear that the wicked witch had really fallen out with her as she left a curt note asking her to get out of t-Girl Towers early on Monday. There were workmen coming. Becky suggested that the reason

Tina wanted her out early was so that she could have them all to herself. Tricia heard that the wicked witch had been out on Friday but had returned to her abode in the North of Manchester.

At least that gave Tricia plenty of time to get ready and she thought it would be a good idea to dummy run her outfit she had planned for Tuesday night. She is a sensible girl. Slightly sexy, slightly foxy but girly; nothing over the top and no high heels. She had to pack what she was going to wear.

She was ready in about an hour and happily walked to the pub. At the bar were Megan, Becky and Georgina; a recipe for an early night as she would get far too drunk to make Naps. They had a natter but were quite sensible and disappeared into town for a couple of hours. Tricia needed some nail varnish remover and, on the train coming up, had found a coupon for some cheap perfume which she wanted to exchange in Superdrug. Sadly they had sold out. Tricia doesn't sell out so easily. She carried on shopping until heading for the Vine where she had agreed to meet up with Megan and Becky to watch the rugby.

The Vine though was packed solid. Tricia decided to have a beer to see if the girls would turn up or give up. She was sitting on a stool in the pub with a party of about five behind her when she heard:

"Its ok, of course she's a girl, you are stupid sometimes".

Tricia was later to meet the girl who made the remark in the ladies and they had a giggle.

"That's the trouble with blokes, they're so gullible; you look great though".

Tricia smiled and happily returned to Paddys where she met up with Megan and Becky to continue an alcoholic day. As sure as eggs are eggs Tricia's night ended in an alcoholic haze although she did have the wherewithal to get an egg sandwich from Sainsbury's.

Why?

Sunday was wonderful because Tricia spent a lot of time in town where it is much more fun than the village. She started by meeting Georgina and Saskia in Paddys where she learned the truth about gay saunas. Apparently only about a fifth of the building is actually dedicated to the sauna. There are coffee bars, relaxation areas and shagging rooms as well. Tricia wondered why the wicked witch didn't just go straight to the gay sauna and ignore the pretence of everything else completely. But Tricia is becoming a bitch and should try to be more considerate. Anyway, she had a bit of a day of football ahead.

She watched United win in Coyotes and was having a smoke on the step outside when a guy she knew from somewhere greeted her.

"You're Tricia aren't you, I've seen you in Naps".

"Yes, what can I do for you" said the silly girl.

"What are you doing this afternoon, honey?"

"Nothing much, why?"

"I can fix you up with some Charlie if you like".

Tricia immediately said no. She is such a good girl! Why should she ever want to snort some cocaine? At least that's what she thinks he meant.

After the match Tricia went into Manchester which after a while was heaving with City and United supporters. It takes a very brave girl to walk through aggressive gangs of guys on her own. She had a burger in Burger King where she watched a young boy watching her. He really wasn't sure but she was pretty convincing. Convincing enough she thought to watch the second half of the City match in the Waldorf. She thought she saw a spare bar stool so elegantly and gracefully plonked her posterior on it and ordered a drink. A minute or so later a middle aged United fan returned from the bar and looked at her.

"Oh sorry, have I pinched your seat" Tricia said innocently.

The coin slowly dropped. The man went ashen faced. Her voice had given her away again.

About five minutes after that Tricia, studiously watching the match, felt his eyes burning into her. He walked behind her then back in front studying her earnestly.

"Thank God for that", he said to his mate,

"I wouldn't!"

Tricia smiled to herself. It had taken quite a time for him to establish that fact.

Tricia had a quite evening. She had of course to leave Tina to the workmen the following day. She did manage a quiet couple of beers in the Banyan Tree next to the flat but was a sensible girl. She left the flat at 7:15 the following morning lugging all her girly gear.

It took forever for Tuesday night to arrive but arrive it did. The hotel she booked in Sheffield was fine but it was scary putting on her make-up in such stark light. Still she felt she had done a pretty good job of it as she marched through Sheffield City Centre. She could have met any number of people she knew on the way to the pub; she was aware but she was also wary. She had a wonderful night with Lesley and Kim whom were hugely supportive of her. Thanks girls! She walked back to the hotel with Lesley and they shared a couple more beers. She thinks she behaved herself well. She also thinks she is growing up.

She was very happy that night but life is life. There had to be a backlash and there was. The following day at work was terrible for both of us. I didn't want to be there, I wanted to be Tricia. Tricia just wanted to get herself out completely and I was up for it. I don't know why. Maybe it was because I was too close to what I do day to day. I needed some support and got it from Lesley who took me aside and told me not to be so stupid. Thank goodness Lesley dived in to help when I was desperate.

I survived the day and returned, absolutely shattered, to a complete shock. My daughter wishes to meet Tricia in Manchester and is going to bring a camera crew with her to document her reaction. How the heck is Tricia, or me, going to cope with that one!

Lesley and Kim. You added a lot to both our lives that night. Thank you so very much. And we must meet up again in Manchester, and have some fun! I may not be so well behaved though :)

Chapter 96

Ding Dong the Witch is Dead

There is no doubt that being me is such fun. I am not frightened at all any more and going out dressed is now as normal as going out in drab. I don't even need any alcohol to calm nerves. I forgot to pack my girly pills so had to buy some more. I went straight to Boots the chemist in the middle of town. I strutted my stuff as only I can. No worries. And I made up with Tina YAY. I spent loads of time with girls, both real and imaginary which I really enjoyed; but then I suppose that's not surprising as I'm one of them now. And, by the way, we're back on the yellow brick road.

Ding Dong! The Witch is dead. Which
old Witch? The Wicked Witch!
Ding Dong! The Wicked Witch is dead.
Wake up - sleepy head, rub your eyes, get out of bed.
Wake up, the Wicked Witch is dead

Tina and Tricia make up.

Tricia marched purposefully into town on Saturday afternoon. She needed some girly pills desperately. The weather was mild, the sun was shining and she knew how good she looked. Mission accomplished she walked confidently down Canal Street on the way to Paddy's. Half way there she passed a hen party enjoying the sunshine.

"I want those legs!"

She was recognized after two minutes in Canal Street. She hadn't been recognized after half an hour in town. At least that's what she thinks. And yes, her legs were finally back on parade. Tricia relishes the fact that it is now warm enough to wear her mini skirts and short dresses. She will get more attention.

Walking around town she realised that she had indeed changed. This was to reoccur over the weekend. She realised she was thinking about herself now; how she walked, how she looked and not thinking about how others were reacting to her. She was now Tricia the woman not Tricia the t-girl in her own mind. That was good.

In the pub she was accosted by another hen party; twenty strong. Tricia had seen twenty t-girls in the pub before but never twenty girls. They had a great time talking about fashion and make-up; the girly stuff Tricia loves to talk about; and she got plenty of tips. The girls were totally at ease with her and didn't take the Micky at all. Where on earth was Micky? Well if they did it wasn't to her face. They desperately wanted Tricia to come with them down Canal Street but Tricia declined. They should be left to enjoy themselves together. Tricia is merely an interloper. Anyway, she can't remember when she got so many kisses.

Mwaaaaawh!

Tricia moved on to New York, New York when she got chatted up by a guy named Ian, of all names. He was intelligent and fun. She hopes they will meet again. She returned to the Irish Pub but disaster struck. They had run out of Unicorn so, and for a change recently, she decided that Napoleons was an option worth taking.

Things have definitely changed though Tricia doesn't know precisely when they happened. The girls from Birchplace were up so Napoleons was teaming with girls. But Tricia felt strangely different; she didn't feel like she used to; she didn't feel like them. She felt in a way special and they seemed to talk to her in a different way than they used to. Tricia is a bit puzzled by it all but is none the worse for it.

Sunday morning arrived but didn't come, though Tricia did and it heralded some good news. Tricia heard a knock on the door at eleven. It was the wicked witch; but Tricia doesn't want the wicked witch, she wants Tina. The girls discussed their differences of which there were only two.

The first Tricia already knew. She was spending too much of her time away from Tina and should walk into town with her more often. The trouble is Tricia is always itching to get out and Tina takes forever to get ready. That was accepted by both girls. Tricia had a solution. She would go out locally to give Tina time to get ready then come back to the flat and walk in with her. Problem solved.

The second issue however could not be resolved. Tina and Georgina had fallen out badly as we know. Later that day Tricia was to learn that Ray had fallen out with Georgina too, or vice versa. But Georgina and Tricia had not fallen out and there was no way Tricia was going to take sides. She would try to get people back together; impossible task though it likely is. Fortunately Tina accepted this and they shook on it. They walked into town together in the opposite direction from the traffic heading for the big match.

"Alright Gents!"

It was certainly more fun walking in with Tina.

Still no proper beer at Paddy's so Tricia had no issues watching Manchester United play Liverpool in Coyotes with Tina and Steph. And did she have fun? You bet she did. A very attractive lesbian kept bumping into her:

"Has anybody told you how beautiful you look?"

Tricia didn't know how to reply or what to think.

She went to the bar to get her second beer (two for a fiver) and ordered using sign language. The girl behind the bar, grinning used sign language back before:

"You are allowed to talk you know".

"Yes, but sometimes my voice gives me away".

"Ha-ha-ha, I can see that

"Hmmm, you can hear that?"

Coyotes is great fun

And Man United won

Two-one

The girls went back to Paddy's where Georgina was on her seat at the bar. You could cut the atmosphere with a knife. How could Tricia possibly build a bridge between these two? Georgina and Tricia were discussing families with Paul behind the bar.

"No, said Tricia, "Tina doesn't have any kids".

"Thank god for that. Can you imagine hundreds of little Tina's crawling around".

Paul thought that was very funny. Georgina and Tricia weren't so sure.

Tricia needed some more cash. I reluctantly agreed to let her draw another twenty quid as she was having such fun and needed something to eat. Having withdrawn the money she was waiting to cross the main road when a young Caribbean walked up behind her and pinched her backside. The first time she'd been goosed in public.

"You look dead sexy"

She thought she probably did. She thought she probably is. That's what Tricia thinks. She wonders, however, if it's related to how much she drinks.

Chapter 97

You Were Meant for Me

Yay. It's Easter so I've six full days to be myself; to develop myself. I know I'm getting better all the time but I need some female traits. I'm not sure what they will be yet but I will think about them. Things like this are so much easier when you are wearing a pretty dress and loads of slap. I'm also trying to develop myself sexually so there will be a lot of buzzy bee over the next six days. I've started wearing flowers in my hair again. Am I going back to being a girly girl again? Actually I think I always have been. By the way, girly girl or not, I adore being Tricia. More so now than ever before.

> You're like a plaintive melody
> That never lets me free
> But I'm content
> The angels must have sent you

In which Tricia refuses all advances. She is such a good girl after all. But we all knew that, didn't we?

It was early spring and the sun, at last, appeared on the horizon. Across the United Kingdom things were at last beginning to stir. And what a stir. The bee, buzzing contentedly, hovered around the tulip. The tulip make little pretence of restraint. She slowly and gracefully opened allowing the bee to enter. Deeper and deeper the bee penetrated, buzzing all the time. The tulip loved the feeling of the bee throbbing gently inside her. Tricia couldn't help thinking how wonderful nature was.

Tricia herself was to buzz her way through six long days in Manchester. All was well in her world. She needed a strategy however to ensure she survived all six days. She therefore decided that the best way to do this involved no daytime drinking at all. Well, not until Easter Saturday. Easter Saturday was the day United played Chelsea which would probably decide the Premiership. No chance then. Tina would be out then but would be absent for the rest of the time. Finances are a rough thing. But as rough as Tina? Now now; Trish, it doesn't suit you to be a bitch.

Wednesday night, as we should know by now, is the night the girls come out but with Easter around the corner it was quiet with only a few people out. Tricia didn't mind. Megan and Becky were out (as we know), so naturally a long hop fuelled conversation ensued. Becky was hanging onto her job, Megan enjoying hers. Megan picked a hair from Becky's top.

"Don't you hate that? Hair on your clothes, ugh".

Tricia thought it a surprisingly feminine thing for Megan to do and say but then thought again.

"Hang on Megan, what about my jacket?"

Megan roared with laughter.

"Ha, ha. Sorry Trish. Everything is fine if the hairs have been fed and watered".

It was far too quiet so Tricia went home for an early night. There were days ahead of her. She was unimpressed by the t-girls knitting in the corner. On her way home she wondered though. What is wrong with knitting? If that's what you want to do then do it. That is Tricia's philosophy and she knows she is in no position to judge others.

Thursday arrived and with it Tricia's first challenge. Could she stay out of the pub all day? She's a canny girl though. She knows she can't but she also knows that if she goes pubbing she'll never get out at all. So she goes into town, does a bit of shopping and heads for the Vine. Well, to be truthful she bought a paper which was quite fun. Some young guys weren't entirely sure she was what she was so kept doubling back around the aisles to get another look at her. Tricia as we know knows precisely what she is and would have answered any questions they posed if they posed any. We also know that posing is one of Tricia's specialist subjects. And she's getting better!

Tricia is pretty good; but not quite good enough. She walked around town without a murmur and was quite happy until she was passing Wetherspoons on the way to the Village. She was picked up by a scruffy drunk. Why she still doesn't know.

"Dirty tranny, dirty tranny, dirty tranny"

Tricia held her head high, looked him in the eye, and winked. He shut up. Tricia could understand the tranny bit, but dirty? She had only had a bath a day ago so it can't be that, and she's now such a good girl, so it can't be that either. A puzzle.

At the pub Tricia immediately found herself in trouble. An extremely drunk mollusc with skin like leather plonked himself in the seat opposite her.

"You're a sexy bitch. Fancy a shag. You're gorgeous".

The mollusc was muttering under his breath. Even drunk he was not brave enough to look her in the eye. Tricia knew what to do. She could remember from my past. She remembered Geoff Boycott. Nothing would get past. She ignored him as completely as she could. Even his offer of some tobacco. Then she was rescued.

"Come and sit with us honey".

So she moved to make the table a five and the mollusc left, unsatisfied, as ever.

Tricia had a great time with Collette and Dee (a couple) and Dave and Gareth (also a couple). Collette, an extremely loud scouser did most of the talking. She explained that she could have got a job in espionage. Tricia wasn't sure; with a gob as wide as the Mersey tunnel? In any case it didn't matter. She refused to sign a form which required her to state she was straight. Those were the days.

Collette did though compliment Tricia, somewhat surprisingly on one thing. For once Tricia was properly tucked and anybody looking down South wouldn't have noticed a thing.

"My God" said Collette "My clit's bigger than yours Trish".

"We all have our cross to bare" grinned Tricia, well proud of herself. Good girl Sindiy!

So, what do you do on a Thursday night in the village when you suspect it will be quiet? Why you go and watch the Liverpool match in a lesbian bar of course. Tricia loves being with the girls but in this instance she wasn't. There was a drunken middle aged man trying to engage her in conversation. Tricia had a net earlier as we know so just re-took her guard and continued blocking. The middle aged man gave up the small talk and got to the basics which were apparently far from small but very basic.

"I've got the hots for you. Come upstairs and suck my dick you horny bitch".

Tricia has seen it all before though so shook her head, smiled, and continued to watch the game. Ten minutes later the middle aged man rushed upstairs alone re-appearing a further five minutes later.

"Honey, I've just thrown up upstairs. They are going to throw me out. Be a sweetie and meet me in the pub on the corner will you".

Sure enough the bouncer, a five foot three inch lesbian; that's wide as well as tall, came to the table and frogmarched him out of the pub.

The bouncers returned and was about to take away his pint when she looked at Tricia.

"You might as well have a lager on the little shit".

So Tricia did.

She was about to take her first few gulps when there gaggle of noise followed by laughter from a group of young lesbians in the corner.

"I will if you will but you have to do it tonight. That's the bet".

With that, and somewhat sheepishly, a rather attractive young woman removed her top and her jeans and ran around the pool table three times in just her bra and panties. Tricia was mildly annoyed. The heaving and bouncing of her wonderfully firm breasts was distracting her from the football. How she wished. Maybe one day. Tricia, for not the first time in her young life, was jealous.

The village was in fact starting to get extremely busy as tomorrow was to be Good Friday so today was really a Friday. Tricia enjoyed the walk down Canal Street before settling down again in the Irish pub; a pub definitely not on a corner. She didn't fancy being snogged buy a man she didn't fancy who had just thrown up. She was having a ciggie outside when some young gays left the pub.

"Ok, so I don't know my geography; but I know that's a bloke".

Tricia was clearly drinking too much again but settled down with Tim (not Katrina) and Trevor (not Amanda). Is a £40 a day budget too much really? It probably is but it works for Tricia, and me.

So Good Friday arrived and Tricia again avoided Paddies until six. She had a couple in the Vine, did some shopping and went for an Indian buffet. On the huge table opposite nobody from family fat recognised what she was they were so busy stuffing themselves. Tricia simply couldn't believe the number of times they refilled. Tricia was full up after one starter and two main courses. That too will cut down her drinking.

She had an early hurdle back in the pub to jump first. A man again plonked himself down next to her (what was it this week) and proceeded to chat her up. He was quite a catch. He had a job, very rare in the village. His name was Pete and he was a fireman. Tricia didn't need to ask about the size of his hose. She could see it protruding under his belt. It certainly made an impressive sight. But then his hands started to wander and Tricia knew she had to take action. She strategically placed her handbag over her rather smaller hose to protect her innocence. Sorry Pete, not today hon, you're far too pissed.

Eventually she managed to get rid of him but then met a whole host of people. Tricia can remember Chris and Paula. Paula thought what Tricia was doing was great but Chris simply didn't get it. He tried so hard and was certainly doing his best. Chris, if you're reading this it takes time for it to filter through your brain. It may never do, but thanks for trying. She also met a straight couple called Vicky and Gary. Gary was a victim of child abuse, the second person Tricia met that night with that story, and still showed signs of anger. Tricia can see it in his eyes. Tricia suspects that Vicky will need to be very brave to hang onto him.

Crikey, is that the time already? I need to go to bed because there is work to do tomorrow. I do so love writing up Tricia's adventures though, and it does keep her in me. Will we, can we, merge together as personalities? I'm beginning to think not. Tricia solved a work problem for me yesterday. I think we have different qualities based on our different life experiences. I'm tired now so can't really think about it; but its interesting.

Chapter 98

Goodnight Sweetheart

It took me ages to remember why Phoebe was called Phoebe but I did in the end by the way. She was in a BBC1 sitcom. Actually Iain found the program a little lame but he did like Phoebe. Did he want to be her? You bet. It is now the end of Easter so more drinks and more fun. It is going to be so hard to go back but I will manage. There are major financial problems brewing in Iain's life as his boiler has gone and he needs to buy a new one; but with what? Fortunately for me (his other boiler?) Unicorn is still being brewed in my life.

> Good night, sweetheart, till we meet tomorrow.
> Good night, sweetheart, sleep will banish sorrow.
> Tears and parting may make us forlorn,
> But with the dawn, a new day is born.

A chapter that's as all over the place as Tricia was.

Easter had by now arrived and was in full swing and Tricia, looking dead sexy in her purple gear, swinging her handbag freely, immediately got beeped by a car horn while walking into town. Tricia knows the difference between a beep and a BEEP by now so she waved and smiled. She was sure the guys in the car didn't know. Or did they? Further into the village Tricia found another admirer. This time of the female variety.

"I love your coat, where did you get it? And look, you're wearing the same earrings and the same rings as me".

Tricia was well chuffed. The girl could only have been 28 at the most.

The previous night Tricia had arranged to meet Vanda in the pub at one o'clock, to take her around town, to help her buy some clothes and a wig. Tricia was a little late to get to the pub (a lady's prerogative?) but was there by ten past. No sign of Vanda but Georgina was holding fort so she plonked herself on a barstool. Two o'clock, still no sign of Vanda. Three o'clock, still no sign of Vanda. Tricia gave up in despair. She had to move or she would be rooted to the barstool. It was time for a walk around town, something to eat, anything to get out of the pub.

So Tricia did exactly that. She is a good girl some of the time (all of the time?) She browsed the shops for well over an hour then had a meal in KFC before, of all things, sitting down in the middle of the concourse at Manchester Piccadilly station to enjoy her coffee. The sitting duck didn't hear a dickey bird, not a murmur; silence. Tricia, like me, enjoys silence sometimes.

Back in the pub she meets up with Lesley again. Tricia hasn't met up with Lesley , ooh for at least a week at most. There were some techniques they needed to discuss. Tricia worries where she is going but knows that Lesley has it all available to her. Her boyfriend loved her to love him every morning and she loved to be the one doing the loving. Tricia and Lesley decided to walk around the village however and it was only then that problems surfaced. Her boyfriend only lived with her part time and had children from another marriage. How he kept that going Tricia doesn't know. Lesley wants more but it's difficult to see how. It's so hard being a woman when there are men on the planet. They are both lovely people and Tricia hopes it will work out …. and that she can see more of them.

Tricia strode into Napoleons without a care in the world so she got in. The first time in a long while she thinks. She had a very entertaining time. She met Jo, a nurse, who thought she looked stunning and couldn't believe she wasn't TS. She met Gavin, only twenty seven poor dear, who was totally mixed up. Is he gay? Is he straight? What happens if he fancies Tricia; is he gay and straight? Far too hard for the both of them so Tricia went upstairs to have a dance.

The dance-floor was solidly packed but there was an argument going on just outside, by the bar.

"If you are going to be a prostitute then you have to learn to dance".

Probably enough said and anyway Tricia had problems of her own to resolve. She noticed she had a ladder in the back of her tights. Naturally she had a spare pair in her handbag as every girl would. Of course not. She treated it as a lesson learned. She spent most of the rest of the night adjusting her tights, so the hole wouldn't show, in the ladies. She hitched them as high as they could go, so that they could be covered by her tiny dress and the hole didn't notice. One day, thought Tricia, and quickly stopped herself.

For some reason Easter Sunday arrived and Tricia awoke early though not particularly bright. It must have been early as she walked in with Tina and can't remember any problems. There was time for a quick one (or two) because the football wasn't on until 12:45. A brilliant, but extremely filthy conversation ensued between Georgina, Tricia, Tina and Lee. Unfortunately Lee and Tricia had to act as interpreters. This feud is hard work. After the game watched in New York New York (first half) and Coyotes (second half) Tina had to go home. United lost, Tina lost and Tricia couldn't help feeling a bit sorry for her. Tricia was therefore left to strut her stuff alone again. Could she cope?

Of course she could. Does anybody ever doubt it? She met Kimberley (no new rug), Ian and Janet; she met Phoebe and Mandy who she was going to meet a lot of over the rest of the weekend; she met Maggi again; she met another Mandy and Val; she met a gay Viking and wasn't sure if it was Katrina or Tim and a new romantic who made his own clothes. A bit of Adam Ant, a bit of Bowie, a bit of Boy George..... brilliant!

Tricia had to go and sit down by herself for a while and was considering how wonderful like can be when it all went wrong. A fight erupted at her side of the bar and a bar-stool and some beer attacked her chicken legs. Fortunately neither they nor she snapped and she met back up with Georgina who had the sense (and opportunity) to disappear out of the way. The assailants were safely frogmarched out of the pub but it gave Tricia a warning. You never know what is around the corner. Tricia decided she absolutely didn't, so went back home sated.

After a good fourteen hours of prolonged sleep; isn't it amazing that when you have a long sleep the bedclothes don't seem disturbed at all; despite how disturbed she probably was. She needed to get ready in a hurry as she had run out of cigarettes. She got dressed in a whirl and put her make-up even quicker. She managed to make herself acceptable? in thirty minutes. It's amazing how fast you can do things if you need to. Tina take note. And remember she could always have gone out as bloke if I wanted. I just didn't. Hmmm.

After so long in the pub the previous day, you wouldn't have thought that Tricia would have returned. But return she did.... with a vengeance; even though she is not a naughty person. Again Mandy and Phoebe were there and Tricia can vaguely remember trying to show Phoebe how to walk. Oh Tricia! Phoebe in fact was a girl in the same frame of mind as Tricia. She was happy to go out into straight-world, take her chances and face them up. She told Tricia how she got her name, but can Tricia remember after all these beers? Of course she can, it was from an English sitcom called Goodnight Sweetheart. You see she is such a good girl (or it may be her notes) ha-ha.

Tricia did have a problem which frustrated her all day however. She had lost the lid of her lippy and she knew what happened when her make-up wasn't properly protected. She is certainly learning. She searched and she searched, but no joy. Resigned, she got back to her life but really worried about her sugar plum lipstick. It was almost her defining feature now there were only occasional flowers in her hair. She was having a cigarette outside the pub when an elderly family crossed her path.

"You should try her bag" said the old lady's son.

Tricia briefly held her bag which was resplendently pink; the exact colour of her coat, and her lipstick.

"There you are honey, a perfect match. Now try on the shoes".

Tricia declined. The lady was only about five foot tall and her shoes can only have been size three. Tricia could perform miracles, but not of those sort.

Tricia continued talking to Phoebe, Mandy and Georgina until Ray and Phil popped by on their regular journey for a quickie.

"You are the queen of The Irish Pub" said Phil to Tricia.

Tricia wasn't so sure. How could she be the Queen of all those Queens? She was happy enough just being a princess.

Gradually the day turned into night and the night ... Tricia started talking to a group of middle aged ladies from Burnley; Ros, Brenda and Irene. Oh how they all laughed, and how they plied Tricia with drinks all night. It was certainly not wise, but when has that ever bothered Tricia?

At the end of the evening, night, morning, whatever, Georgina brought out the new accoutrements which were bought by Patrick earlier in the day. They consisted of salt and pepper pots of various colours but they looked remarkably like dildos. There is now likely one salt pot missing. Tricia can give you a clue as to where it can be found. Whatever you do, don't look in Georgina's direction. You may get a glare; after all she can be the bitchiest of bitches. On the other hand you may get a smile. Life can be fun sometimes.

Chapter 99

Danny Boy

Even six days at Easter wasn't enough for me. I was so desperate to get back to Manchester again and be myself I was aching all over. I am improving, I am improving, I am becoming more girly but I am also skint. Never mind, there is some backpay coming my way soon. No new pretty dresses for me this week, they will have to wait. I will have to enjoy myself in the village again. I will, I have so many friends. This, by the way, is one of my favourite songs of all.

> Oh Danny boy, the pipes, the pipes are calling
> From glen to glen, and down the mountain side
> The summer's gone, and all the flowers falling
> T'is you, T'is you must go and I must bide.

Tricia is a very brave girl, again.

With the clocks going back there is now no mad panic for Tricia to get to Manchester. She has until at least eight before the light goes and that is plenty of time. She can now get shaved, dressed, do her make-up and nails and be out in forty five minutes. Although if truth be told, she was out all weekend.

Walking in and feeling sexy she gets a tinkle from a passing bicycle which pleases her so she grins back. Already! This is fun. She gets stopped halfway up Canal Street (she assumes its up and not down) by a group of girls.

"You look stunning"

Fun indeed and its only Friday night. Tricia though prefers Friday to

Saturday. Friday is chilled, Saturday has an edge to it and sometimes the atmosphere can be quite tense.

This Friday there were loads of t-girls out but not Tina who was still broke. Tricia bumped into Grace and Amanda and decided to go to Naps again. She stopped off in Thompsons on the way with Amanda as she hadn't been in on a night time before. She didn't really enjoy it though. The trouble with Thompsons she felt was that it was far too transient. People kept coming and going. It was like a stopping off place for a beer before the serious part of the evening begun. Still, it was extremely busy so trade must have been good.

It was busier in fact than Napoleons which was extremely quiet for a Friday night. Tricia left early knowing that it would likely fill up later. She wanted to enjoy a long weekend and needed her beauty sleep. She could remember times when she blew herself out on a Friday night and so ruined the rest of the weekend.

There was to be a huge event happening in Tricia's life in a couple of week's time so she had some planning to do. She got up bright and early enough to hit Paddys at opening time. On the way she walked in using her old route, all the way along the towpath. She was evaluating possible filming locations. Her danger song, which she hadn't heard for a while, came into her head before the Rain Bar. There were two drunken men singing their hearts out on the bench opposite. This might be interesting, thought Tricia, who could see two people ahead walking towards her so she knew she would be safe.

"Oh Danny Boy......"

Tricia took a deep breath.

The singing stopped and the swearing started as Tricia walked past them. Tricia prepared herself for a blast of insults. And a blast of insults was indeed what she got but not the way you would think. She was insulted for being an English girl; or English bitch as they put it. She smiled and they promptly picked up where they had left off with their Republican song,

"Oh Danny Boy...."

Only a few yards further up the canal, under Oxford Road, were two huge explosions on the street above. A barge was passing the other way under the bridge.

"What on earth was that?" said the sailor?

"No idea" said Tricia "I think a car must have backfired".

The look on the sailor's face had to be seen to be believed. Tricia's voice had given her away again.

In the pub all was not well. Paul hadn't been seen for a week; he was on a massive bender. Lee was doing sterling service behind the bar as always but glasses were building up on the other side. Enter Georgina stage left, well barstool left actually. She agreed to act as pot girl. Not a bad choice actually as she was far too young to serve drinks. She was to perform this task all weekend.

Tricia had a couple of beers and then an errand to run. The Grand National was due to start after four and she was determined to have a bet. Not many women, never mind t-girls enter a betting shop which, despite recent improvements, is still one of the last bastions of male chauvinism. Tricia slipped out of the pub, took another deep breath and entered the seedy world of Ladbrokes. The funny thing is that the blokes were so busy studying the form that failed to study the mare's form. The filly placed her first bet. She didn't win the race but she thinks she won the war. A confident young lady left the bookies very happy with her afternoon's work.

The day was to follow a familiar pattern after the wager. Tricia returned to Paddy's to bump into Kimberley. Then Steph arrived loaded down with Ritz crackers of all things. Her Mum apparently likes them. Actually so does Tricia; but six boxes?

Georgina was still around and plenty of gays were in so Tricia carries on her merry way drinking far too much. She ends up outside Napoleons at midnight. She lights up a cigarette. She notices that she is gently swaying in the breeze. Then she wakes up. She realises there is no breeze so she walks home. Sometimes she can be such a good girl.

The good news though is that after another relatively early night Tricia was hot to trot on the Sunday. Not just her but Tina was around too; although in drab as a gay male. Don't ask, Tricia doesn't understand either.

There was a hugely entertaining lunchtime session with John the farmer butting in when he felt necessary. Tricia didn't realise they held sheep shearing competitions. There was a huge debate about which five programs constituted "Watch with Mother". The consensus was:

Monday

Andy Pandy

Tuesday

????

Wednesday

The Flowerpot Men

Thursday

Tales From the Riverbank

Friday

The Woodentops

So what was on Tuesday? All sorts of programs were proposed: Twizzle, Sooty and Sweep, Camberwick Green, Trumpton, Tinga and Tucker to name a few. The internet said it was Story Book, but Tricia can't remember Story Book. She asked her Mother who came up with Rag, Tag and Bobtail which Tricia does remember.

Another Sunday, another match day. Tricia likes the end of the football season as there are matches on every week. The girls try New York, New York but they couldn't find the channel so Coyotes called again. United won, Chelsea could only draw so the title was back in the balance. That didn't really matter though. Tricia walked upstairs to the ladies and noticed a large mirror on the wall opposite. She strutted her stuff as she walked through and couldn't help but notice a not unattractive young woman wiggling her way towards her. Her wiggle is certainly improving and that is without the sky-scraper heels she longs to wear. She must do something about that when she can find some funds. She has an idea.

Tina had to leave after the game but when Tricia returned to Paddy's; as well as Georgina the pot girl, Megan, Becky and Josie were in. So you can imagine what happened next. Tricia did get home safely and woke up to a familiar buzzing noise. But where was it coming from? It had disappeared far too deep inside her. Fortunately I managed to force it out and arrived to work rather earlier than is normally the case on Monday morning. I'm not sure I was much use though.

Chapter 100

Busy Doing Nothing

It is soon to be the big day; the scary day. Iain may give some clues as to what its about in this chapter and I bet he won't spill the beans. I had to sort out areas where we could or couldn't film and had been warned about the difficulties. You get moved on if you film in public places and you need to respect other peoples' feelings. I do anyway so that's ok. The boiler at home (no, not me) has gone and we need a new one which will cost a huge amount. My laptop has given up the ghost too so I need a new one of those and my camera has broken too. I need to somehow get some funds. Is this the time to do what I must? That is scary too as I like security. Iain needs to get away from his job though. By the way the weekend was very quiet.

> We're busy doin' nothin'
> Workin' the whole day through
> Tryin' to find lots of things not to do

Tricia takes a breather.

It was to be a remarkably quiet weekend for once. Tricia had some thinking and some planning to do but nothing special happened to her. Tina, on the other hand, is Tina so all sorts happened to her. Georgina was stranded in Berlin as a result of an earthquake in Iceland. What was worse was she was with her daughter so she had to dress as a bloke. The poor girl; I can't imagine how she is surviving.

Tricia surpassed herself on Friday night. She had to get to Napoleons so couldn't drink too much in Paddy's. She is a clever girl and knew that a

Chinese buffet would cut down her drinking. It was uneventful but it worked. The business end of the weekend, Tricia decided should happen tonight which would leave her free to play on Saturday and Sunday.

She had walked in all the way along the canal just like she used to. There was no way any filming was to take place in the flat. She found the perfect place to start filming. On the canal at Bridgewater which was both picturesque and quiet. That sorted she needed to find out if they could in Paddy's and Naps. She had a chat with Patrick and Steve. Yes, they could film in the pub but only when it was quiet. So a lunchtime filming session was favourite. She tried in Naps.

"No".

She tried to make him change his mind but knew it was fruitless. She also found out that Gilly's had closed which was a pity. The camera crew would have loved it there. She must check the New Union tomorrow. She is pretty sure that will be ok. She texted all her friends to set up meetings and left herself free to do .... Well absolutely nothing really; except drink. And as we know Tricia can drink for England. No Tina on Saturday afternoon so Tricia had to make do with Pete, a debt collector. Fortunately Pete quite fancied Tricia otherwise she could have been in big trouble.

"But honey", said Tricia, "you don't do violence do you? I'm beginning to feel a bit scared".

"No Tricia. I just warn them. If they don't listen then there will be trouble. I never touch them though".

"And do they listen?"

"Sometimes and when they do I am happy because I've saved a difficult situation".

"And when they don't?"

"I have to report them".

"Ouch"

"Definitely ouch. But its their fault. They shouldn't have borrowed the money if they couldn't pay it back".

"Circumstances change though. Don't I know what".

Tricia wasn't at all sure about being screwed by a debt collector. What if she couldn't pay him back? Sooner or later Tricia knew that some lucky man or woman would have their wicked way with her. All that buzzing was bound to pay dividends. Would it pay for anything else though? Like designer handbags, shoes or beautiful dresses. Tricia decided she needed to be careful, so channelled her thoughts in other directions.

So she minced to the New Union to check that the room for the camera crew was all set up. Indeed it was and yes, they could film there. It was no different than her local though; it had to be quiet. Then she trotted off to get some scoff before returning later to Paddy's for a few more beers and a quiet night. Tina arrived, promptly pulled and was later to come as Tricia was to hear. For now though Tricia was quiet happy, perched on a barstool discussing sweet nothing with Waldorf and Statler, Andy and Charles.

Sunday was football day again so Tina arrived at the flat early. She had enjoyed the night in the Rembrandt but with whom? Tina didn't know his name but he was apparently a good screw. Despite the fact that Tina was already dressed, Tricia still managed to be ready before her and was promptly sent out to get some milk for the coffee.

Walking in with Tina on match days is certainly fun. Tina has this habit, you see, of sprinting across roads leaving Tricia behind. So for a while Tina walks ten yards in front of Tricia. This means that Tina gets spotted first. By the time the motorists have recovered from that shock they are prepared. They notice Tricia and deliver her a volley load of abuse. Tina gets away scot free. Tricia doesn't understand. When she walks in on her own, even during match days, she gets no abuse whatsoever. Tina though is quite happy with the arrangement.

"I ought to drag you around on a long lead Trish".

"Tina, will you never stop dreaming about being a Domme.

Actually Tricia quite likes the attention. It makes a change; and she never thought she'd say that.

For what its worth United won and Chelsea only drew so the Premiership was open again. The girls retired happy to the pub where Tina pulled again leaving Tricia to talk sweet nothings with Tim and Julia. Julia gave her a little secret. Apparently girls walk around the house on tiptoes to prepare themselves for high heels. Tricia took that on board. It may solve her high heel problem. And she must get back to her exercises every morning. She knows what to do but never gives herself enough time to do it. And neither, may I add, do I.

Tricia later learned that Tina had enjoyed the night in a room above the Rembrandt, but with whom. Actually it was a different guy and another room two doors away from the bloke the night before, Tina did nip back to the first guy's room for some breakfast but he couldn't provide. Tricia can understand why.

Tricia managed to do very little over the weekend but at least had prepared for the following one. Very scary but very interesting too. She is sure she will survive…. But will I? We shall see.

Chapter 101

Don't Tell Mama

Yay! Mayday so a bank holiday and another extended stay for me. Who would have believed that Megan, of all people, would be proud enough to show off her body? I didn't think she wanted it!

Anyway a break for me in more ways than one. Iain's boiler broke so he had to use his contingency funds. He is so good to me he has allowed me a little budget for myself. So I get to buy some high-heels and a maxi dress. You see, I am dead fashionable. The shoes have about a two and a half inch heel and are part of a cunning plot by me to get used to my three and a half inch stilettos. Bit by bit you see.

Tina has cleared some of the lounge so we now actually have somewhere to sit. There are also many workmen in t-Girl Towers so I have to be careful. When I told my Mum by the way, she phoned the Samaritans but all is well now. Fortunately for me though she doesn't know the half of it.

> So please, Sir
> If you run into my Mama
> Don't reveal my indiscretion.
> Just leave well enough alone.

The Gas Man Cometh

Now, what you need to know is that the previous weekend one of my daughters came up to Manchester to meet Tricia. She had never even seen a picture of her. She came up with her boyfriend and some of their mates armed with cameras. We agreed to meet half way from t-Girl Towers on the canal. When we did she was hugely emotional but recovered quickly enough, in no small part due to Tina who supported Tricia and lightened things up a bit. My daughter enjoyed the rest of the weekend and had a great Friday night in the village. I was a little worried about the Monday but she was fine and we instantly got back to a Father/Daughter relationship. What happened though was very personal and I think should be left like that. My daughter will though be up again in a while and all is well. Only two more daughters to go then. But that was last weekend.

This weekend was a ridiculous weekend in many ways. The most ridiculous part of it was that the Council were replacing the heaters at the flat. So Tricia would get a brand new heater in her room which would provide precisely the same amount of heat as her old one. Zero!

The bad news of the weekend was that Tina's Mum wasn't well. She was however to get better, gladly. She must be a martyr to have looked after Tina all these years. Except that she doesn't know anything about Tina. Tina tried to explain to Tricia that her parents were too old and couldn't take the shock. Tricia wasn't convinced though. She knows that family love is unconditional. There would be a hard time for a while but equilibrium would eventually be restored.

My work was to prevent Tricia getting up to Manchester until the Saturday morning, but she left bright and early and was safely ensconced in her local by two. There she was joined by Megan, Becky and Shaleen. Megan and Shaleen had a story to tell and Tricia likes stories. They had been up since four in the morning posing naked for Spencer Tunick in various parts of Manchester with lots of other people. Dew was on the ground and it was apparently more difficult to walk in bare feet than in Tricia's four inch stilettos. Tricia did think about volunteering, but she would have to do without her wig and make-up so she saw no point. Neither did anyone else come to that, which was fortunate for all concerned. Megan described it as almost a spiritual occasion and really enjoyed it. They apparently passed a vagrant drinking a bottle of cider on the way. He must have wondered what they had put in that particular bottle. Tricia wondered whether Megan would show her family the pictures;

"No way Tricia, she'd freak".

Tricia is sure she wouldn't.

They were to be joined by Kimberley (good) and Crystal Chandelier and the limpet (not so good). Kim was shortly to have a throat operation to remove her Adam's apple and was a little apprehensive. Still Tricia felt, it would be lovely not too have that thing protruding out of your throat, and it may make the voice higher. She will see how Kimberley gets on. It was about at this point that the limpet pounced. Fortunately for Tricia, unfortunately for Kim, he was sitting next to Kimberley. The iron lips clamped on Kimberley. Tricia wasn't sure whether she would like the attention or abhor it but it didn't take long for her to find out. She was smoking a cigarette at the front when Kimberley burst through the door.

"Tricia, can you do anything? I can hardly breathe. It's taken me about five minutes to prise him off me. I don't like it one bit".

"Leave it with me hon, I'll take the brunt. I know how to handle him so let's swap seats".

Tricia is a good girl sometimes. As we know the limpet fancies Tricia rotten and repeatedly tries to clamp his lips around hers. Tricia's mouth closed strategy aligned with a few sharp whacks on his knees managed to curb his ardour and his ardon. It was hard work though.

It was time for Tricia to go shopping so she makes a sharp exit and was to spend quite a while around town. Sadly she received no comments. She was quite miffed. She did buy herself an in trend (so she says) maxi dress and some gorge new black shoes with two and a half inch heels. Tricia's cunning plan is to get used to wearing them before moving up to the higher heels she has got. Her aim is that by the end of the month she will be so good she can even dance in these heels. She has optimistic targets which are just about SMART.

Back at the pub Tricia bumped into Kenny and Angela who tell her she is amazing and Tina invented a new term for smoking at the front. It is now called door whoring.

"I'm off for a fag Trish, I'm going door whoring".

There is some truth in that though, provided you can push the rent boys out of the way. Tricia's own door whoring got interesting that evening. First she got accosted by a woman beggar. Tricia learnt that if you are a girl, it's far harder to get rid of a woman beggar than if you are a bloke. Tricia did eventually get rid of her though.

Now, there are three elderly gentlemen who often come to Paddys Goose, particularly on a Sunday. One is Chinese and is a butler to another. The third would appear to be a friend. Tricia has spoken to them before and always smiles to them. They drink pots of tea in the pub. The Chinese gentleman reads a Chinese newspaper while the two friends chat. All very mysterious; almost like the Maltese Falcon. Anyway, they were leaving the pub while Tricia was door whoring. The man with the butler smiled at Tricia.

"You look very beautiful and very happy".

"Thank you. I hope you had a good evening".

"We always do. Never forget, all the world's a stage and you are merely an actor upon it".

"I think I know that and I promise I won't forget".

Tricia occasionally needs reminding of vitally important things.

For once Tricia left the pub and went to meet Tina and Jaimie at the Outpost where they were playing pool. Underneath the Outpost is something very interesting, Tricia learnt; but you'll have to wait for that. The Outpost was very friendly but was full of bears and didn't have honey Tricia liked. She will probably go back though and will definitely go downstairs.

Sunday night was the cricket World Cup twenty twenty final which England were involved in. Tricia couldn't find anywhere it was on. Eventually she went to Piccadilly Station where there is a pub called the Sportsman. She new it would be on there and it was. She was enjoying the game when a guy wandered across for a chat.

"I dress at home but would love to come out like you"

"Then do it hon".

"I can't"

"You can do anything. Aren't I proving that?

England won, everybody was happy"

Tricia returned to that flat for the final time that weekend to find a note left by Tina.

'Trish, just so you know, the cooker is in the microwave. Please destroy this note'.

Some parts of Tricia's life simply cannot be explained.

Chapter 102

Pretty Woman

God am I looking forward to this weekend. Its going to be hot, very hot, almost as hot as me ha-ha. So I can wear my new maxi dress on Saturday to show what a fashionable young lady I am and I have washed my yellow Grecian goddess dress so I can wear that again tonight.

Saturday should be fun. I have been set a challenge by a website that knows me. I need to buy a pretty flowery tea dress, a tan satchel and tan court shoes. I have seen a gorge tea dress on the Debenhams website. My plan is to wear my new outfit on Sunday. I will look such a girly-girl but then that's exactly what I am and I love it. I also need some more perfume and will be practicing a new girly walk during the weekend.

Now, and by the way, I might have chosen the 'the green green grass of home' and I might also meet some gorgeous hunk during the weekend. If I do I may even charge him for my enjoyment.

I can watch the film again and again though.

Hang on, its only Friday lunchtime. I should be in Iain space.

> Pretty woman, walking down the street
> Pretty woman, the kind I like to meet
> Pretty woman
> I don't believe you, you're not the truth

Tricia the girly girl

Tricia was so looking forward to a hot, sunny weekend. She had her wardrobe planned and a task to do. She loves doing tasks, provided they involve girly stuff. I washed her sexy yellow dress and bra in the week (Tricia asked me to mention that yellow is so in fashion). It is a dress that fits her like a glove. But there's the rub, and there will be plenty of those this weekend. She felt fantastic and knew she likely looked fantastic. She was however to suffer from two wardrobe malfunctions which were absolutely nothing to do with her wardrobe. Firstly, and Tricia can't understand why, her right chicken fillet kept slipping down out of her bra. Last week her new yellow bra fitted perfectly and was really comfortable. What could have changed? Tricia got on with her life and kept re-adjusting herself.

The second malfunction involved Sindiy who absolutely refused to stay where she belongs. Tricia would put her back in her cradle, walk about ten paces, then out she would pop again. The trouble was that her dress fitted her like a glove; but that was no excuse for a finger appearing in Tricia's never regions. She wished it fitted her like a mitten.

Her aim was to go to Napoleons, but as chance would have it she needed some cigarettes so went to the village shop. There she bumped into Jaye who told her not to bother. There were only four people in the night club. So Tricia went home on the stroke of midnight when the pub closed. She arrived safely with both gold slippers.

Saturday was glorious. The sun blazed down all day and, fashionable girl that she was, provided Tricia with the perfect opportunity to wear her purple hooped maxi dress. She was going shopping and was going to adore it. She found and bought the pretty tea dress after visiting about twenty stores. She found a dead in-trend tan satchel in New Look; a bit pricey but never mind however she didn't buy it. She needed the shoes to go with it. She tried every shop she knew but couldn't find any. There were plenty of flats, peep-toes and gladiators but no court shoes of any colour. She ran out of time so will have to try again on Sunday when she must also get some perfume.

Let's forget about Tricia for a while and ask a pertinent question. Has Georgina been a good girl? Well, Tricia knows she will from now on. She is ensconced in a chastity belt and has sent the keys to a friend in Bradford but, and here's the rub (or not in Georgina's case) she did not put any stamps on the envelope. So will they get there? Will Georgina ever be free? Time will no doubt tell; its clever is time.

Tricia met up with Megan, Becky and Tina and they went to the top of Spirit; the penthouse, where they had a lovely time watching the sun setting over Manchester and smoking far too much. It was wonderful to be able to smoke with a drink. Tina and Tricia did end up in Napoleons this time, which was slightly busier, but Tricia had far too much to drink so failed to pull. Not to worry, Tricia had a cunning plan for Sunday when she would continue her task.

Tricia had decided that her walk needed improving. It was not girly enough. So she put on her pretty floral tea dress and her black peep-toe shoes with heels. She looked a pretty picture, a real girly girl. She practiced her walk in Tina's room where she could see how she looked in the mirror. She liked it.

To be truthful Tricia's new walk is really a parody of a woman. I can't imagine any real girl would walk like this. She lifts her arms higher but keeps her elbows next to her body. Her wrists, pointing downwards, flop limply with every step. She thrusts her chicken fillets out as far as they can go and shortens her stride. The effect of all this, and her reason for doing it (if reason is the word) is that her backside starts to wiggle frantically from side to side. Dead sexy she thinks. She walked in through the canals again to practice. The funny thing was that she seemed to get away with it and received no comments whatsoever.

She was a bit early for the pub so went to the bus station for a fizzy drink, her bootie wiggling from side to side like there was no tomorrow. Still no comment. She had a couple of beers in Paddy's before her shop and could see the effect of the walk in the mirrors on the wall. She loved the way she looked and the way it made her feel. It also made her think more about how she stood up and sat down.

She minced into town but was not to suffer any joy with the tan court shoes. It must be the wrong time of the year. More luck with the perfume though. She found some Vera Lang 'Look' knocked down from £60 to £25. Very strong it was too. So Tricia was now smelling like a girly-girl as well as looking and walking like one. She thought she would get loads of comments in town but she didn't get any at all. She seemed to pass better than before. Maybe real girls walk the same way as Tricia after all.

Tricia received a text from Tina who was going to be in the pub at four. She quickly got herself something to eat then wiggled her way back to Paddy's.

Tina was sharing a beer with Amanda (not Trevor, a different one). Last night they shared a bed. I will let you decide who played the bloke's part as I am far too confused. The girls had a few beers and a chinwag then met Chamin. Chamin was a young frustrated cross dresser who Tricia knew would look fantastic if he plucked up the courage. Tricia agreed to help him and he knows where to find her. I hope he does. It will make a change.

So an interesting weekend but no nookie for Tricia. She didn't mind. She is still very happy just being herself. She is going to push herself harder now and attempt more tasks. She loves her new girly walk, her pretty floral tea dress and her strong perfume. She is going to become as girly as she can.

I have a problem though. I'm totally destroyed on a Monday morning and can hardly walk. The high heels do indeed take a toll.

Chapter 103

Friends

This is an amazing weekend. It has just been a bundle of fun from start to end and I'm nearly at the end in more ways than one. There are two downsides though. Napoleons seems to have gone right downhill. Next week I think I'll try Baa-Bars instead. I enjoy the company of lesbians. It's maybe because I am one myself.

Though I love shopping I don't seem to be able to find what I want at the moment. That's maybe not so bad however as it means I get to look in more shops. I can't believe how much I love it.

Oh and by the way it is wonderful to have so many great friends.

> But, I'll be there for you, (when the rain starts to fall)
> I'll be there for you, (like I've been there before)
> I'll be there for you,
> Cos you're there for me too.

The one where Tricia becomes the pie-eyed piper of Manchester.

It was to be a normal day in Tricia's not so normal life. The girls had spent the previous night in The Irish Pub and Naps but Naps was full of straights. All they seemed to want to do was feel Tricia's boobies. What is the world coming to? If truth be told however, Tricia quite likes getting her chicken fillets squeezed. What if they were real though? Wouldn't that be fun?

Earlier the girls were sitting on bar stools in the local as normal. And also as normal Tina was all over a totally drunk middle aged man. There was a gentle gabble of conversation, a lovely atmosphere. Above the din the middle aged man was overhead by all around the bar.

"I know who you remind me of"

All conversations stopped. This might be interesting.

"Jennifer Aniston, you know her from Friends".

The whole bar area burst into hysterical laughter. Lee behind the bar in particular couldn't believe what he had just heard.

"But she's about the second most beautiful woman in the world, how can you possibly compare ..." the rest was never uttered as he burst into laughter again.

"Who's she Trish? I've never seen Friends". Tina was stuck in the seventies again.

"Google her hon, you might like what you see".

Beer goggles are wonderful!

Tina awoke around eleven the following morning, half dressed and half drunk, and burst into Tricia's room singing a song by the most famous American crooner of all. Tricia didn't know the song but after a while, using a process of elimination, established the singer to be Bing Crosby. At least the song distracted the gentle buzzing noise coming from under the blankets.

Although half dressed Tina was still going to take longer than Tricia to get ready. So Tricia, looking very grey to suit the weather, got her girly umbrella, bought a paper and had a pint in the Banyan Tree. She is a good girl who heeds advice you see. She said she would be back at half one but knew Tina still wouldn't be ready. She got back at quarter to two and Tina still wasn't ready.

At five past two the girls got into the lift and walked to Paddy's together. Tricia thinks that when they walk to the pub together they should hold hands. That is what girly-girls do when they are close friends isn't it? She has however failed to convince Tina of this. When she suggested they held hands in town she got a stream of abuse. Tricia suspects that Tina is not quite such a girlie-girl as she.

Anyway, at the pub the girls bump into a Squaddie called Sean. He is about to be posted to Catterick but, in a couple of months, would be off to Basra poor thing. Sean immediately fell in love with Tina's boots; he couldn't keep his hands off them. And, funnily enough, Tricia.

"Its you I really want darling".

"You'll have to work hard to get into my knickers hon".

Tricia isn't sure whether that statement is entirely true. She suspects that up to pint eight they do indeed have to work very hard, but between pints nine and ten she'll likely drop her panties for anyone. After pint ten she's so drunk she is incapable. The rain had stopped by now though allowing Tricia to do some shopping in town leaving Sean and Tina's boots to go to the New Union to play a game.

Tricia was still looking for tan shoes and was now quite happy to settle out of court. She knows they are on trend, trendy girl that she is. She was on her way to the Arndale, wiggling her posterior as only girlie-girls do when she got a quizzical look from a young girl. Tricia winked. The young girl rushed up to her.

"Are you a man or a woman?"

"I'm a woman of course". Tricia knew her voice would give her away.

"Where are you going?"

"To the Arndale to get some clothes and shoes".

"Do you mind if we come with you?"

"We?"

Tricia looked behind her where there was some children patiently waiting. There were six of them in all with ages ranging from ten to fifteen. The young girl became the spokesperson for the group and would ask Tricia questions any of them thought up. They were very polite and, despite telling them all about Iain they called her Tricia all the while.

"Do you mind if we help you shopping Tricia?"

"Not at all hon" and Tricia, with her little gang of children behind, dived into Shout. The children picked the things out they thought would look good on Tricia. They tried to be so helpful. A young boy (about ten) picked up a very girly dress which was almost girlie enough for Tricia.

"I think you'd look lovely in this Tricia".

"Careful hon, or you'll end up like me. Its not quite me though".

Tricia and her party went up to Evans to try and get the tan shoes. Still no joy but the children were. They were really helpful. Tricia was however to get a shock when she swanned out of the shop. She was greeted by another four children. There had obviously been some texting going on. The caterpillar wended its way through the shopping centre stopping occasionally for photos and questions.

Tricia heard a young boy mumble "we can't ask Tricia that"..

The self-appointed spokesperson came back alongside Tricia.

"Excuse me Tricia, but would you mind if I ask you a very personal question?"

"Of course not, but I may choose not to answer".

"Do you sleep with men?" She covered her mouth with her hand in embarrassment.

"Of course not honey, I'm a girl" Tricia paused.

"Men sleep with me".

She could hear her answer being relayed down the line with astonishment.

Tricia had a lovely time with the children but realised when enough was enough and somehow managed to dissuade them from going to Canal Street where there are lots of girls like Tricia.

Back at Paddies with Becky, Megan and Steph and some interesting snippets in the front smoking area also known as Bloom Street. George with the beard (bushy isn't the word for it, more like tropical rainforest) and the walking stick was trying to use the aforementioned walking stick with a purpose not intended. He was trying to look up Tricia's pretty dress. Megan went mad at him.

"There are boundaries and you are crossing them", she screamed.

"I don't why he bothered anyway", said Tricia coyly.

"Everybody knows there's nothing up there". Tricia winked.

A hen party joined Steph and Tricia for a smoke. They were all dressed as Pirates.

"Where are your parrots girls?" asked Tricia, "have they flown away?".

"We can't help much with the parrots Trish but we've got a cockatoo". Steph was very fond of puns.

Inside the pub the girls were discussing chastity belts of all things. How did they work? They understood how it might for a bloke as it could be tucked away underneath; much like Tricia does every morning after putting her panties on. But how can it work for a woman? A bloke would have to sit down to pee, but how could a woman pee at all. How could she survive being locked in it for nine months while her husband was away at the Crusades? Although Tricia wishes to be a girlie-girl, she is dead glad that the medieval days are over.

That night Tricia again bumped into Mad Wendy. Wendy is a very attractive middle aged woman and dresses in a similar fashion to Tricia. She is someone who Tricia aspires to being like. She is also, as her name suggests, totally manic. But they both like each other a lot and have a laugh together.

"But what if we were to make love together Trish?"

"What, like a pair of lesbians?"

"Yes, it might be fun"

"Have you ever been the bloke before?.... because don't look here".

"Hmm" said Wendy, "No, but that would be fun".

Wendy had to leave as her last bus was due. But not before she'd exchanged phone numbers with Tricia.

Wendy's leaving sadly left Tricia at the mercy of the limpet. She now has a tactic which works. She keeps her lips firmly shut. If the limpet gets his tongue inside her mouth she hasn't got a chance. He can't cling on when her lips are sealed. Tricia thinks she needs a chastity belt for her lips when the limpet is around.

The following day a very tired Tricia decided on another couple of challenges. Where on earth do you buy hats from? Next weekend she has a seventieth birthday party in The Irish Pub to attend and wishes to look her best. She thinks she will wear SGD2, very SJP. She wants to sparkle as only she can. But Tricia didn't want to pay too much. After all, how often is she going to get to wear a hat? So she tried the charity shops but no joy again. She is really struggling with shopping at the moment but she is loving the struggle.

The second challenge was to take a video of her new girly walk to see how it could be improved. Brave girl that she is she decided to do the video in Piccadilly Gardens when it was packed. She set her girlie pink camera on a bench and got up to strut her stuff. A passing woman (well she passed better than Tricia) promptly picked up the camera.

"Excuse me, you've left this behind".

Tricia sighed.

"No I haven't I'm filming. Oh, never mind".

Tricia picked up the camera from the woman and waited. She was to get the video filmed about five minutes later and was quite pleased with what she saw. There is still room for improvement though. Tricia could get more girly still and that is what she wants to do.

Back to the pub and more girlie talk with Kimberley and Janet; and cricket talk with Ian. Kim has just had an operation to remove her Adam's apple and is shortly to do speech therapy training so she is well on her way. Janet, who has just started swinging, wants a fling with a t-girl. Ian wants to watch. Will Tricia fit the bill? If so who on earth is going play the role of bloke. Now there's one for our girly-girl to ponder.

Oh, and Tricia can officially announce that Jennifer Aniston looks decidedly rough in the morning, unshaven and without her make-up.

Chapter 104

Easter Parade

I suspect nothing could beat last weekend but who knows? That is why life is such fun! Anyway I have a birthday party to go to and I was determined to buy a hat. That may be fun too.

Did I? Of course I did. You all know I'm a girl of my words. By the way the song is pretty obvious.

> In your Easter bonnet, with all the frills upon it
> You'll be the grandest lady in the Easter parade
>
> I'll be all in clover and when they look you over
> I'll be the proudest fellow in the Easter parade

Hold onto your Hats

Tricia had a birthday party to go to, lucky girl. The birthday party was in her local pub and was for Dave. She intended to look her best; she wished to make an impression. As we know she decided that she needed a hat. She had been networking and the real girls told her to try Peacocks. Tricia likes Peacocks and often gets dresses from there so that is where she started.

Armed with her handbag and her shopping list which consisted of:

One birthday card

One suitable present

One hat

Tricia hit the stores at two o'clock on Sunday June 6th. The sun was shining and Manchester was packed. She found a coffee mug for someone of seventy by chance and the card was straightforward so the essentials were sorted. Now, thought Tricia, for the fun bit.

Tricia wiggled into Peacocks trying to keep her stride shorter and her back straighter. She saw the hats to her left and immediately noticed the one she wanted. It was very, very pink which was good. Not only was it a girlie-girl colour but it also matched the flowers on her pretty dress. She tried it on and checked herself in the mirror. She looked lovely; but how much was it going to set her back?

In fact it was only a fiver. Absolutely perfect for a girl of little means. But for a fiver she was not going to get a box to put it in and the hat would crumple if it was placed in her handbag which held the kitchen sink. Tricia considered her options and decided there was only one. She had to wear it! Having paid, Tricia put the hat on at a jaunty angle, checked herself in the mirror, she still looked dead gorgeous, and walked out into the Arndale Centre.

Tricia couldn't believe it, this really was fun. There were shoppers everywhere; thousands of women but not one of them wearing a hat like hers. People were pointing, looking and grinning at her. She was the centre of attention. She loved it and grinned back. No winking now, back as straight as it will go and look stately Tricia. For the first time in her life she was a ladee!

She stepped out of the Arndale and into the open air. After a minute or so the inevitable happened. Tricia should have seen it coming but was too busy enjoying herself. A gust of wind sheared the hat off Tricia and off it went on its way, merrily bounding down the pavement. Tricia sighed. Well at least it wasn't her wig this time. Her new girly walk with even smaller strides broke into a trot (we know she is hot to trot) and with her arms swinging down straight, her chicken fillets thrust out as far as they would go and her backside wiggling like an over-wound pendulum she must have made a ridiculous sight. She would catch up with the hat, bend down keeping her knees together in a such a short dress and her back straight, then another gust of wind would blow the hat further. She would then have to compose herself again, stand up straight, and trot off again after the hat. To get herself going Tricia noticed that she wiggled her hips a couple of times to loosen them before moving.

Eventually the hat was recovered and was gracefully perching again on top of Tricia's wig. She was more careful walking back to the pub. If she felt a breeze coming she held on to it. The wind caught her unawares however as she was turning into the road where the coach station is. It crept up behind her removed the hat and this time, on its rim, blew it further. Tricia, showing the determination if not the technique of a middle distance runner followed it all the way to Bloom Street using her peculiar waddle. What the people waiting for coaches thought didn't worry her. She was simply grateful that she managed to retrieve the hat.

At the pub, hat proudly perched on Tricia's head; Tricia met Tina, got the card signed and gave it and the present to Dave with a kiss on both his cheeks. There were numerous comments about her hat including ones which suggested that she shouldn't be wearing it indoors.

The party got into full swing but without the t-girls. They were nowhere to be seen. In fact they were sitting in the corner on bar stools in front of a big mirror trying Tricia's hat on. They could not be prised away. They learnt how many different ways the hat could be worn.

"Hey Trish, if you do it that way you look like a cowgirl" Tina was being complimentary as always.

"Tina, turn the rim up, yes that works, very Joan Collins!"

"Ooh Steph, you look lovely with it like that, almost Audrey Hepburn".

Almost indeed.

Then the food came out, the hat returned to Tricia and the girls rejoined the party and had a wonderful time.

Tricia thought and thought hard. She decided that she had never had more fun for a fiver. She decided she was going to get another, far more ornate hat. She would scour the charity shops far and wide. Hats are brill, and she's almost ready for Ladies Day at Ascot. Wouldn't that be fun? Would she be able to get into the Ladies Enclosure? Then she thought again. Maybe Chester would be more appropriate; with all the Chavs and the Wags.

And it's closer too.

Chapter 105

Suicide is Painless

Dear All,

By the way, to this day I still love MASH. I'm always in favour of a good munch. As I am writing this there is a gentle hum of buzzing in the background. No, not helicopters; I also enjoy buzzy bee. I feel empty now without him inside me. The trouble is that Tina keeps barging into my room when he is buzzing away. I think I'm going to have to get a sign to put on my door so Tina knows not to come in. The sign might as well be permanent however.

Hugs,

Trish xx

> Suicide is painless
> It brings on many changes
> and I can take or leave it if I please.

Tricia is on the lash and gets the horn….. again.

Tricia was re-applying her make-up in the unisex toilet for the umpteenth time in the night

"Would you like some of my lippy hon?"

The small guy next to her couldn't immediately reply. He was struggling to get into his rubber hood.

"Not for me darling, I'm not into that".

"Careful hon, you'll kill yourself wearing that"

"I've often wondered how much fun suicide would be".

Though in general small in stature, Tricia noticed something quite alarming about the man in the rubber suit next to her. She reverted back to her schooldays and covered her mouth with her hand to hide her embarrassment.

"Would you mind if I asked you something very personal hon?"

"Not at all, but I may choose not to answer".

"Is that part of your outfit?"

Tricia's cheeks, although powdered in rouge, could get redder still.

"You may touch but not feel"

"Ooooh my goodness!" Tricia rushed out into the bar. That, she felt, would be far too painful for a sixteen year old girl to handle.

Outside she bumped into Geraldine, or at least half Geraldine. Geraldine was wearing a very pink tutu and tights. Her lower half, Tricia thought, looked beautiful. The trouble was her top half. Tricia had never seen such a hairy chest and beard!

"Hey Trish, come here". Steph was talking to a domme.

"This is Tricia; it's her first time so she's a virgin".

Tricia giggled as only virgins can.

"Good, then I'll warm up my new crop on her; bend over girl".

So, in the middle of the night, in the middle of a crowded bar Tricia bent over and lifted her skirt. To be truthful her skirt was that short it hardly needed lifting at all. But she took her spanking with aplomb. It was horrible and stung like anything on her legs but was quite delightful on her backside. Her backside was starting to get very used to twitching.

"You'll do dear; but next time it will be the dungeon, and I won't be practicing.

Tricia had seen the dungeon. Whipping posts, a wrack, torture devices of all kinds; torture devices she was sure she'd come to love.

Just then a young girl flip-flopped in wearing a very short skirt. Tricia could take no more. How on earth could someone get turned on by wearing flippers? A drunken Tricia left earlier than was ideal but would return. She had met the resident Dommes who had showed an interest in her. Not only had she a fully paid up member but she was also now a fully paid up member of Club Lash. Thanks Steph, and roll on July 9th. Tricia may just get a bit braver. Tricia may just see if she can get into the dungeon.

It was the start of the World Cup. Owing to some bad management on Tricia's behalf, she and Tina had to watch the opening match in drab. That didn't stop Tricia practicing her girly walk to and from the Binary Bar though. It eased her into the weekend. And it didn't stop Tina and Tricia discussing outfits.

"You have to wear a belt with that dress Trish".

"No hon, that's an absolute no-no. I need to wear flats as well.

"No girl should ever wear flats! Heels are sexy and turn men on.

Tricia knows though, she reads all the fashion magazines. A maxi dress with a belt and heels? Never!

Following the game the girls dressed up and looked as they should. Immediately things started to improve. Tricia was standing on the roundabout with an equally attractive girl, both dressed to the nines and showing lots of leg. Tina had of course already sprinted across the road, not walking like a girl at all. A passing car of young lads blew their vuvuzehlas at the girls. That was one horn Tricia didn't mind getting.

It was extremely hot walking in even though it was late afternoon. Far too hot in all that slap to walk in direct sunshine. For once in their life they therefore walked in on the shady side of the street. Tricia is starting to hate the heat. She just can't stop her face, especially her beard, glowing (that's what girls do isn't it?) She is using as much powder now as she is using batteries. Even so, it tales half an hour in the pub for the glowing to stop. Sometimes beads of sweat will collect and drop onto her pretty dress. And we all know how much slap she uses!

"Trish, I've got some money to spend. Why don't we go into town. We never go into town"

"Hon, I go into town all the time. But where is the money coming from? I thought you were stony".

"It's the rent money".

"Oh dear!"

"But I absolutely must get a new wig".

"Then do it properly hon, don't get cheap rubbish".

"I know what I'm doing Tricia".

Tricia wondered, but nevertheless the girls strutted into town. Tricia had something to buy as well. After all it is the world cup, and England may reach the quarter finals. First stop though was for Tina's wig.

Tricia knows Tina is getting better at street walking but she is still very edgy. She is listening for comments all the time and may react and blow a fuse. Tricia now concentrates on herself and doesn't worry about the outside world. She wishes to look her girly best at all times. She wishes to walk as girlies walk, smell as girlies smell; eventually she will learn to talk as girlies talk. She knows what she is though and it doesn't worry her about who else does.

For once Tina was prepared. She had brought her old wig with her and even knew its name. Tricia shook her head but kept her mouth shut. Experiment Tina, don't go for the same look every time. The girls are so different but in many ways the same. Yes, they did have a Cher wig but no, not in the same colour. They brought out a wig which was very, very blonde. Tricia was puzzled. How can you possibly have a Cher wig which is blonde? Tina can; but it will take time to wear it with confidence.

The girls made their way into the Arndale and into shop after shop. Tina was amazed at the number of sexy cheap dresses on offer. Since she was in straight town she wasn't on offer herself for once. Tricia found her purchase but will keep it under wraps for now. At least until the quarter finals.

Tina and Georgina have now made up but it is still a love hate relationship. Tricia thinks that isn't bad it's more fun like that. In the ladies at the pub there is a picture of a crossdresser with a beard. Georgina thought about writing 'Tina' on it but didn't. Tina wrote 'Georgina' instead. In kohl. It was all cheap stuff but as cheap as Tina who now has a new moniker. She is known as Martini. 'Any time, any place, Anywhere!'

England versus USA. Tricia, Tina, Megan, Becky, Amanda, Steph, everyone. Tricia knows it ended up one all, but can't quite remember how it got there. She had a bust up with Megan of all people but realised she had drunk too much. She was a good girl and got a cab home that night. Megan and Tricia made up the following day.

There was still one more shopping day left for Tricia who looked fantastic in her stripy gray mini dress. Her legs were proudly on display and with her new girly walk she gets lots of attention; beeps from cars and wolf whistles. A different kind of attention than she was used to. She bought herself an England kit for the next world cup match on Friday. A pair of sexy red hot pants and white top which boldly states 'Englands No 1 striker". Quite apt thought Tricia who woke up the following morning alongside a lesbian. Peter must have left in the early hours, thought Tricia. Anyway, that really is apt. Isn't Tricia a lesbian herself now?

Chapter 106

Postman Pat

The weekend, though wonderful, was completely overshadowed at 10.15 on Monday morning. It was Iain who found out so I'll let him tell you. I'm so excited I could wee myself. Even better, I'm off work the week before so I have a whole week to prepare. And prepare I will. All those girlie things I'm going to have to do! How Iain is going to get through the rest of this week goodness only knows.

But England are out of the World Cup. Dreadful but expected. I could defend better in my high heels. My bikini was all ready to be revealed if we won. It will have to wait for another occasion to be unveiled to the unsuspecting world. By the way, what on earth is this all about?

> Postman pat
> Postman Pat
> · Postman pat and his black and white cat.
> Early in the morning, just as day is dawning,
> he picks up all his post bags in his van.

Tricia goes straight.

Tricia had this weekend, then a week at work, then the next week off. So nine days as Tricia culminating in Sparkle weekend. She was dead looking forward to that but she was looking forward to this weekend. She was going to practice and practice her girly walk so lots of time around town. She also needed to update her summer coffin so was on the lookout for short dresses and mini skirts.

My other, non-twin daughter was coming up for the weekend with some mates for a hen party and got to meet Tricia, Trish was gradually getting out farther and Father. In fact they were to meet up at the front of Paddys Goose where Tricia was practicing something else; the art of girlie smoking.

Tricia knows the rules. The cigarette needs to be viewed as a phallic object which gives her the chance to impress any man present of her ability with her lips and tongue. Firstly though she needs to pretend to have lost her lighter. In Tricia's case this is a fairly easy task as it is likely to be buried at the bottom of her handbag which holds the kitchen sink or mixed in with her make-up. So she needs to find a man with a lighter. That is not difficult when you are in the smoking shelter. Having found him she turns in towards her target to accept the light and leaves her hand behind, touching his wrist for a few moments too long after her cigarette is lit. She will then take a couple of puffs (yes, that is puffs) inhaling deeply with her cigarette perched firmly between the ends of her middle and index fingers. After each puff (yes, that is puff) she gives a little girlie whimper. While she is not smoking she holds her cigarette high, at shoulder level, with her wrists bent upwards to display her perfectly manicured nails. She will then engage her man in conversation looking deeply into his eyes. What she is really doing of course is mimicking the sex act; but she knows that. That is why she chooses her man carefully. Tricia's practicing and posturing were to pay off in due course as we shall see. But that comes later.

It was time for town and to practice Tricia's girlie walk. Tricia's walk has become slightly less girlie but girlie enough and far more natural. She doesn't have to concentrate so hard on it so it is a lot easier. She can still feel her backside wiggling frantically and loves it when the sun is in front of her as she can see her silhouette in the shadows. There were to be no problems at all in town where Tricia bought a couple of tops, a dress and some more jewellery.

She met up with Tina back in Paddy's and they met up with a colourful character called Johnny no socks, also known as Roadduck. There was a slight disturbance to the conversation when a pissed guy wandered across and asked Tricia if she wanted him to suck her. He got a very tart reply from the tart she was becoming. And we know she's so becoming.

"Honey, inside I'm all woman, so no, you don't suck me".

Now for something completely different and a first in Tricia's young life. After a long chat with her daughter and friends Tricia was walking home outside the village. She heard someone wolf whistle from behind so turned around and smiled. The man approached her and gave her a quick peck on the cheek.

"You look dead gorgeous. Can I walk with you?"

"Where are you heading, and you know what I am?"

"I need to get the bus at four so I've a few hours to kill. I find you very attractive".

Now, it turned out that Bob was a postman in Stockport. That is hardly a surprising fact. What was more surprising however was that he was totally straight and had never been with a t-girl before. Tricia used her by now finely honed value set to make her decision.

'Will it be fun?' Yes.

'Will it harm me?' No.

So Tricia and Bob walked back to T-Girl Towers arm in arm for a bit of how's your Father.

To be truthful what went on was pretty tame compared with Tricia's recent sexual encounters. Bob wasn't one hundred per cent sure of being with a t-girl and Tricia didn't wish to push him too far. She did however very much enjoy a two hour session of heavy petting with a straight guy. At half three Bob got dressed and went off to catch his bus. Tricia remained in her sexy undies and went off to find her buzz. A lovely night.

After a long lie in, which gave Tina time to get ready, Tricia changed into her England supporters gear. She removed her sexy undies and put on her England bikini. She had a new white top which had 'I love cute boys" written on it (it should be fun cruising Canal Street wearing that thought Tricia) and tiny red shorts. For some reason which Tricia didn't quite understand, Paddy's refused to show the match. It was something to do with potential violence, though Tricia suspected there was more chance of violence through alcohol than football; and as the match kicked off at three in the afternoon that shouldn't happen. So the punters left the pub and moved en masse to New York New York. What they witnessed could only be described as dismal. There was more chance of Tricia wearing trousers again than stripping down to her bikini. At least the bar were saved that. But if the goal that wasn't a goal was allowed who knows?

Back outside the pub on a fag break Tricia was dodging the rent boys and lamenting the state of English football with Alf (no, not Sir Alf). A car stopped in front of them, the driver looked Tricia up and down and then drove off again.

"I thought he was stopping for you" said Alf.

"I think he most probably was. Maybe I'm not quite ready yet".

Tricia's sexual appetite seems to be growing and growing at the moment.

I was a little tired, a little emotional and a little miserable as I arrived at work, on time on the Monday morning for once. After reading my work emails to check nothing was urgent I opened Tricia's hotmail account. After all I hadn't any access to a computer all weekend. And there it was. Yay!

Now, you don't know this because after Tricia's failure last time I have been keeping it close to her chicken fillets. Two weeks ago, encouraged by the workmates who knew, Tricia decided to enter the 'Tranny of the Year' contest at Sparkle. Two years later on Tricia felt she might just be good enough. And she was. The email read:

~~~~~~~~~~~~~~~~~~~~~~~~~~~~~~~~~~~~~~~

From: Sparkle
Sent: 27 June 2010 11:05:01
To: tricia.dale@hotmail.co.uk

Hi Trish. Congratulations you're in the contest.

Firstly I would like to thank you for taking part in this years competition.

I will hope to see you between 9 pm and 10.30 pm the Friday night before the contest upstairs In AXM Bar, wear you can pick up your sash and ask any questions about the competition.

If you can't make it we will be having a quick rehearsal at the Place Apartments Hotel we will be meeting downstairs in the bar at 12.45 pm. Please don't be late, as it wont run for very long. Rehearsals take place on the first floor landing at 1:00 pm. You don't have to be dressed for this, but bringing your heels may be a good idea.

Can you kindly confirm your definitely entering and if you will be picking up your sash on the Friday night or Saturday Afternoon MANY THANKS

I would just like to take this opportunity to give you a few tips and explain a little more about the judging.

Outfit –

Make sure your you can walk in it and are able to clime stairs, something outrages may well impress the Judges but might may not help you to look as convincing as you can, so you really have a choice here, ether going all out to win the best outfit prize, or go for good marks in both convincing and outfit sections. Outfits that are both glamorous and feminine emphasizing all the right curves would be my choice.

Shoes, do not make the mistake of wearing to high a heel if this spoils your walk, as this will ruining your chances in the style and deportment section.

Accessories, jewellery needs to be on the large size or sparkle other wise it will not be seen. Props are also fine from a parasol to a pram (but not to big and no real babies)

Style and deportment –

Your walk, arm movements, turns and how you carry your self is what you will be judged on.

Try to use the next week to practice your walk even watch a few catwalk models on you-tube if you can, this will give you a good idea on how to do your turns and poses

Convincing –

This is that all important transformation, looking as feminine as possible, Its how far you can go to hide your masculine origins . Your figure will plays an important part here, the use of good breast forms hip and bottom pads, corsets (with out upsetting your movement) or just wearing the right outfit to flatter your shape. A good hair style and makeup will also carry extra marks.

Make up, should be bolder than you normally wear but don't go over the top if is not your style. False eye lashes are great , lip liner and a little extra blush will help your features stand out, remember you will not be seen that close up.

Congeniality –

Myself and one other secret judge will pick this winner, we will be looking out for that stand out entrant it may be that there just a lot of fun or helpful and kind to there fellow contestants. 5 extra points will be added to there score, which could make all the difference. (each section is marked out of 12 to prevent these marks overpowering the end totals)

I hope that helps a little if you have any questions you can ring me on 0000000000

The Winner will be the person with the best combined score.

And please remember this competition is about having fun and getting involved, so try not to take things to seriously but that does not mean that you shouldn't try your damnedest to win!!

Kind regards Sparkle team.

~~~~~~

This was my entry:

From: tricia.dale@hotmail.co.uk
To: Sparkle
Subject:TOTY 2010
Date: Thu, 17 Jun 2010 20:31:32 +0100

Hi,

Please find attached my entry form and my photo for the tranny of the year competition. The photo was taken by one of the kids who were following me around Manchester so does link to my entry. Its not of the highest quality but I think shows me as what I am. I can provide other pictures if you need.

I would love to be invited into the competition. Even the thought of preparing for the event fills me with excitement. I am a Manchester girl during the weekend but live in Chesterfield and work in Sheffield during the week. Something has to pay for my wardrobe! I am out to all who need to know including my three daughters and my ex-partner. I am very very happy.

I came into this for three reasons:

1. To get myself out there

2. To document everything that happened while doing so (I have a blog which I am converting into a book)

3. To help others like me get out there.

The competition may provide me with an opportunity to help others. That is now the only thing I am really serious about. I love my life, am very happy in it and can't wait for weekends to arrive.

I hope you view my application favourably and look forward to hearing from you soon.

I am Tricia I am she
I am who I want to be

Hugs,

Trish xx

Tricia's entry read:

TOTY 2010 Contestant Entry Form

NB. We have simplified the entry form this year to make things easier for everyone!

Any false or misleading information could result in disqualification.

Name	Tricia Dale
Age	52
Where are you from?	Chesterfield and Manchester
Describe yourself in three words?	Out, Proud, Happy

> I walk along canals and locks
> I watch a young girl feed the ducks
> The sun is high, the breeze is strong
> This is a place where I belong
> I buy a beer, I feel so calm
> I'm looking pretty, I'm feeling fine
> Dressed to kill and made-up too
> Now what does Tricia want to do?
> Buy some shoes or buy a dress
> She's waited too long to impress
> Fifty years to be here
> Celebrate with another beer?
> To the boutiques she will go
> Her vulnerability will be on show
> But boys and girls, its fine to talk
> That t-girl there walks the walk
> She struts her stuff, she feels so proud
> She needs to scream, to shout out loud
> I am Tricia, I am she
> I am who I want to be.

It has taken me just over two years, a tremendous amount of determination and commitment and lots and lots of practice to become the person I am today. I knew I was getting there when I was walking in the local neighborhood about a year ago. I passed a gang of young children playing in the street. I carried on walking and heard the pitter patter of tiny footsteps behind me. A little girl, around six years old, patted me on the backside.

"Excuse me, but you're not a real girl are you?"

I put my perfectly manicured finger to my lips. "Sssshhh, don't tell anyone".

I carried on walking. As I turned the corner a shrill voice shrieked out

"I've told someone". Instead of being offended I burst out laughing.

I've since dressed on coaches, trains, buses and trams. I've dressed in Manchester, Liverpool, Sheffield, Blackpool, Carlisle and London. I've even been round the Houses of Parliament dressed. The world awaits!

At weekends I live in a flat in South Manchester with no gas or electricity; my long dresses hang in an upright open coffin. I'm therefore well aware that money can't buy happiness, but being true to yourself can. I am also the pied, or more likely pie-eyed piper of Manchester. A few weeks ago in Piccadilly Gardens a girl wasn't sure about me so I gave her a wink.

"Are you a girl or a boy?" she asked

"I'm a girl of course". I knew my voice would give me away. What I didn't realise was that she was with her mates. Luckily for me they were lovely, polite kids. They followed me shopping asking me questions all the while. We went into Evans to look for shoes. When I came out I was amazed to see there were more kids waiting for me. I now had about ten teenagers following me. There had obviously been some texting going on. Eventually the inevitable happened.

"Tricia, do you mind if I ask a very personal question?"

"Of course not, but I may choose not to answer".

The girl put her hand to her a mouth in embarrassment. "Do you sleep with men?" and gave a girly giggle.

"No I don't honey, I've told you I'm a girl............. men sleep with me!"

Please post completed entries along with a recent, good quality photograph (which must show your face and be to a maximum size of 500kb) to Sparkle TOTY 2010.

Deadline for receipt of completed entries is Friday 18th June 2010.

So Tricia is going to be in a beauty CONTEST. Oh what fun! She very much doubts she will win; there are some brilliant and convincing trannies out there, but she will do her best though and will certainly enjoy it. One thing is for sure though. She will put in a far better performance than the England soccer team!

Chapter 107

Manic Monday

I should have been preparing for the beauty competition but, as frequently happens in life, something gets in the way. It was large but it was lovely. So, and by the way:

> It's just another manic Monday (oh-woe)
> I wish it was Sunday (oh-woe)
> 'Cause that's my Funday (oh-woe)
> My I don't have to runday (oh)
> It's just another manic Monday.

Meditor Rumpo (Latin)

Tricia was sitting in the pub preparing her week. A cock up by me at work meant that I had to go back on the Friday, the day before the beauty contest! But actually even Tricia thought that was probably a good thing. It would take her mind off things and keep her off the beer. She needed to be as fit as she could on the Saturday. She had at least done what I told her and prepared a list of what needed buying. It was as follows:

New Wig (Mon)	£100
Prom dress (Tue)	£100
Shoes (Tue)	£50
Sexy underwear (Wed)	£20
Jewellery to match prom dress (Wed)	£20
Body waxing (Thu)	£50

Eyebrow shaping (Thu)	£20
Nails (Sat)	£20
Spray tan (Sat)	£20
Pedicure (Sat)	£10
False eyelashes (Sat)	£10
Total	**£420**

I had given Tricia a budget of £500 so she had a little money spare. She really was going to be a girly-girl this week and do all the things real girly-girls love to do. She was so looking forward to it! She was going to really enjoy herself. Her planning had been done back at work in Sheffield by Lesley and it was to be complimented in Manchester by another Lesley. So she was in good hands.

Her jobs this weekend she decided had to be about planning – which she was doing, rallying around all the support she could get from her friends and practicing her catwalk. She worked out that she had only Friday, Saturday, Wednesday and the following Friday to practice. She was going to practice upstairs at Napoleons on the dance floor with mirrors all around. And the dance floor with mirrors all around only opened on those nights. On Friday night she was such a good girl and did all three jobs, even leaving Napoleons at a relatively early time. She did get accosted on the dance-floor by a group of girls though.

"Why are you walking? This is a dance-floor".

"Can't you see I'm not just walking, I'm cat-walking. I'm in a beauty contest next week".

"Wow, cool!"

The girls had great fun practicing themselves and showing Tricia how to do it.

You see Tricia had a problem. Wherever she had walked in the past, she had a handbag to carry. She was not going to carry a handbag on the catwalk though. So what should she replace it with. The girls showed her. Hand on hip, or two hands on hips. Tricia would need to practice more but this was a good start and the girls were a great help and great fun.

So all went swimmingly on the Friday night but as we know things often go astray in Tricia's complicated life and they were about to again.

Neil was originally from Manchester but had emigrated to Bulgaria where he owned some property. He was back in Manchester until Tuesday to see his parents who were very ill. Georgina introduced them and they got chatting and chatting and chatting.

"Are you going to Naps Trish?"

"Yes, but not for too long. I've a competition next week and need to practice my catwalk on the dance-floor with the mirrors.

"I'll see you later then". Neil winked and kissed her.

Tricia actually left the pub earlier than normal as she wanted to catwalk when the dance-floor was free. She had been practicing for a good couple of hours (interspersed with beers and ciggies of course) and was pretty much oblivious to everything and everybody. After yet another catwalk session, she was beginning to get tired, she walked down the stairs and was stopped at the bottom by Neil.

"You have done enough for one night. Go and have your cigarette than join me".

Tricia thought; she should be practicing. Tricia fought. No she didn't,

"Ok hon, I'll join you in five".

They continued their long dialogue from earlier but not for so long this time.

Neil had a room booked at Munro's down the road. He knew what he wanted. Tricia, the sexually re-awakened Tricia, knew precisely what she wanted.

Not so good the following morning though. Neil had disappeared leaving Tricia in the hotel room alone. No note, no explanation. Should she wait? What should she do. Tricia was well miffed. She loves her sex in the morning as we know and now she'd have to go back to buzzy bee. Then she put her sensible hat on. Last night she will not forget for a long time. So she shrugged her shoulders and got on with her life, with a smile on her lips and some lovely memories in her heart.

Tricia spent a quiet Sunday. She did a fair bit of shopping, but it was window shopping. She was looking for ideas for her outfit. She had a few beers in the evening but not too many. She was back to being the girl with the sensible head.

She was still being sensible on Monday. She went shopping in the morning, booked a wig fitting for the following day, then went to the pub for a couple, just a couple of beers. She met Georgina as expected who had some good advice.

"Tricia, you're on holiday so why don't you treat yourself to a hotel room for a few nights. It's cheap mid-week and you will have hot running water and electrickery".

"Thanks hon, I'll think about it".

Tricia was about to leave when..... Well, you've probably guessed already who turned up.

"I'm sorry Trish, please don't say anything. My parents are on their last legs and I promised I would see them. I've managed to work something out though. I'd love to spend another night with you and just one phone call will sort that out".

"I think I'll have a cigarette and a think hon".

Tricia knew the answer was yes. She didn't need the cigarette to decide that. It was the how that concerned her. She didn't want to bring him back to T-Girl Towers; she wanted better than that. It was then that she remembered Georgina's wise words. That is what she would do. She had a plan and the rest of the afternoon, evening and best of all night with her new boyfriend. She skipped back into the pub.

"Hon, the answer is yes of course, but I need to set something up first".

She kissed him passionately.

"Lets have a chat for a while, there is no rush".

It was about an hour and a half later that Tricia, arm-in-arm with Neil, walked into Eazysleep. I had worked out the deal.

"Would you be happy if I paid £50 for three nights. I know your rooms will be empty otherwise". It was agreed so Tricia picked up the key and Neil and her went up to the room for a bit of foreplay.

"Let's save the best for later hon. Why don't we go for a meal, have a couple of beers and a chat and the come back for some fun. Does that sound good?"

"I like that".

So after a gorgeous curry, after three drinks and lots and lots of cuddles upstairs at Spirit, Neil and Tricia returned to their new love-nest. Tricia was very impressed that Neil was not at all phased, and looked after her, when they were outside the village together. They had a wonderful curry and a final nightcap before retiring for the night.

Neil had to get up early in the morning to get to Manchester Airport and then Sofia. They had one more passionate moment before he rushed out of the bedroom, had a shower, put on his clothes and then remembered.

"Trish, we need to swap numbers"

He shouted out his phone number and Tricia dialled it with a smile fixed firmly on her face.

Where on earth is this going?

Chapter 108

Stationery Traveller

By the way no lyrics this time. I had my laptop with me as I was up all week and had it playing random tracks at the hotel. This song came on and immediately hit me; it was so haunting. Iain says it is the antithesis of me. If there is one thing I must not be it is a stationary traveller. I played it all week when I was putting my make-up on. The week when I was preparing to be a beauty queen. Oh what fun! Actually I enjoyed the build-up almost as much as the competition itself.

Finally Tricia prepares.

After kissing Neil goodbye Tricia had work to do. She had got behind. She had to walk back to the flat, pick up some more clothes, jewellery and make-up and laptop and then get a taxi back to her hotel. She had to do all this before her wig fitting which was at 14:00. She hurried back to T-Girl Towers and rushed around quickly getting her stuff together. It had to be a capsule wardrobe this time as she only had a hold-all to put things in and had her laptop to fit in as well. She managed it with time to spare so she could have a shower back at the hotel. She is unused to such luxury. At the hotel Tricia got out her laptop, went downstairs to get the network password and bingo, she was on the internet. She put her laptop onto a Genesis shuffle then went for her shower. Genesis were not playing when she came out though.

'What's all this about' thought Tricia who checked her laptop. It still said Genesis shuffle but the next song was one by Camel. She shrugged her shoulders and started dressing herself. The Camel song started and immediately entranced her. She set it to replay as she began her make-up. She was to play it for the next two days while she got ready to go out. But the wig shop awaited for now.

"What I would like" said Tricia "is something similar but slightly longer than my current wig, about the same colour but maybe a little lighter and maybe streaked".

"How much have you got to spend?"

"I've budgeted about £100".

"You don't want much!"

And the very helpful shop assistant rummaged through the shop getting all the wigs that she thought would suit Tricia.

Just as before the one that Tricia chose she tried on very early and it was kept to one side. All options explored Tricia tried it on again and really liked it. It was definitely lighter, longer, streaked and less stark than her other wig and it came in at £90; under budget. Tricia enjoyed the whole experience and found it fun talking to the saleswoman about the impending beauty contest.

Tricia's next task was to book her beauty treatment. It did, as she suspected turn out to require two sessions. Tomorrow was reserved to buy her prom dress and shoes so she booked the Thursday for the serious treatment and the Saturday morning for the glam stuff. She had already discussed what she needed with Lesley in Sheffield.

- Full wax,

- Shaping of eyebrows,

- Manicure and acrylic nails on fingers,

- Pedicure and painted nails on toes,

- False eyelashes,

- Spray tan on legs.

Tricia had a chat with Lilly. Two sessions it had to be as she couldn't spray tan immediately after waxing the legs. So the waxing and eyebrows to be done on the Thursday morning; the rest on Saturday morning. Both appointments were booked for 10.30 to make it easy for Tricia to remember. By the Saturday Tricia would have her prom dress so Lilly could match the nails to that. As she was leaving Lilly surprised her.

"Before Thursday you must exfoliate or I won't do the waxing".

"What on earth is exfoliate?"

"You've never heard of it?"

"No, never" Lilly was well amused.

"Go to the chemist and ask. You'll need a quite harsh exfoliator and get some for your face while you're at it. You will be surprised".

So Tricia trudged back whence she had come to the big Boots opposite the Arndale shrugging her shoulders. It was hard work being a beauty queen. She could only ask because she did not know.

"Excuse me, I am getting a full wax on Thursday and I need an exfoliator. My beautician told me that it needs to be harsh."

My beautician, thought Tricia, what is the world coming to?

"I know exactly what would be best".

The saleslady took Tricia to a place in the shop she had never been before and gave her a big bottle of yellow goo.

"Its sugar based. Before you start put some on the back of your hand and rub in using little circles so you can gauge the pressure you need then use it all over your body." The saleslady demonstrated.

"How often should I use it?"

"Once a week. And if you are getting a waxing do it the night before, not in the morning. It will really help."

A puzzled Tricia paid for the exfoliator (un-budgeted) and left to go to the pub where she spent a quiet evening. She can be a good girl sometimes.

Wednesday was shopping day for Tricia. Lesley (Sheffield) had lent her some dresses to try but the black one wasn't really her; the electric blue one was but it was size ten so slightly too tight at the shoulders. A pity because it meant that more of Tricia's allowance would need to be spent. At least she had budgeted for it. Tricia didn't really mind as she adores clothes shopping and went into shop after shop, not seeing anything which said buy me until she went into Pastiche and saw the dead gorgeous silver and peach princess dress. It fitted her well and came in under budget at £65 so she skipped out the shop and up to Evans where she found some strappy silver heels at £40. A match made in heaven.

Now, if you have been paying attention, you will be aware that Wednesday night is Concorde night and that Concorde night means that the dance-floor with mirrors all around will be open at Napoleons; the perfect opportunity for Tricia to practice her catwalk in her new silver heels. First though Tricia had her exfoliation to do for the first time. She took her time and was very thorough before, joy of joys, a shower to wash the sugar off. She was amazed at how good her skin felt afterwards. It was positively alive.

Just then Neil phoned from Bulgaria. Would Tricia like to go over there to meet him? Tricia wasn't sure. She would like to fly as Tricia, indeed she is flying as Tricia but not in a plane. According to Dave and Georgina she will be fine getting through customs if she wears a white butt-plug. Tricia wasn't sure of that either. Then the third amazing thing happened that night. Tricia had no trouble at all walking in her silver heels even though they were higher. She is clearly learning.

Thursday already? What happened to the week? Tricia was up early for her as she had to be at the beauticians for half past ten. She was anticipating agony with the waxing but was surprised at how easily the hair came off; even when she was double teamed. It must have been the exfoliation which did the trick. She wore her pretty flowery tea dress as it was easy to get on and off. A wise choice as it would be perfect for the spray tan as well on Saturday, it was so short. Tricia had to check out of the hotel and go back to t-Girl Towers. She enjoyed her stay though and it was vital for the shower following her exfoliation. She is determined to exfoliate every week from now on. It will be part of my beauty regime on Thursday nights. Both our lives are changing dramatically.

Tricia went back into town on Thursday afternoon to shop for her underwear. She wanted to be gorgeous all over on the Saturday. She quickly found a very pretty, slightly padded, peach bra and pantie set. She was careful to make sure that the straps of her bra would be hidden by the silver in her frock. She checked and if she took her time they would. Shopping and outfit therefore completed, she might though look for some more silver jewellery on Saturday morning.

Time for a few more in Paddies for one final time before going to work tomorrow. A conversation took place between the bar staff, Georgina and Tricia.

"You know what they say" said Lee,

"One man's meat is another man's poison".

"Actually", said Georgina,

"One man's meat is another man's pleasure".

Tricia felt that a day away from all this would do her good. She would be back in Manchester the following night however. She had her sash to pick up after all.

Tricia had thoroughly enjoyed the last week which cemented her desire to be Tricia all the time. But how? She loved being beautified, shopping for her prom dress and heels, finding the ever so pretty bra and pantie set, trying on her wigs. She simply adored everything about being a girl. Then of course there was the other part of being a girl earlier in the week. The hanky-panky with Neil. But the best was still to come. How will she manage at being a beauty queen in front of a thousand people? Tricia doesn't know. But she is looking forward to it immensely.

Chapter 109

She's Always a Woman

OMG OMG OMG. This was the best day of my life so far. I loved it, I loved it, I loved it! The night before I was v.v. good girl and did what Iain told me; what Iain's Dad drilled into him. Write a list; get organised. I owe Iain's Dad because he gave me my name and, when he died, he set me free. I think I would have loved him as much as Iain did. My list consisted of the following:

09:00 – Wake up (set alarm beforehand).

10:00 – Walk into town.

10:30 – Spray-tan, nails and false eyelashes at beauticians.

11:30 – Look for silver jewellery and peach flower for hair to match prom dress and shoes.

12:15 – Paddys Goose for pint one.

12:45 – Go to Place Apartments for rehearsal.

13:00 – Tranny of the Year rehearsal.

14:00 – Paddys Goose for pint two.

14:30 – To the Britannia to change into prom dress (beauty queen).

15:30 – Paddys Goose for pint three.

16:00 – Go around the gardens, look at the stalls and visualise myself as beauty queen.

17:00 – Paddys Goose for pint four.

17:30 – Meet for competition.

18:00 – Be a beauty queen.

The worry I had was how many pints should I have for my optimum performance. I knew that Iain performed best between pints three and four when he entered competitions which didn't require running like darts or snooker. But then Iain never played them in front of an audience of a thousand. And he didn't wear a dead gorge peach dress with high silver heels either. I thought four was probably right; I didn't want to fall off either my heels or the stage.

Anyway, after doing my list in Paddy's I had to go to AXM to pick up my beauty queen sash which I was to wear all weekend. Tina, who was giving me a lot of support, came with me. We eventually sorted out where we needed to be in AXM and I picked up my sash.

"Hello Trish, nice to meet you. Do you have any questions about the competition?"

I had four.

"Nice to meet you. How many girls have entered?"

"About thirty, but they won't all turn up".

"Will I have to sit on stage?"

"No, but you'll have to climb up and down stairs to get on and off stage, catwalk and pose to the audience".

"What will be used from the profile I sent you?"

"The relevant and funny bits will be picked out and used but if you want something specific or different let me know tomorrow lunchtime".

"Can I address the audience?"

"No, we couldn't have that. We would have girls singing and all sorts. It would turn into the X-Factor and we only have so much time".

"Ok thanks, I understand. I'll see you tomorrow at the Place Apartments at one".

"Lovely, thanks Trish".

I hung around with Tina for a while and chatted to some of the girls with beauty queen sashes the same as mine. They seemed a nice enough bunch. We went back to Paddy's Goose for one final pint before my final catwalk practice in the mirrors at Naps. 'Just polish up what you've practiced Trish and remember you've got higher heels on'. I left promptly at one, ignoring the glances of the admirers. Tomorrow was too big a day to risk anything else.

I woke up before nine. OMG OMG OMG is this really going to happen? I was like an eight year old girl playing the part of a princess in her first play; soo excited! I quickly got dressed. I knew I had to wear the same dress as I wore for Thursday because that would be perfect for the spray-tan. I didn't mind though. I love my pretty floral tea dress. I had to take my prom dress and heels with me and had arranged with my ex, who was hugely supportive and brought supporters and banners stating 'Trish' with her, to change in her hotel room which was just down the road from the village. It is all about planning. Iain's Dad was right, Iain was right. I am learning.

An idea was forming in my mind while I was getting ready to go the beauticians. If I could point out something from my profile, why don't I get the compare to read my poem out. It is very powerful and very me. Its ending is perfect:

"I am Tricia, I am She"

"I am who I want to be".

It seemed perfect and different. I will discuss it at the practice session.

So I arrived promptly at the beauticians and had a wonderful time being made beautiful. I showed Lilly my dress and she knew exactly what to do. She attached long acrylic French nails and painted a diagonal line in peach across the tip of each nail. Next was the pedicure. I had spent ages on my feet, powdering, spraying and exfoliating during the week so it wasn't to difficult for Lilly. They too were painted peach to match my dress. The spray-tan was easy. It was a bit like being in a shower with paint coming out of the nozzle instead of water. Finally false eyelashes which I have never been able to master. Fortunately I didn't have to. So my skin was ready, my nails were ready, inside I was ready. But outside. Could I really catwalk in front of a thousand people? You bet I could. YAY YAY YAY. I couldn't wait.

I had time for a quick shop around town to show off my tanned chicken legs and bought another silver ring and a necklace before hitting the pub for the first pint of the day. Georgina was, as ever, in her element, on her stool; but a bit miffed that there were so many t-girls in the village. But a fun little chat and some encouragement before I had to go to the Place Apartments for the rehearsal. I took my sash out of my bag and put it on for the occasion. I left my prom dress and heels behind the bar to be picked up later.

At the rehearsal the girls were very friendly and supportive. I was very friendly and supportive. I didn't know what was to come but it turned out not to be as bad as I thought it would. There was a practice catwalk marked out on the floor and I had to strut my stuff, posing at each corner before posing for the judges, then back through the middle, a final pose (milking the applause) then back and off stage. I can do this I thought; I'm going to love it. So I volunteered to go first. It suddenly hit me how much I adored being a girl.

I discussed the possibility of using my poem as I still liked the idea. We felt it was a little long so cut out a bit by agreement but the good new was that the compare would read it out for me. I had a voice at least, even if it wasn't my own (thank goodness).

Back to the pub to pick up my dress and heels and to consume my second pint of the day. Georgina was, as ever, in her element, on her stool; but a bit miffed that there were so many t-girls in the village. Then off to the Britannia, to my ex-partners hotel room around the corner where I could put on my gorge pink prom dress and heels and touch up on my make-up. Many thanks to Louise, Woo and Trudy who really helped me.

Then Tina, of all people, threw a spanner in the works. She phoned my mobile.

"Trish, its Sparkle and I really need the brown Cher wig".

"Then go and buy it".

"I can't, I'm still at the flat but you are in town".

"I'm not, I'm at the Britannia getting ready".

"But I really want it".

"Honey, in about two hours time I am entering a beauty contest in front of a thousand people. I can't be worrying about brown Cher wigs at this time".

"Oh can't you".

"No I can't. I've everything planned out. In any case I would get the wrong one".

"Oh Trish!"

"Oh Tina!"

"So its a no then".

"Its a no. I can't believe you even asked on this of all days".

Aaaaarrrgh! Calm down girl. Walk back to the pub for a pint. Then to the Gardens for a bit of visualisation. Then another pint and then, my dear, you are going to be a prom queen. No pressure there then.

The contestants (including me) met as agreed at 17:30 next to the bus next to the stage. The girls were really friendly and we chatted to each other for the half hour before the competition begun. I felt good. I knew I looked good. I was a little nervous but knew from Iain's cricketing days not to worry about that. Nerves keep you alive and on edge. Eventually we lined up in order. I was outside left (number eleven). Beauty queens are not known for their brains so it was a major task to get them in the right order; particularly since some girls had not turned up so there were gaps in the numbers.

I was now really looking forward to it. The queue gradually shortened. Each girl got great support from the audience and hugs and congratulations backstage from the other contestants after they had finished. Eventually I walked up the steps and waited at the back of the stage.

"You'll have to do this slowly Trish. I forgot to take the verse out of your poem".

"That's ok. I know the poem backwards so I can use it to pace my catwalk".

"Number eleven. Tricia Dale from Manchester".

"Good luck"

I walked on stage to huge cheers and flash-lights going off everywhere. This was brill. I loved being in the spotlight; I loved being the centre of attention. I enjoyed it all so much I didn't concentrate enough on my catwalk which I think let me down in the end. The poem went down really well and I got a massive cheer from the audience as I did my final pose and walked off-stage. Backstage the girls all applauded and congratulated me. But the competition was like that. We all had a wonderful time and were hugely supportive of each other. It didn't really matter who one; in fact we likely all did.

I think I might have got the audiences vote, and others agreed but I forgot the golden rule of being a beauty queen. I didn't sleep with the judges. Never mind , it was such fun and it wasn't finished yet.

At the end of the competition we were supposed to come on stage; dance at the back for one song; wave goodbye to the audience and go back off-stage. I climbed the stairs after the girl playing inside left, waited for the others and started dancing. Then I noticed an opportunity that I simply couldn't miss. There was nobody on the catwalk. So, barging girls out of the way left, right and centre, I danced down the catwalk on my own to the cheers of the audience. Oh what fun! I'm dead glad I'm such a confident dancer. All that training in Naps definitely paid off. Walking around the park after we had finished, I got applauded all the way. And there is a video of me looking so girly back-stage. I so love being Tricia.

I think I do this bit now so, by the way, this one is very, very me.

Oh--she takes care of herself

She can wait if she wants

She's ahead of her time.

Tricia the Beauty Queen.

OMG OMG OMG I can't believe the video. Is that really me? Is that what I have turned into? How can I possibly live my life as a male now? I think we are at the cusp. I think the see-saw is about to tilt the other way. I am determined to do something very, very, brave. And the song really is Tricia.

Chapter 110

I'm Coming Out

A chapter set in Sheffield for once and not at the weekend. Actually it takes place at Iain's desk at work on Friday 16th July. Spurred on by being a beauty queen, I decided it was time I came out to the office. I had kept my ceramic nails on all week and was going to tell anybody who challenged me. Would you believe that nobody did so I had to force myself out? The song, by the way, is from an episode of Ugly Betty and just had to be used. The thread was simply called 'Fun' and the song lyrics were included on the attachments. There was also some banter in the office. Iain had previously told his line manager, HR, and Janet in his team that this was going to happen.

> I'm coming out
> I want the world to know
> Got to let it show

Fun.

Hi All,

Well, we don't have any do we! But I'm about to change that.

I don't know, but you lot are either very blind, very kind or very scared. I think it's the former but I may be wrong. You see, I wanted a bit of fun this week because I knew it would be hard. So I put on a pair of long, flamboyant fingernails. Since you haven't noticed, I have had to endure them all week (actually its easier to type than you think).

I needed the nails for last Saturday but decided to keep them on. The question I am posing therefore is:

"Why did I need long fingernails on Saturday?"

To help you I will drop in a few clues in the form of songs (first one attached). The lyrics to the songs are hugely important so read carefully and don't sing too loudly or you'll disturb Fozzie!

You may guess the answer or ask me further questions but I will only reply to the first person that answers back. Please keep everyone copied in so they know what is going on. If there are no replies I will send another song to keep you going.

To spice things up there is a box of fudge, unfortunately my daughter nicked one, for the winner which is behind Julie's desk.

Have fun!

I will :)

Iain

Attached:

Film and/or Musical: The Wizard of Oz

Song: Somewhere Over the Rainbow

Every good story should begin with this song. It has taken me a long, long time to get to the other side of the rainbow. I'm not there all the time but am some of the time. Everybody should be on the other side of their rainbow or have a rainbow to get to the other side of. Have you? What is at the end of your rainbow? If you haven't got one yet, stay with me and I'll teach you how.

Iain

I didn't notice so I must be blind. Judy Garland has got a lot to answer for, but I am aware of what she is an icon for, so is this what you are getting to?

Peter

No, but a good start Peter. I'm off to lunch now so I'll leave you another clue.

Attached:

Film and/or Musical: South Pacific

Song: Happy Talk

Before you can get to the other side of the rainbow you have to have a dream. I had a dream a long, long time ago and thought it was truly a dream because dreams don't happen do they?

Actually they do if you really want them to.

Have you got a dream?

I think you want to either go to Australia for a holiday or emigrate?

That's from the song clues but I don't know where the long fingernails fit in except Koala's (Australian emblem) have long claws ?

Ian

No, I'm very happy where I am.

Shabs, the nails are peach - not pink - and that is important.

Fozzie, I didn't perform in South Pacific.

I'm being very kind to you because I said I would only reply to the first email sent.

Tricia Dale

What was I doing at six o'clock in the evening on Saturday?

:)

Iain

Attached:

Film and/or Musical: Pinocchio

Song: When You Wish Upon a Star

To get to the other side of the rainbow you not only have to have a dream but you need to wish it come true with all your strength. Some dreams are very hard to realize. My dream was very hard to realize. It has taken me over a year to wish but my whole life has been spent dreaming.

Oh, go on then. I'll help you out.

I don't want to take home the fudge because it will spoil my figure

Iain

Attached:

Film and/or Musical: Carousel

Song: You'll Never Walk Alone

To get to the other side of the rainbow you not only have to have a dream, you not only need to wish it come true with all your might, but you also need to keep going, despite others trying to blow you off course. This is particularly true if you dream the type of dreams I do. Dreams which other people don't understand.

Film and/or Musical: West Side Story

Song: Somewhere

There is a place where I live out my dream, where I am at the other side of the rainbow. I'll let you know soon where that place is but not just yet. In time there will be a place for people who dare to dream the types of dream I dream. But that is a long, long way away.

~~~~~~

Some day I'll wish upon a star

And wake up where the clouds are far behind me

~~~~~~

Were you outside when you used these 'long peach fingernails' on Saturday at 6 o'clock?

Steve

Oh yes

Saturday is usually the night when you go out on the town, anything to do with getting ready to go out?

I think I'm pretty well out now :)

It's something to do with the World Cup. Peach is an orange colour which can denote Holland. But they played on the Sunday.

So, you were at an official reception give by the Uruguayan Ambassador before their match against Germany on Saturday evening.

Mike

It has nothing whatsoever to do with the World Cup. And the final was appalling!

Oops forgot, another song ....

I am a dozy bitch sometimes

Tricia Dale

Hope you're having fun.

I am :)

Attached:

Film and/or Musical: West Side Story

Song: One Hand, One Heart

I just love West Side Story. Its my favourite musical of all time and I listen to it again and again.

There are two sides to me you see. There is the side you know and the side you don't. The difficult thing for me to do, and I'm still trying, is to merge the two sides into one. I'm not now sure whether this is possible.

~~~~~~

Somewhere over the rainbow way up high

There's a land that I've heard of once in a lullaby

~~~~~~

Were you at a Gay Pride do somewhere (over the rainbow)?

Mitun

Yes I was, but that's not the answer.

The question is why my nails

Were all those songs played on Saturday night?

Steve

None of the songs were played on Saturday night (from my recollection, which is hazy)

Here we go again and this time looking at your email, it may be it the text 'dozy bitch' which is not one you would normally apply to the male gender. Am I moving in the right direction?

I think you may be on the way :

Attached:

Film and/or Musical: West Side Story

Song: Gee, Officer Krupke

I just love West Side Story. It's my favourite musical of all time and I listen to it again and again.

The difficulty for people who dream the type of dreams I dream is that we are not accepted as the norm. Everybody thinks there is something wrong with us, but I promise you there isn't. People and society don't like things that are different and we are very different; as is the place where I mainly live my dreams which is called a village although it's in the middle of a big City.

You got married.

No, I couldn't imagine that. Togetherness is hard.

D*mn, thought I had it there. So many songs refer to vows, not being alone, togetherness etc.

Rocky Horror Picture Show ?

Also peach was important

Is punk important?

Steve

Nope

Hi Iain.

Still puzzling over the **pair** of nails, wouldn't a full set have been better?

Regards, Map.

Ha-ha!

So, which digits are they on – bearing in mind I can't see you from here

I've two hands - but ten nails. They are on all ten

Did you need to wear ten long peach false nails for the look, or to actually use ?

For both

This is longer than the Forsythe Saga, but let's summarise

You were at a gay parade, but not gay

You were wearing long painted nails

You were coming out

Therefore you must have something that as per your last song, people think as a 'social disease' but in reality it is just a life style

I was definitely wearing long painted nails.

I have been out a while.

So essentially, you are nowhere further than you were at the beginning

Hopefully this will help you

I will be leaving later today but will still be going to Manchester.

I so love my nails :)

Attached:

Film and/or Musical: Seven Lively Arts.

Song: Every Time We Say Goodbye

I'm getting close to letting you know my secret so I'll give you some more clues. My dream tends to start happening about two hours after I leave work on Friday at 15:30 on the dot. It could happen anywhere, indeed it has happened in London, Liverpool and even Sheffield; but it generally happens in Manchester. My dream tends to end about two hours before I return to work at 10:00 on Monday morning. Every Monday morning it gets harder and harder to leave. So I dream my dream during the week and live it, on the other side of the rainbow, at the weekend. Does that help?

~~~~~~

Where troubles melt like lemon drops

Away above the chimney tops

That's where you'll find me

~~~~~~

Were you in fancy dress as Frank N Furter? (Has someone already asked that?)

Mitun

Nope

Were you "out" as Iain, or did you use a Saturday name?

Are the ear-rings also involved?

Yay, well done Mark. But you haven't answered the question!

Attached with pic of Tricia in maxi-dress

Film and/or Musical: Calamity Jane

Song: Secret Love

Here goes, its time to open up my closet. The nicest way to get into the village in Manchester from my flat (where I live at weekends) is to walk along the canal paths. I love doing this; it gives me time to think. About half way there is a bar called Duke's 92 where I often stop and have a beer. Piccy is of me (Tricia) at t-Girl Towers where I stay during the weekend.

The poem is called Arrival

I walk along canals and locks
I watch a young girl feed the ducks
The sun is high, the breeze is strong
This is a place where I belong
I buy a beer, I feel so calm
I'm looking pretty, I'm feeling fine
Dressed to kill and made-up too
Now what does Tricia want to do?
Buy some shoes or buy a dress
She's waited too long to impress

Fifty years to be here
Celebrate with another beer?
To the boutiques she will go
Her vulnerability will be on show
But boys and girls, its fine to talk
That t-girl there walks the walk
She struts her stuff, she feels so proud
She needs to scream, to shout out loud
I am Tricia, I am she
I am who I want to be.

~~~~~~~~~~~~~~~~~~~~~~~~~~~

Somewhere over the rainbow skies are blue

And the dreams that you dare to dream

Really do come true

~~~~~~~~~~~~~~~~~~~~~~~~~~~

Ok you're half way there so can now respond individually to me. I will let you all know who the winner is with some more pictures of me looking even more glam. So it's worth staying on.

Careful with the blog - its very very scary!!!!

I'll give you a huge hint. Think of the game Monopoly,

Hugs,

Trish xx

Well I wouldn't wear peach with purple stripes !

You're a keyboard player ?

Beauty Pageant

Yay, Fozzie wins.

I didn't because I forgot the golden rule. You have to sleep with the judges ha-ha.

Don't I look dead gorge though,

Hugs Trish xx

PS Next week I will be Iain again;

but in few hours .... :)

Life is fun!

Don't worry, family all know and are supportive. Please help supporting me,

Iain

Attached are piccies of Tricia in the beauty contest.

So I have now told my work colleagues, indeed my workplace as I included all areas who knew me in the distribution list. I heard there was a bit of an email frenzy that afternoon but I can't imagine why. The questions are, I suppose, how will it be taken and where will my disclosure lead me to? I don't know the answer yet but I do know one thing. It will be great fun finding out!

Now, what was the last song which no-one got to see?

THE END?

Lightning Source UK Ltd.
Milton Keynes UK
UKOW05f0020040214

9 781456 785970